THERAPEUTIC
MODALITIES
in Sports Medi

THERAPEUTIC MODALITIES
in Sports Medicine

Third Edition

WILLIAM E. PRENTICE, Ph.D., P.T., A.T., C.

**Professor, Coordinator of Sports Medicine Specialization,
Department of Physical Education, Exercise and Sport Science
Clinical Professor, Division of Physical Therapy,
Department of Medical Allied Health Professions,
Associate Professor, Department of Orthopaedics
School of Medicine
The University of North Carolina,
Chapel Hill, North Carolina**

**Director, Sports Medicine Education and Fellowship Program
HEALTHSOUTH Rehabilitation Corporation
Birmingham, Alabama**

with 201 *illustrations*

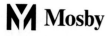 Mosby

St. Louis   Baltimore   Berlin   Boston   Carlsbad   Chicago   London   Madrid
Naples   New York   Philadelphia   Sydney   Tokyo   Toronto

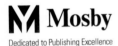

Editor-in-Chief: James M. Smith
Acquisition Editor: Vicki Malinee
Assistant Editor: Christy Wells
Project Manager: Carol Sullivan Wiseman
Senior Production Editor: Shannon Canty
Senior Designer: Betty Schulz
Cover Design: GW Graphics & Publishing
Manufacturing Supervisor: John Babrick

Printed in the United States of America
Composition by Graphic World, Inc.
Printing/binding by R.R. Donnelley & Sons Company

Mosby–Year Book, Inc.
11830 Westline Industrial Drive
St. Louis, Missouri 63146

Library of Congress Cataloging in Publication Data

Therapeutic modalities in sports medicine / [edited by] William E. Prentice. — 3rd ed.
    p. cm.
    Includes bibliographical references and index.
    ISBN 0-8016-7922-2
    1. Sports injuries — Treatment. 2. Sports physical therapy.
  I. Prentice, William E.
  RD97.T484 1994
  617.1′027 — dc20
                                                   94-20591
                                                       CIP

96 97 98 / 9 8 7 6 5 4 3 2

Contributors

Gerald W. Bell, Ed.D., P.T., A.T., C.
Associate Professor
Department of Physical Education
University of Illinois
Urbana, Illinois

J. Marc Davis, P.T., A.T., C.
Athletic Trainer/Physical Therapist
Division of Sports Medicine
Student Health Service
The University of North Carolina
Chapel Hill, North Carolina

Craig Denegar, Ph.D., P.T., A.T., C.
Associate Professor of Physical Therapy
Slippery Rock University
Slippery Rock, Pennsylvania

Phillip B. Donley, M.S., P.T., A.T., C.
Director, Chester County Orthopaedic and Sports Physical
    Therapy
West Chester, Pennsylvania

Susan H. Foreman, M.Ed., P.T., A.T., C.
Assistant Athletic Trainer
University of Virginia
Charlottesville, Virginia

Daniel N. Hooker, Ph.D., P.T., ScS, A.T., C.
Coordinator of Athletic Training and Physical Therapy
Division of Sports Medicine
Student Health Service
The University of North Carolina
Chapel Hill, North Carolina

Clairbeth Lehn, P.T., A.T., C.
Athletic Trainer/Physical Therapist
Division of Sports Medicine
Student Health Service
The University of North Carolina
Chapel Hill, North Carolina

William E. Prentice, Ph.D., P.T., A.T., C.
Professor, Coordinator of Sports Medicine Specialization
Department of Physical Education, Exercise and Sport
    Science
Clinical Professor, Division of Physical Therapy
Department of Medical Allied Health Professions
Associate Professor, Department of Orthopaedics
School of Medicine
The University of North Carolina
Chapel Hill, North Carolina

Ethan N. Saliba, Ph.D., P.T., A.T., C.
Instructor, Currey School of Education
Assistant Athletic Trainer
University of Virginia
Charlottesville, Virginia

Preface

Professional athletic trainers and physical therapists use a wide variety of therapeutic techniques to treat and rehabilitate sports-related injuries. A thorough treatment regimen often involves the use of therapeutic modalities. At one time or another, virtually all sports therapists make use of some type of modality. This may involve a relatively simple technique, such as using an ice pack as a first aid treatment for an acute injury, or more complex techniques, such as the stimulation of nerve and muscle tissue by electrical currents. There is no question that therapeutic modalities are useful tools in injury rehabilitation. When used appropriately, these modalities can greatly enhance the athlete's chances for a safe and rapid return to athletic competition. Unfortunately, the sports therapists' rationale for using a particular modality is too often based on habit rather than on logic or analysis of effectiveness. For the sports therapist, it is essential to understand the scientific basis and the physiologic effects of the various modalities on a specific injury. When this theoretical basis is combined with practical experience, it has the potential to become an extremely effective clinical method.

What role should a modality play in injury rehabilitation? An effective treatment program includes three primary objectives: (1) management or reduction of pain associated with an injury, (2) return of full nonrestricted range of movement to an injured part, and (3) maintenance or perhaps improvement of strength through the full range of motion. Modalities are by no means the most critical factor in accomplishing these objectives. Therapeutic exercise that forces the injured anatomic structure to perform its normal function is the key to successful rehabilitation. However, therapeutic modalities certainly play an important role in reducing pain and are extremely useful as an adjunct to therapeutic exercise. The use of therapeutic modalities in any treatment program is an inexact science. If you were to ask ten different sports therapists what combination of modalities and therapeutic exercise they use in a given treatment program, you would probably get ten different responses. There is no way to "cookbook" a treatment plan that involves the use of modalities. This book will attempt to present the basis for use of each different type of modality and allow sports therapists to make their own decisions as to which modalities will be most effective in a given situation. Some recommended protocols developed through the experiences of the contributing authors will be presented.

The sports therapist continues to gain acceptance in the medical community as a highly qualified and well-educated paramedical professional concerned with the treatment and rehabilitation of athletic injuries. It is essential for the programs educating student trainers and therapists to provide classroom instruction in a wide range of specialty areas including injury prevention, care and management, injury evaluation, and therapeutic treatment and rehabilitation techniques. Detailed instructions in the use of therapeutic modalities should be of primary concern to those who intend to pursue a career in sports medicine.

The use of therapeutic modalities in the treatment of athletic injuries by individuals with various combinations of educational background, certification, and licensure is currently a controversial issue. Formal classroom instruction in the use of therapeutic modalities is included in all physical therapy programs and is also provided in the majority of athletic training education programs. Physical therapists who are licensed to practice can legally use modalities in their patient treatment programs. Likewise, many states have also granted licensure to athletic trainers, thus allowing them to legally incorporate therapeutic modalities into their treatment regimen. Specific laws governing the use of therapeutic modalities vary considerably from state to state. How should modalities be used by athletic trainers who are not licensed by the state in which they are working?

The use of therapeutic modalities has traditionally been in the hands of physical therapists and athletic trainers. The laws of the various states place limitations on this use. The reader should be aware that a modality must be used within the limits allowed by the law of his or her particular state. I do not intend for the reader to interpret anything in this book as encouraging him or her to act outside the scope of the law of his or her state.

I hope that this text will be a useful tool in the continuing growth and professional development of all individuals concerned with and interested in the field of sports injury rehabilitation. The following are a number of reasons why this text should be adopted for use.

COMPREHENSIVE COVERAGE OF THERAPEUTIC MODALITIES IN A SPORTS-MEDICINE SETTING

This text provides a theoretically based but practically oriented guide to the use of therapeutic modalities for the individual who routinely treats sports-related injuries. It is intended for use in advanced courses in sports medicine in which various clinically oriented techniques and methods are presented.

The third edition of this text has been expanded and updated to provide more comprehensive coverage of various modalities. In particular, the chapters on electrical stimulating currents, diathermy, and ultrasound have undergone major revisions to reflect the most current information available. The revised discussion of electrical stimulating currents reflects the current state of knowledge relative to their effects at the subsensory cellular level. I believe this chapter provides a new basis for various theories and explanations regarding how electrical currents may be used therapeutically.

New chapters have been added on iontophoresis and electromyographic biofeedback, in addition to a new chapter that provides guidelines for determining when and how therapeutic modalities should be incorporated into a treatment program. The appendices provide a comprehensive list of manufacturers and distributors of various types of therapeutic modalities and related equipment.

This text begins by classifying the modalities in a logical order in relation to the electromagnetic and acoustic spectra. Guidelines for selecting the most appropriate modalities for use in different phases of the healing process are presented. Pain is discussed in terms of neurophysiologic mechanisms and the role of therapeutic modalities in pain management. Detailed discussions of various therapeutic modalities, including the electrical stimulating currents, iontophoresis, biofeedback, shortwave and microwave diathermies, infrared modalities, low-power laser, ultraviolet therapy, ultrasound, traction, intermittent compression, and massage are presented with emphasis on (1) the physiologic basis for use, (2) clinical applications, and (3) specific application techniques. Although therapeutic modalities are important and necessary tools that should be used in dealing with physical problems of all varieties, this text will deal specifically with why and how these modalities are best used in the treatment and rehabilitation of sports-related injuries.

BASED ON SCIENTIFIC THEORY

This text discusses various concepts, principles, and theories that are supported by scientific research, factual evidence, and previous experience of the authors in dealing with sports-related injuries. The material presented in this text has been carefully researched by the contributing authors to provide up-to-date information on the theoretical basis for using a particular modality in a specific injury situation. Additionally, the manuscript for this text has been carefully reviewed by sports therapists, both athletic trainers and physical therapists, who are considered experts in their field to ensure that the material reflects factual and current concepts for modality use.

TIMELY AND PRACTICAL

Certainly, therapeutic modalities used in a clinical setting are important tools for the sports therapist. This text fills a void that has existed for quite some time in the educational curricula, particularly for the student of athletic training. It provides the student with a comprehensive resource that should be used in student instruction on the theoretical basis and practical application of the various modalities.

During the preparation of this third, as well as previous editions of this text, the editor received much encouragement from sports-medicine educators and students regarding the usability of this text in the classroom setting. It should serve as a needed guide for the sports therapist who is interested in knowing not only how to use a modality but also why that particular modality is most effective in a given situation.

The authors who have contributed to this text have a great deal of clinical experience dealing with sports-related injury. Each of these individuals has also at one time or another been involved with the formal classroom education of the student trainer or therapist. Thus this text has been directed at the student of sports-injury rehabilitation who will be asked to apply the theoretical basis of modality use to the clinical setting.

PERTINENT TO THE SPORTS THERAPIST

This text deals specifically with the use of therapeutic modalities in the sports-medicine setting. Several other texts are available that discuss the use of selected physical modalities with patient populations other than athletes. The sports-medicine emphasis makes this text unique. With the expansion of material in this third edition, I now believe that this is the most comprehensive text on therapeutic modalities available in any specific discipline.

PEDAGOGICAL AIDS

The aids this text uses to facilitate its use by students and instructors include:

Objectives. These goals are listed at the beginning of each chapter to introduce students to the points that will be emphasized.

Figures and Tables. Essential points on each chapter are illustrated with clear visual materials.

Summary. Each chapter has a summary that outlines the major points covered.

Glossary of Key Terms. Each chapter contains a glossary of terms for quick reference, and a comprehensive glossary is located before the appendices.

References. A list of up-to-date references is provided at the end of each chapter for the student who wishes to read further on the subject being discussed.

Appendices. A chart of trigger points, a comprehensive list of manufacturers of therapeutic modality equipment, and a list of units of measure are provided.

LABORATORY MANUAL

In recent years, I have received numerous requests from educators, clinicians, and students to prepare a supplemental laboratory guide to accompany this text. With this third edition, a separate laboratory manual has been developed by William S. Quillen to facilitate and demonstrate the material presented in this text. This manual includes practical laboratory exercises designed to enhance the students' understanding of therapeutic modality use. This manual illustrates the principles and theories of modality use through practical demonstrations and experiences.

ACKNOWLEDGMENTS

If you have never been involved in the production of a textbook, it is difficult to understand the magnitude of such an undertaking. Dozens of individuals have been involved with this project from its inception, and all have contributed in their own way, but a few deserve special thanks.

Christy Wells, my developmental editor at Mosby, has been responsible for coordinating the efforts between the publisher and me. She has offered a great deal of assistance in the completion of this text.

Shannon Canty, my production editor on this and several other projects, has been diligent in her attention to essential details in the production process. As always, I rely heavily on, and appreciate, her expertise.

When assembling a group of contributors for a project such as this, it is essential to select individuals who are both knowledgeable and well respected in their fields. It also helps if you can count them as friends, and I want to let them know that I hold each of them in the highest regard, both personally and professionally.

The following individuals have invested a great amount of time and effort in reviewing this manuscript. Their contributions are present throughout the text. I would like to thank each one of them for their valuable insight.

Timothy Carver
Oberlin College

Magie Lacambra
Arizona State University

Xristas Gaglias
South Dakota State University

James Zachazewski
Massachusetts General Hospital

Ron Courson
University of Alabama

And finally, I would like to thank my wife Tena and my sons Brian and Zachary for being understanding, patient, and supportive while I pursue a career and a life that I truly enjoy.

William E. Prentice

Contents

Therapeutic Modalities in Relation to the Electromagnetic and Acoustic Spectra

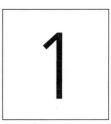

William E. Prentice

OBJECTIVES

After completion of this chapter, the student will be able to do the following:

- Discuss what radiant energy is and how it is produced.

- Describe the relationship between wavelength and frequency.

- Indicate how the sports therapist can make use of electromagnetic radiations to affect the biologic tissues of the body.

- Discuss the physiologic effects produced by each therapeutic modality.

- Differentiate between the electromagnetic and acoustic spectra.

There is considerable confusion among sports therapists regarding the relationship of the various therapeutic modalities to the **electromagnetic** and **acoustic spectra.** Electrical stimulating currents, shortwave and microwave **diathermy,** the **infrared** modalities, **ultraviolet** therapy, and low-power lasers are all therapeutic agents that emit a type of energy with wavelengths and frequencies that can be classified as electromagnetic radiations. **Ultrasound** is a form of radiation with a wavelength and frequency of vibration best classified as acoustic energy rather than as an electromagnetic radiation. Each of the modalities that make use of these varying types of energy will be discussed in the following chapters.

RADIANT ENERGY

Radiation is a process by which energy in various forms travels through space. Most of us are familiar with the effects of radiation from the sun. Sunlight is a type of radiant energy, and we know that it not only makes objects visible but also produces heat. The sun emits radiant energy as a result of high-intensity chemical reactions. Radiant energy in the form of sunlight travels through space at about 300,000,000 m/sec and eventually

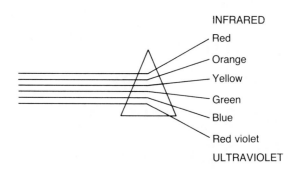

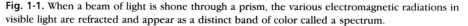

Fig. 1-1. When a beam of light is shone through a prism, the various electromagnetic radiations in visible light are refracted and appear as a distinct band of color called a spectrum.

reaches earth where its effects may be felt or seen. The sun is not the only object capable of producing this radiant energy.

All matter produces energy that radiates in the form of heat. The sun produces radiation through chemical reactions. When a sufficiently intense chemical or electrical force is applied to any object, radiant energy in various forms can be produced by movement of electrons. Many of the therapeutic modalities discussed in this text produce radiant energy (i.e., the infrared modalities, the diathermies, ultraviolet, lasers, and the electrical stimulating modalities).[2,8]

If a ray of sunlight is passed through a prism, it will be broken down into various regions of colors (Figure 1-1). Each of these colors represents a different form of radiant energy. The colors appear because the various forms of radiant energy are **refracted** or change direction as a result of differences in wavelength and frequency, thus resulting in distinct bands of color called a spectrum. These color variations that we can detect with our eyes are referred to as visible light or luminous radiations. It becomes apparent when looking at this colorful display that there is a region of red at one end of the spectrum and a region of violet at the other end. When passed through a prism, the type of radiant energy refracted the least is red, whereas that refracted the most is violet.[8]

This beam of sunlight passing through the prism is also propagating forms of radiant energy that are not visible to our eyes. If a thermometer is placed close to the red end of the spectrum, heat will be detected. Likewise, a photographic plate placed close to the violet end of the spectrum will indicate chemical changes. The form of radiant energy that produces heat and is located in the spectrum beyond the visible red portion is referred to as the infrared radiation region. The form of radiant energy that produces chemical changes and is located beyond the violet end of the visible spectrum is called the ultraviolet radiation region (Figure 1-2). Ultraviolet, infrared, and visible light rays are produced by heat. As the temperature increases in a particular substance, the vibration of molecules tends to increase the activity of the electrons. The movement of electrons produces electromagnetic waves. The higher the temperature, the greater the frequency of electromagnetic waves produced. These electromagnetic waves produced by heat are usually absorbed by many objects and have little penetration.[7]

Other forms of radiation beyond the infrared and ultraviolet portions of the spectrum may be produced when an electrical force is applied.[8] Beyond the infrared

Region	Clinically Used Wavelength	Clinically Used Frequency*	Estimated Effective Depth of Penetration	Physiologic Effects
Electrical stimulating currents	3×10^8 Km to 75,000 Km	1–4000 Hz	Effects may occur anywhere between electrodes	Pain modulation, muscle contraction, relaxation, ion movement
Commercial radio and television				
Shortwave diathermy	22 m 11 m	13.56 MHz 27.12 MHz	3 cm	Deep tissue temperature increase, vasodilation, increased blood flow
Microwave diathermy	69 cm 33 cm 12 cm	433.9 MHz 915 MHz 2450 MHz	5 cm	Deep tissue temperature increase, vasodilation, increased blood flow
Infrared Cold packs (8° F) Cold whirlpool (63° F) Hot whirlpool (99° F) Paraffin bath (117° F) Hydrocollar (170° F) Luminous IR (1341° F) Nonluminous IR (3140° F)	111,000 A 99,514 A 93,097 A 90,187 A 82,457 A 28,860 A 14,430 A	2.7×10^{12} Hz 3.01×10^{12} Hz 3.22×10^{12} Hz 3.32×10^{12} Hz 3.63×10^{12} Hz 1.04×10^{13} Hz 2.08×10^{13} Hz	1 cm	Superficial temperature decrease Vasoconstriction—decreased blood flow Analgesia Superficial temperature increase Vasodilation—increased blood flow
Red	**Laser**			
Visible light	GaAs 9100 A HeNe 6328 A	3.3×10^{13} Hz 4.74×10^{13} Hz	5 cm 10–15 mm	Pain modulation and wound healing
Violet				
Ultraviolet UV-A UV-B UV-C	3200–4000 A 2900–3200 A 2000–2900 A	9.38×10^{13}–7.5×10^{13} Hz 1.03×10^{14}–9.38×10^{13} Hz 1.50×10^{14}–1.03×10^{14} Hz	2 mm	Superficial chemical changes Tanning effects Bactericidal
Ionizing radiation (x-ray, gamma rays, cosmic rays)				

*Calculated using $C = \lambda \times F$, C = velocity (3×10 m/sec), λ = wavelength, F = frequency.

Fig. 1-2. Electromagnetic spectrum.

portion of the spectrum lie several large regions of radiations known as the diathermies; these include radio, television, and nerve and muscle stimulating currents. Beyond the ultraviolet end of the spectrum lie the high-frequency ionizing and penetration radiation regions (i.e., x-ray, alpha, beta, and gamma rays).

ELECTROMAGNETIC RADIATIONS

All of these various classifications of radiations collectively constitute the electromagnetic spectrum (see Figure 1-2). All the electromagnetic radiations lying within this spectrum have several common theoretical characteristics[1,3]:

1. They may be produced when sufficiently intense electrical or chemical forces are applied to any material.
2. They all travel readily through space at an equal velocity.
3. Their direction of travel is always in a straight line.
4. They may be reflected, refracted, absorbed, or transmitted, depending on the specific medium that they strike.

The luminous, infrared, and ultraviolet rays in sunlight travel in waves through a vacuum or through space at a velocity of about 300 million m/sec and all reach the earth at about the same time. These rays are emitted from chemical reactions taking place on the sun, and each type of radiation has individual physical characteristics. The different regions of the electromagnetic spectrum are differentiated by analyzing the wavelengths and frequencies of the radiations within this spectrum. Despite the fact that the electromagnetic radiations produced by the different modalities all share the same physical characteristics as any other type of electromagnetic radiation, when these radiations come in contact with various biologic tissues, the velocity and direction of travel will be altered within the various types of tissues.

WAVELENGTH AND FREQUENCY

Wavelength is defined as the distance between the peak of one wave and the peak of either the preceding or succeeding wave. **Frequency** is defined as the number of wave oscillations or vibrations occurring in 1 second and is expressed in hertz (Hz) units.

Each of the various types of radiation in the electromagnetic spectrum has a specific wavelength and frequency of vibrations. Since it is accepted theoretically that all forms of electromagnetic radiation are produced simultaneously, travel at a constant velocity through space, and reach earth at the same time, it follows that longer wavelengths must have shorter frequencies and shorter wavelengths must have higher frequencies.

$$\text{Velocity} = \text{Wavelength} \times \text{Frequency}$$
$$C = \lambda \times F$$

Thus an inverse or reciprocal relationship exists between wavelength and frequency. Velocity is a constant 3×10^8 m/sec.[9] Therefore if we know the wavelength, frequency can be calculated.

LAWS GOVERNING THE EFFECTS OF ELECTROMAGNETIC RADIATIONS

When electromagnetic radiations strike or come in contact with various objects, several things may happen. Some rays may be **reflected,** while others are **transmitted** through the tissues where they may be refracted. Still others penetrate to deeper layers where they may be **absorbed** (Figure 1-3). Generally, those radiations that have the longest wavelengths tend to have the greatest depths of penetration, regardless of their frequency. It must be added, however, that a number of other factors, which will be discussed later, can also contribute to the depth of penetration.

The purpose of using therapeutic modalities is to stimulate a specific body tissue to perform its normal function. This stimulation will only occur if energy produced by the electrotherapeutic device is absorbed by the tissue. The **Arndt-Schultz principle** states that no reactions or changes can occur in the body tissues if the amount of energy absorbed is insufficient to stimulate the absorbing tissues. The goal of the sports therapist should be to deliver sufficient energy in one form or another to stimulate the tissues to perform their normal function while realizing that too much energy absorbed in a given period of time may seriously impair normal function and, if severe enough, may cause irreparable damage.[3]

If the therapeutic energy is not absorbed by the tissues, then according to the **Law of Grotthus-Draper,** it must be transmitted to deeper layers. The greater the amount of energy absorbed, the less transmitted and thus the less penetration.[1,6] The transmitted energy tends to (1) travel in a straight line, (2) come in contact with a tissue that reflects or turns away the energy, or (3) have its angle of transmission changed or refracted within the tissue. Radiant energy is more easily transmitted to deeper tissues if the source of radiation is at a right angle to the area being radiated. Thus the smaller the angle between the propagating ray and the right angle, the less radiation reflected and the greater the absorption. This principle, known as the **cosine law,** will be extremely important in the chapters dealing with the diathermies, ultraviolet light, and infrared heating, since the effectiveness of these modalities is based to a large extent on how they are positioned with regard to the patient (Figure 1-4).

The intensity of the radiation striking a particular surface varies inversely with the square of the distance from the source. For example, a source of radiation that is 2

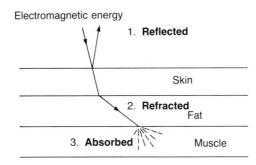

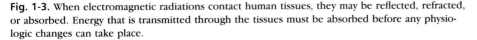

Fig. 1-3. When electromagnetic radiations contact human tissues, they may be reflected, refracted, or absorbed. Energy that is transmitted through the tissues must be absorbed before any physiologic changes can take place.

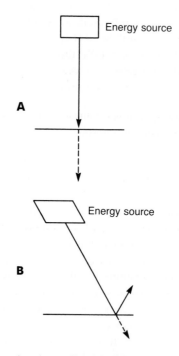

Fig. 1-4. The cosine law states that the smaller the angle between the propagating ray and the right angle, the less radiation reflected and the greater absorbed. Thus the energy absorbed in *A* would be greater than in *B*.

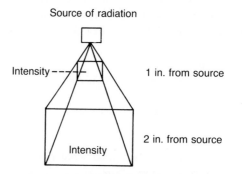

Fig. 1-5. The inverse square law states that the intensity of the radiation striking a particular surface varies inversely with the square of the distance from the source.

inches away from the surface will have one quarter of the intensity of a source of radiation that is 1 inch from the surface. This principle, known as the **inverse square law,** will obviously be of great consequence when setting up a specific modality to achieve a desired physiologic effect (Figure 1-5). Regardless of the path this transmitted energy takes, the physiologic effects will only be apparent when the energy is absorbed by a specific tissue.

All physical modalities emitting electromagnetic radiations are subject to the relationship between absorption and transmission of energy. The modalities that emit radiations with relatively longer wavelengths have the ability to transmit energy through the superficial tissue layers, thus penetrating it to the deeper tissues where it is absorbed.

THE APPLICATION OF THE ELECTROMAGNETIC SPECTRUM TO THERAPEUTIC MODALITIES

The therapeutic modalities discussed in detail in later chapters (with the exception of ultrasound, massage, traction, and intermittent compression) all emit radiations with physical characteristics that may be classified as electromagnetic radiations.

Figure 1-2 represents the electromagnetic spectrum and places all of the modalities in order based on wavelengths and corresponding frequencies. It is apparent, for example, that the electrical stimulating currents have the longest wavelength and the lowest frequency and, all other factors being equal, should therefore have the greatest depth of penetration. As we move down the chart, the wavelengths in each region become progressively shorter and the frequencies progressively higher. Shortwave and microwave diathermy, the various sources of infrared heating, and the ultraviolet regions have progressively less depth of penetration.

It should be mentioned that the regions labeled as radio and television frequencies, visible light, and high-frequency ionizing and penetrating radiations certainly fall under the classification of electromagnetic radiations. However, they do not have application as therapeutic modalities and, while extremely important to our everyday way of life, warrant no further consideration in the context of this discussion.

Electrical Stimulating Currents

The electrical stimulating currents that affect nerve and muscle tissue have the longest wavelengths and the lowest frequencies of any of the modalities. The wavelengths of electrical stimulating units are extremely long, ranging somewhere around 15,000 km. Clinically used frequencies range from 1 to 4000 Hz. Most stimulators have the flexibility to alter the frequency output of the device to elicit a desired physiologic response. The nerve and muscle stimulating currents are capable of (1) pain modulations either through stimulation of cutaneous sensory nerves at high frequencies (TENS) or through production of β-endorphin at lower frequencies (electroaccutherapy), (2) producing muscle contraction and relaxation or tetany depending on the type of current (alternating or direct) and frequency (Russian currents), (3) facilitating soft tissue and bone healing through the use of subsensory microcurrents (MENS), and (4) producing a net movement of ions through the use of continuous direct current and thus eliciting a chemical change in the tissues (iontophoresis, see Chapter 6).[9] The electrical stimulating currents and their various physiologic effects will be discussed in detail in Chapter 5.

ELECTROMYOGRAPHIC BIOFEEDBACK. Electromyographic biofeedback is a therapeutic procedure that uses electronic or electromechanical instruments to accurately measure, process, and feed back reinforcing information via auditory or visual signals. In sports medicine, it is used to help the athlete develop greater voluntary control in terms of either neuromuscular relaxation or muscle reeducation after injury. Biofeedback is discussed in Chapter 7.

Shortwave and Microwave Diathermy

The diathermies are considered to be high-frequency currents because they have more than a million cycles per second. When impulses of such a short duration come in contact with human tissue, there is not sufficient time for ion movement to take place. Consequently there is no stimulation of either motor or sensory nerves. The energy of this rapidly vibrating electrical current produces heat as it passes through tissue cells, resulting in a temperature increase. Shortwave diathermy may be either continuous or pulsed. Both continuous shortwave and microwave diathermy are used primarily for their thermal effects, while pulsed shortwave is used for its nonthermal effects.

The electrotherapeutic shortwave and microwave devices have preset frequencies and wavelengths that cannot be altered. Shortwave diathermy units are set at either 13.56 MHz (1 MHz = 10 million Hz) with a corresponding wavelength of 22 m or 27.12 MHz with a wavelength of 11 m.[3]

Microwave units have shorter wavelengths than do shortwave diathermy units and are set at wavelengths of 33 or 12 cm with respective frequencies of 915 or 2450 MHz. The depth of penetration with microwave units is a bit deeper than with shortwave units because the amount of energy when using microwave units is concentrated in one spot rather than spread out over a large area.[3] This will be discussed in more detail in Chapter 8.

Infrared Modalities

Perhaps the greatest confusion over the relationship between electromagnetic radiations and therapeutic modalities is associated with the infrared region. We tend to think of the infrared modalities as being the luminous and nonluminous infrared bakers or lamps only, when the largest number of modalities used by sports therapists emit radiations with wavelengths and frequencies that clearly fall within this infrared region. Cold packs, hydrocollator packs, whirlpools, paraffin baths, and contrast baths are all infrared modalities.[4]

Earlier it was stated that any object heated (or cooled) to a temperature different than the surrounding environment will dissipate heat through radiation to the other materials with which it comes in contact. The infrared modalities are used to produce a local and occasionally a generalized heating or cooling of the superficial tissues. It is generally accepted that the infrared modalities have a maximum depth of penetration of 1 cm or less. The infrared modalities can elicit either increases or decreases in circulation depending on whether heat or cold is used. They are also known to have analgesic effects as a result of stimulation of sensory cutaneous nerve endings.

The infrared region of the spectrum is located adjacent to the red end of the visible light region. The wavelengths of the infrared modalities are obviously much shorter than are those of the electrical stimulating currents and the diathermies and are expressed in Angstrom (Å) units; 1 Å is equal to 10^{-10} m.

Both the infrared and ultraviolet wavelengths are temperature dependent. Those modalities with the lower temperature have the longer wavelength. This means that an ice pack will have a longer wavelength and thus a greater depth of penetration than will a hydrocollator pack. Temperatures used with the infrared modalities range from 0° C with ice to more than 3000° C with infrared lamps. The wavelengths in this temperature range fall between 10,000 and 105,000 Å with corresponding frequencies ranging between 2×10^{12} and 4×10^{13} Hz.

An Angstrom is an extremely small unit of measure, and thus the differences in depth of penetration are not great between any of the infrared modalities. The critical factor is the superficial increase or decrease in tissue temperature that elicits the same physiologic response regardless of wavelength.

Laser

Of the modalities discussed in this text, the low-power **laser** is certainly the newest used by the sports therapist. The word laser is an acronym for *light amplification by stimulated emission of radiation*. Laser is a form of electromagnetic radiation that is classified within both the infrared and visible light portions of the spectrum.

Lasers are either high-power or low-power. High-power lasers are used in surgery for purposes of incision, coagulation of vessels, and thermolysis, owing to their thermal effects. The low-power or cold laser produces little or no thermal effects but seems to have some significant clinical effect on soft tissue and fracture healing, as well as pain management through stimulation of acupuncture and trigger points.

Two types of low-power lasers are used by sports therapists: the helium-neon laser (HeNe) and the gallium-arsenide laser (GaAs). The HeNe laser has a wavelength of 632.8 nm and a direct depth of penetration to 0.8 mm, although there may be some indirect effects up to 10 to 15 mm. The GaAs laser has a wavelength of 910 nm and can penetrate indirectly as much as 5 cm. The laser as a therapeutic tool will be discussed in Chapter 10.

Ultraviolet Therapy

The ultraviolet portion of the electromagnetic spectrum is adjacent to the violet end of the visible light region. As stated previously, the radiations in the ultraviolet region are undetectable by the human eye. However, if a photographic plate is placed at the ultraviolet end, chemical changes will be apparent. Although an extremely hot source (7000° to 9000° C) is required to produce ultraviolet wavelengths, the physiologic effects of ultraviolet radiation are mainly chemical in nature and occur entirely in the cutaneous layers of skin. The maximum depth of penetration with ultraviolet radiation is about 1 mm. The ultraviolet range extends between 2000 and 4000 Å. The ultraviolet region is subdivided into three different areas: near ultraviolet or UV-A (3200 to 4000 Å), middle ultraviolet or UV-B (2900 to 3200 Å), and far ultraviolet or UV-C (2000 to 2900 Å). Clinically used ultraviolet frequencies range between 7×10^{13} and 7×10^{14} Hz.[2,5,8] Although rarely used by the sports therapist, the application of ultraviolet therapy is discussed in Chapter 11.

THE ACOUSTIC SPECTRUM AND ULTRASOUND

One additional therapeutic modality frequently used by sports therapists is ultrasound. Ultrasound devices produce a type of energy that must be classified as acoustic rather than electromagnetic energy. Ultrasound is frequently classified along with shortwave and microwave diathermy as a deep-heating, "conversion" type modality, and all of these are capable of producing a temperature increase in human tissue to a considerable depth. However, ultrasound is a mechanical vibration, a sound wave, produced and transformed from high-frequency electrical energy.[3] Ultrasound must be considered a type of acoustic vibration rather than a type of electromagnetic radiation.

Acoustic and electromagnetic radiations have very different physical characteristics. When acoustic vibrations are produced, they travel at a velocity that is significantly lower than that of electromagnetic radiations. Electromagnetic waves travel at approximately 300 million m/sec, while sound waves travel at speeds from hundreds to several thousand m/sec.

The relationship between velocity, wavelength, and frequency is a bit different with acoustic energy than with electromagnetic energy, even though the inverse relationship between wavelength and frequency still exists. The distinction is that the velocity of travel is much greater for electromagnetic energy than for acoustic energy. Therefore wavelengths are considerably shorter in acoustic vibrations than in electromagnetic radiations at any given frequency.[3] For example, ultrasound radiation traveling in the atmosphere has a wavelength of approximately 0.3 mm, while electromagnetic radiations have wavelengths of 297 m at a similar frequency.

We stated that electromagnetic radiations are capable of traveling through space or through a vacuum. As the density of the transmitting medium is increased, the velocity of travel significantly decreases as a result of refraction, reflection, or absorption by the molecules in the medium. Acoustic vibrations will not be transmitted at all through a vacuum, since they depend on conduction through molecular collisions. The more dense the transmitting medium, the greater the velocity of travel. In human tissue, ultrasound waves have a much greater velocity of transmission in bone tissue (3500 m/sec), for example, than in fat tissue (1500 m/sec).

Frequencies of ultrasound wave production are between 700,000 and 1,000,000 cycles per second. Frequencies up to around 20,000 Hz are detectable by the human ear. Thus the ultrasound portion of the acoustic spectrum is inaudible. Ultrasound generators are generally set at a standard frequency of 1 megahertz (1000 KHz). The depth of penetration with ultrasound radiation is much greater than with any of the electromagnetic radiations. At a frequency of 1 mHz, 50% of the energy produced will penetrate to a depth of about 5 cm. The reason for this great depth of penetration is that ultrasound radiation travels very well through homogeneous tissue (e.g., fat tissue), while electromagnetic radiations are almost entirely absorbed. Thus when therapeutic penetration to deeper tissues is desired, ultrasound radiation is the modality of choice.[5,7]

Therapeutic ultrasound radiation has traditionally been used to produce a tissue temperature increase through thermal physiologic effects. However it is also capable of enhancing healing at the cellular level as a result of its nonthermal physiologic effects. The usefulness of therapeutic ultrasound radiation in the sports medicine arena will be discussed in greater detail in Chapter 12.

SUMMARY

1. Radiant energy may be produced when a sufficiently intense chemical or electrical force is applied to any object.
2. Electrical stimulating currents, shortwave and microwave diathermy, the infrared modalities, and ultraviolet therapy are all classified as portions of the electromagnetic spectrum according to corresponding wavelengths and frequencies associated with each region.
3. All electromagnetic radiations travel at the same velocity; thus wavelength and frequency are inversely related.
4. Radiations may be reflected, refracted, absorbed, or transmitted in the various tissues.
5. Those radiations with the longer wavelengths tend to have the greatest depth of penetration.
6. The purpose of using any therapeutic modality is to stimulate a specific tissue to perform its normal function.
7. Ultrasound radiation is part of the acoustic spectrum and is best propagated through dense tissue such as biologic tissue; thus it is extremely effective in reaching deep tissues.

GLOSSARY

absorption Energy that stimulates a particular tissue to perform its normal function.

acoustic spectrum The range of frequencies and wavelengths of sound waves.

Arndt-Schultz Principle No reactions or changes can occur in the body if the amount of energy absorbed is not sufficient to stimulate the absorbing tissues.

cosine law Optimal radiation occurs when the source of radiation is at right angles to the center of the area being radiated.

diathermy The application of high-frequency electrical energy that is used to generate heat in body tissue as a result of the resistance of the tissue to the passage of energy.

electromagnetic spectrum The range of frequencies and wavelengths associated with radiant energy.

frequency The number of cycles or pulses per second.

infrared The portion of the electromagnetic spectrum associated with thermal changes located adjacent to the red portion of the visible light spectrum.

inverse square law The intensity of radiation striking a particular surface varies inversely with the square of the distance from the radiating source.

Law of Grotthus-Draper Energy not absorbed by the tissues must be transmitted.

radiation The process of emitting energy from some source in the form of waves. A method of heat transfer through which heat can be either gained or lost.

reflection The bending back of light or sound waves from a surface that they strike.

refraction The change in direction of a sound wave or radiation wave when it passes from one medium or type of tissue to another.

transmission The propagation of energy through a particular biologic tissue into deeper tissues.

ultrasound A portion of the acoustic spectrum located above audible sound.

ultraviolet The portion of the electromagnetic spectrum associated with chemical changes located adjacent to the violet portion of the visible light spectrum.

wavelength The distance from one point in a propagating wave to the same point in the next wave.

REFERENCES

1 Draper D, Sunderland S: Examination of the Law of Grotthus-Draper: does ultrasound penetrate the subcutaneous fat in humans? *J Ath Train* 28(3): 246-250, 1993.

2 Goldman L: *Introduction to modern phototherapy,* Springfield, Ill, 1978, Charles C. Thomas.

3 Griffin J, Karselis T: *Physical agents for physical therapists,* Springfield, Ill, 1988, Charles C. Thomas.

4 Lehmann J, editor: *Therapeutic heat and cold,* ed. 2, New Haven, 1982, Elizabeth Licht.

5 Lehmann JF, Guy AW: *Ultrasound therapy.* Proc Workshop on

Interaction of Ultrasound and Biological Tissues. Washington, DC, HEW Pub. (FDA 73:8008), Sept, 1972.

6 Licht S: *Therapeutic electricity and ultraviolet radiation,* New Haven, 1959, Elizabeth Licht.

7 Schriber W: *A manual of electrotherapy,* Philadelphia, 1975, Lea & Febiger.

8 Sears F, Zemansky M, Young H: *University physics,* Reading, Mass, 1976, Addison-Wesley.

9 Stillwell K: *Therapeutic electricity and ultraviolet radiation,* Baltimore, 1983, Williams & Wilkins.

SUGGESTED READINGS

Goodgold J, Eberstein A: *Electrodiagnosis of neuromuscular diseases,* Baltimore, 1972, Williams & Wilkins.

Jehle H: Charge fluctuation forces in biological systems, *Ann N Y Acad Sci* 158: 240-255, 1969.

Koracs R: *Light therapy,* Springfield, Ill, 1950, Charles C. Thomas.

Licht S, editor: *Electrodiagnosis and electromyography,* ed. 3, New Haven, 1971, Elizabeth Licht.

Scott P, Cooksey F: *Clayton's electrotherapy and actinotherapy,* London, 1962, Bailliere, Tindall and Cox.

Guidelines for Using Therapeutic Modalities in Rehabilitation

2

William E. Prentice

OBJECTIVES

After completion of this chapter, the student will be able to do the following:

- Discuss how therapeutic modalities should be used in rehabilitation of sports-related injuries.

- Understand the physiologic events associated with the four phases of the healing process.

- Discuss specific modalities that can be used effectively during each phase of healing, and provide a rationale for their use.

- Identify indications and contraindications for using the various modalities discussed throughout this text.

Therapeutic modalities, when used appropriately, can be extremely useful tools in the rehabilitation of the injured athlete. Like any other tool, their effectiveness is limited by the knowledge, skill, and experience of the person using them. For the sports therapist, decisions regarding how and when a modality may best be used should be based on a combination of theoretical knowledge and practical experience. Modalities should not be used at random, nor should their use be based on what has always been done before. Instead, consideration must always be given to what should work best in a specific clinical situation.

In any rehabilitation program, modalities should be used primarily as adjuncts to therapeutic exercise and certainly not at the exclusion of range-of-motion and strengthening exercises. Rehabilitation protocols and progressions must be based primarily on the physiologic responses of the tissues to injury and on an understanding of how various tissues heal. Thus the sports therapist must understand the healing process to be effective in incorporating therapeutic modalities into the rehabilitative process.

There are many different approaches and ideas regarding the use of modalities in injury rehabilitation. Therefore no "cookbook" exists for modality use. Instead, sports therapists should make their own decisions from the options in a given clinical situation about which modality will be most effective.

UNDERSTANDING THE HEALING PROCESS

Clinical decisions on how and when therapeutic modalities may best be used should be based on recognition of signs and symptoms, as well as some awareness of the time frames associated with the various phases of the healing process.[1,10] The sports therapist must have a sound understanding of that process in terms of the sequence of the various phases of healing that take place.

Once an acute injury has occurred, the healing process consists of the inflammatory response phase, the fibroblastic-repair phase, and the maturation-remodeling phase. Although the phases of healing are presented as three separate entities, the healing process is a continuum. Phases of the healing process overlap and have no definitive beginning or end points.[6]

Inflammatory Response Phase

Once a tissue is injured, the process of healing begins immediately[2] (Figure 2-1). The destruction of tissue produces direct injury to the cells of the various soft tissues. Cellular injury results in altered metabolism and the liberation of materials that initiate the inflammatory response. It is characterized symptomatically by redness, swelling, tenderness, and increased temperature.[3,9]

Inflammation is the process through which **leukocytes** and other **phagocytic cells** and exudate are delivered to the injured tissue. This cellular reaction is generally protective, tending to localize or dispose of injury by-products (e.g., blood and damaged cells) through phagocytosis, thus setting the stage for repair. Locally, vascular effects, disturbances of fluid exchange, and migration of leukocytes from the blood to the tissues occur.

The vascular reaction involves vascular spasm, formation of a platelet plug, blood coagulation, and growth of fibrous tissue.[13] The immediate response to damage is a vasoconstriction of the vascular walls that lasts for approximately 5 to 10 minutes. This spasm presses the opposing endothelial linings together to produce a local anemia that is rapidly replaced by hyperemia of the area due to dilation. This increase in blood flow is transitory and gives way to slowing of the blood flow in the dilated vessels, which then progresses to stagnation and stasis. The initial effusion of blood and plasma lasts for 24 to 36 hours.

Three chemical mediators, *histamine, leucotaxin,* and *necrosin* are important in limiting the amount of exudate, and thus swelling, after injury. Histamine released from the injured mast cells causes vasodilation and increased cell permeability, owing to swelling of endothelial cells, and then separation between the cells. Leucotaxin is responsible for margination in which leukocytes line up along the cell walls. It also increases cell permeability locally, thus affecting passage of the fluid and white blood cells through cell walls via diapedesis to form exudate (plasma). Therefore vasodilation and active hyperemia are important in forming exudate and supplying leukocytes to the injured area. Necrosin is responsible for phagocytic activity. The amount of swelling that occurs is directly related to the extent of vessel damage.

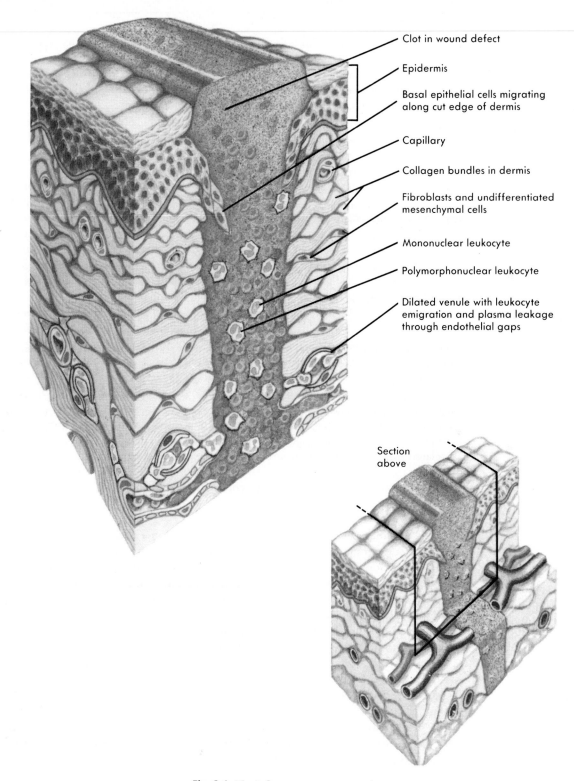

Clot in wound defect

Epidermis

Basal epithelial cells migrating
along cut edge of dermis

Capillary

Collagen bundles in dermis

Fibroblasts and undifferentiated
mesenchymal cells

Mononuclear leukocyte

Polymorphonuclear leukocyte

Dilated venule with leukocyte
emigration and plasma leakage
through endothelial gaps

Section
above

Fig. 2-1. The inflammatory response phase.

Platelets do not normally adhere to the vascular wall. However, injury to a vessel disrupts the endothelium and exposes the collagen fibers. Platelets adhere to the collagen fibers to create a sticky matrix on the vascular wall, to which additional platelets and leukocytes adhere and eventually form a plug. These plugs obstruct local lymphatic fluid drainage and thus localize the injury response.

The initial event that precipitates clot formation is the conversion of *fibrinogen* to *fibrin*. This transformation occurs because of a cascading effect beginning with the release of a protein molecule called *thromboplastin* from the damaged cell. Thromboplastin causes *prothrombin* to be changed into *thrombin,* which in turn causes the conversion of fibrinogen into a very sticky fibrin clot that shuts off blood supply to the injured area. Clot formation begins around 12 hours after injury and is completed within 48 hours.

As a result of a combination of these factors, the injured area becomes walled off during the inflammatory response stage of healing. The leukocytes phagocytize most of the foreign debris toward the end of the inflammatory response phase, setting the stage for the fibroblastic-repair phase. This initial inflammatory response lasts for approximately 2 to 4 days after initial injury.

CHRONIC INFLAMMATION. A distinction must be made between the acute inflammatory response as described above and chronic inflammation. Chronic inflammation occurs when the acute inflammatory response does not eliminate the injuring agent and restore tissue to its normal physiologic state. Chronic inflammation involves the replacement of leukocytes with *macrophages, lymphocytes,* and *plasma cells.* These cells accumulate in a highly vascularized and innervated loose connective tissue matrix in the area of injury.[8]

The specific mechanisms that convert an acute inflammatory response to a chronic inflammatory response are to date unknown. However, they seem to be associated with situations that involve overuse or overload with cumulative microtrauma to a particular structure.[5,8] Likewise, there is no specific time frame in which the classification of acute is changed to chronic inflammation.

Fibroblastic-Repair Phase

During the fibroblastic-repair phase of healing, proliferative and regenerative activity leading to scar formation and repair of the injured tissue begins. (Figure 2-2).[7] The period of scar formation referred to as **fibroplasia** begins within the first few hours after injury and may last for as long as 4 to 6 weeks. During this period, many of the signs and symptoms associated with the inflammatory response subside. The athlete may still indicate some tenderness to touch and will usually complain of pain when particular movements stress the injured structure. As scar formation progresses, complaints of tenderness or pain will gradually disappear.[11]

During this phase, growth of endothelial capillary buds into the wound is stimulated by a lack of oxygen. Thus the wound is now capable of healing aerobically. Along with increased oxygen delivery comes an increase in blood flow that delivers nutrients essential for tissue regeneration in the area.[4]

The formation of a delicate connective tissue called *granulation tissue* occurs with the breakdown of the fibrin clot. Granulation tissue consists of *fibroblasts,*

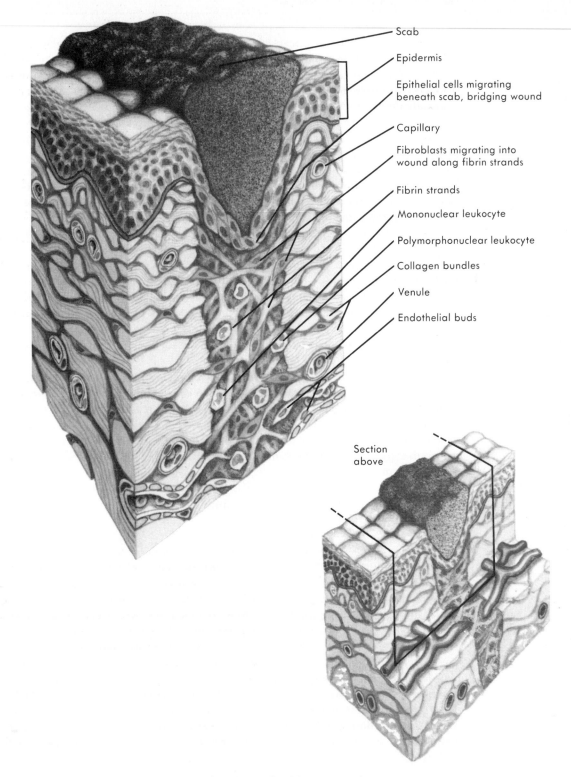

Scab

Epidermis

Epithelial cells migrating
beneath scab, bridging wound

Capillary

Fibroblasts migrating into
wound along fibrin strands

Fibrin strands

Mononuclear leukocyte

Polymorphonuclear leukocyte

Collagen bundles

Venule

Endothelial buds

Section
above

Fig. 2-2. The fibroblastic-repair phase.

collagen, and capillaries. It appears as a reddish granular mass of connective tissue that fills in the gaps during the healing process.

As the capillaries continue to grow into the area, fibroblasts accumulate at the wound site, arranging themselves parallel to the capillaries. Fibroblastic cells begin to synthesize an *extracellular matrix* that contains protein fibers of *collagen* and *elastin,* a *ground substance* that consists of nonfibrous proteins called *proteoglycans, glycosaminoglycans,* and fluid. On about day 6 or 7, fibroblasts also begin producing collagen fibers that are deposited in a random fashion throughout the forming scar. As the collagen continues to proliferate, the tensile strength of the wound rapidly increases in proportion to the rate of collagen synthesis. As the tensile strength increases, the number of fibroblasts diminishes, signaling the beginning of the maturation-remodeling phase.

This normal sequence of events in the fibroblastic-repair phase leads to the formation of minimal scar tissue. Occasionally, a persistent inflammatory response and continued release of inflammatory products can promote extended fibroplasia and excessive fibrogenesis that can lead to irreversible tissue damage.[14] Fibrosis can occur in synovial structures, as is the case with adhesive capsulitis in the shoulder; in extraarticular tissues, including tendons and ligaments; in bursa; or in muscle.

Maturation-Remodeling Phase

The maturation-remodeling phase of healing is a long-term process (Figure 2-3). This phase features a realignment or remodeling of the collagen fibers that make up the scar tissue according to the tensile forces to which that scar is subjected. Ongoing breakdown and synthesis of collagen occur, resulting in a steady increase in the tensile strength of the scar matrix. With increased stress and strain the collagen fibers will realign in a position of maximum efficiency parallel to the lines of tension. The tissue gradually assumes normal appearance and function, although a scar is rarely as strong as normal tissue. Usually by the end of approximately 3 weeks, a firm, strong, contracted, nonvascular scar exists. The maturation-remodeling phase of healing may require several years to be totally complete.

Factors That Impede Healing

EXTENT OF INJURY. The nature or amount of the inflammatory response is determined by the extent of the tissue injury. **Microtears** of soft tissue involve only minor damage and are most often associated with overuse. **Macrotears** involve significantly greater destruction of soft tissue and result in clinical symptoms and functional alterations. Macrotears are generally caused by acute trauma.

EDEMA. The increased pressure caused by swelling retards the healing process, causes separation of tissues, inhibits neuromuscular control, produces reflexive neurologic changes, and impedes nutrition in the injured part. Edema is best controlled and managed during the initial first-aid management period.[16]

HEMORRHAGE. Bleeding occurs with even the smallest amount of damage to the capillaries. Bleeding produces the same negative effects on healing as does the accumulation of edema, and its presence produces additional tissue damage, thus exacerbating the injury.

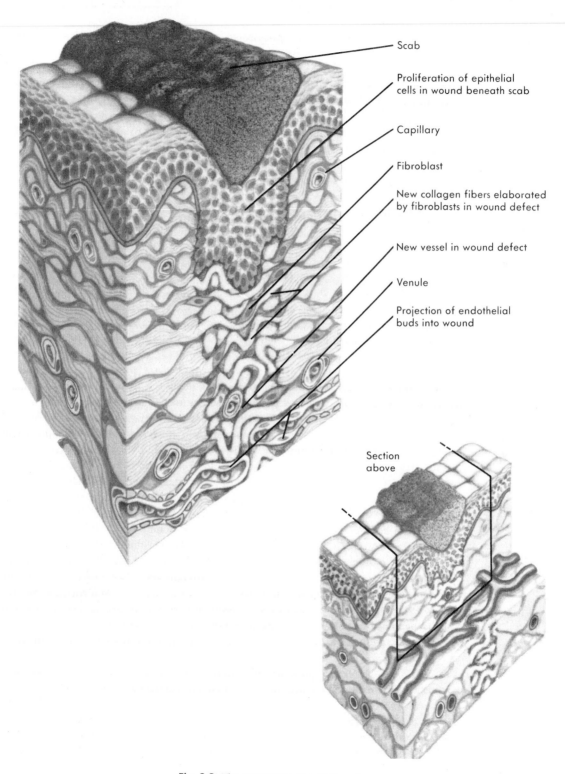

Scab

Proliferation of epithelial cells in wound beneath scab

Capillary

Fibroblast

New collagen fibers elaborated by fibroblasts in wound defect

New vessel in wound defect

Venule

Projection of endothelial buds into wound

Section above

Fig. 2-3. The maturation-remodeling phase.

POOR VASCULAR SUPPLY. Injuries to tissues with a poor vascular supply heal poorly and slowly. This is likely related to a failure in the delivery of phagocytic cells initially and also of fibroblasts necessary for scar formation.

SEPARATION OF TISSUE. Mechanical separation of tissue can significantly impact the course of healing. A wound that has smooth edges that are in good apposition will tend to heal by primary intention with minimal scarring. Conversely, a wound that has jagged, separated edges must heal by second intention with granulation tissue filling the defect, resulting in excessive scarring.[12]

MUSCLE SPASM. Muscle spasm causes traction on the torn tissue, separates the two ends, and prevents approximation. Both local and generalized ischemia may result from muscle spasm.

ATROPHY. Wasting away of muscle tissue begins immediately with injury. Strengthening and early mobilization of the injured structure retard atrophy.

CORTICOSTEROIDS. Use of corticosteroids to inflammation is controversial. Steroid use in the early stages of healing has been demonstrated to inhibit fibroplasia, capillary proliferation and collagen synthesis and to increase tensile strength of the healing scar. Their use in the later stages of healing and with chronic inflammation is debatable.

KELOIDS AND HYPERTROPHIC SCARS. Keloids occur when the rate of collagen production exceeds the rate of collagen breakdown during the maturation-remodeling phase of healing. This process leads to hypertrophy of scar tissue, particularly around the periphery of the wound.

INFECTION. Bacteria in the wound delays healing, causes excessive granulation tissue to form, and frequently causes large, deformed scars.

HUMIDITY, CLIMATE, AND OXYGEN TENSION. Humidity significantly influences the process of epithelization. Occlusive dressings stimulate the epithelium to migrate twice as fast without crust or scab formation. The formation of a scab occurs with dehydration of the wound, and the scab traps wound drainage, promoting infection. Keeping the wound moist allows the necrotic debris to go to the surface and be shed.

Oxygen tension relates to the neovascularization of the wound, which translates into optimal saturation and maximal tensile strength development. Circulation to the wound can be affected by ischemia, venous stasis, hematomas, and vessel trauma.

HEALTH, AGE, AND NUTRITION. The elastic qualities of the skin decrease with aging. Degenerative diseases, such as diabetes and arteriosclerosis, also become a concern of the older athlete and may affect wound healing. Nutrition is important for wound healing. In particular, vitamin C (scurvy), vitamin K (clotting), vitamins A and E (collagen synthesis), zinc (for the enzyme systems), and amino acids play critical roles in the healing process.

INJURY MANAGEMENT USING MODALITIES

Traditionally in a sports-medicine setting, injuries have been classified as being either acute injuries that result from trauma or chronic injuries that result primarily from overuse. This operational definition is not necessarily correct. If active inflammation is present that includes the classic symptoms of tenderness, swelling, redness, and so on, the injury should be considered acute and must be treated accordingly using rest, ice, compression, and elevation. Even if active inflammation persists for months after initial injury, it should still be considered acute. Classification of an injury should be determined according to the existing signs and symptoms that indicate the various stages of the healing process and not according to time frames or mechanisms of injury. Once the signs of acute inflammation are no longer present, the injury may be considered to be chronic. Inflammation may be considered chronic when the normal cellular response in the inflammatory process is altered, replacing leukocytes with macrophages and plasma cells, along with degeneration of the injured structure.

Based on this definition of acute and chronic injury, the rehabilitation progression after injury may be determined by the four phases of healing. These phases overlap, and the estimated time frames for each phase show extreme variability between patients. Table 2-1 summarizes the various modalities that may be used in each of the four phases.

Initial Acute Injury Phase

The acute phase is marked by swelling, pain to touch or with pressure, and pain on both active and passive motion. Modality use in the initial treatment phase should be directed toward limiting the amount of swelling and reducing pain. In general, the less initial swelling, the less the time required for rehabilitation. Traditionally, the modality of choice has been and still is **ICE.**

Cryotherapy produces vasoconstriction, at least superficially and perhaps indirectly in the deeper tissues, and thus limits the bleeding that always occurs with injury. Ice bags, cold packs, and ice massage may all be used effectively. Cold baths should be avoided because the extremities must be placed in a gravity-dependent position. Cold whirlpools also place the extremities in the gravity-dependent position and produce a massaging action that is likely to retard clotting. Although the application of ice immediately after injury to limit acute swelling is important, the initial use of ice is more important for producing analgesia, which occurs through stimulation of sensory cutaneous nerves that, via the gating mechanism, block or reduce pain.

Immediate compression has been demonstrated to be an effective technique for limiting swelling. Compression may be accomplished using elastic wraps. An intermittent compression device may also be used to provide even pressure around an injured extremity. The pressurized sleeve mechanically reduces the amount of space available for swelling to accumulate. Units that combine both compression and cold are more effective in reducing swelling than those units using compression alone. Regardless of the specific techniques selected, cold and compression should always be combined with elevation to avoid any additional pooling of blood in the injured area caused by the effects of gravity.

Electrical stimulating currents may also be used in the initial phase for pain reduction. Parameters should be adjusted to maximally stimulate sensory cutaneous nerve fibers, again to take advantage of the gate control mechanism of pain modulation. Intensities that produce muscle contractions should be avoided because they may increase clotting time.

Ultrasound has been demonstrated to be effective in facilitating the healing process when used immediately after injury and certainly within the first 48 hours. Low spatial-averaged intensities below .2 W/cm^2 produce nonthermal physiologic effects

TABLE 2-1   **Clinical Decision Making on the Use of Various Therapeutic Modalities in Treatment of Acute Injury**

Phase	Approximate Time Frame	Clinical Picture	Possible Modalities Used	Rationale for Use
Initial acute	Injury—day 3	Swelling, pain to touch, pain on motion	CRYO	↓ Swelling, ↓ pain
			ESC	↓ Pain
			IC	↓ Swelling
			LPL	↓ Pain
			ULTRA	Nonthermal effects to ↑ healing
			Rest	
Inflammatory response	Day 2—day 6	Swelling subsides, warm to touch, discoloration, pain to touch, pain on motion	CRYO	↓ Swelling, ↓ pain
			ESC	↓ Pain
			IC	↓ Swelling
			LPL	↓ Pain
			ULTRA	Nonthermal effects to ↑ healing
			Range of motion	
Fibroblastic-repair	Day 4—day 10	Pain to touch, pain on motion, swollen	THERMO	Mildly ↑ circulation
			ESC	↓ Pain—muscle pumping
			LPL	↓ Pain
			IC	Facilitate lymphatic flow
			ULTRA	Nonthermal effects to ↑ healing
			Range of motion Strengthening	
Maturation-remodeling	Day 7—recovery	Swollen, no more pain to touch, decreasing pain on motion	ULTRA	Deep heating to ↑ circulation
			ESC	↑ Range of motion, ↑ strength
			LPL	↓ Pain
			SWD	↓ Pain
			MWD	Deep heating to ↑ circulation
			Range of motion	Deep heating to ↑ circulation
			Strengthening Functional activities	

CRYO, Cryotherapy; *ESC*, electrical stimulating currents; *IC*, intermittent compression; *LPL*, low-power laser; *MWD*, microwave diathermy; *SWD*, shortwave diathermy; *THERMO*, thermotherapy; *ULTRA*, ultrasound; ↓, decrease; ↑, increase.

that alter the permeability of cell membranes to sodium and calcium ions, which are important in healing.

The low-power laser is also effective in pain modulation through the stimulation of trigger points and may be used acutely.

The injured part should be rested and protected for at least the first 48 to 72 hours to allow the inflammatory phase of the healing process to proceed.

Inflammatory Response Phase

The inflammatory response phase begins as early as day 1 and may last as long as day 6 after injury. Clinically, swelling begins to subside and eventually stops altogether. The injured area may feel warm to the touch, and some discoloration is usually apparent. The injury is still painful to the touch, and pain is elicited on movement of the injured part.

As in the initial injury stage, modalities should be used to control pain and reduce swelling. Cryotherapy should still be used during the inflammatory response stage. Ice bags, cold packs, or ice massages provide analgesic effects. The use of cold also reduces the likelihood of swelling, which may continue during this stage. Increases in swelling should not occur by the end of this phase, assuming that the tissue is not subjected to additional trauma.

It must be emphasized that heating an injury too soon is a bigger mistake than using ice on an injury for too long. Many sports therapists elect to stay with cryotherapy for weeks after injury; in fact, some therapists never switch to the superficial heating techniques. This procedure is simply a matter of personal preference that should be dictated by experience. Once swelling has stopped, the sports therapist may elect to begin contrast baths with a longer cold-to-hot ratio.

An intermittent compression device may be used to decrease swelling by facilitating resorption of the by-products of the inflammatory process by the lymphatic system. Electrical stimulating currents and low-power laser can be used to help reduce pain. The use of low intensity ultrasound should continue during this phase.

After the initial stage, the athlete should begin to work on active and passive range of motion. Decisions regarding how rapidly to progress with exercise should be determined by the response of the injury to that exercise. If exercise produces additional swelling and markedly exacerbates pain, then the level or intensity of the exercise is too great and should be reduced. Sports therapists should be aggressive in their approach to rehabilitation, but the approach will always be limited by the healing process.

Fibroblastic-Repair Phase

Once the inflammatory response has accomplished what it is supposed to, the fibroblastic-repair phase begins. During this phase of the healing process, fibroblastic cells are laying down a matrix of collagen fibers and forming scar tissue. This stage may begin as early as 4 days after the injury and may last for several weeks. At this point, swelling should have stopped completely. The injury is still tender to the touch but is not as painful as during the last stage. Pain is also less on active and passive motion.

Treatments may change during this stage from cold to heat, once again using increased swelling as a precautionary indicator. Thermotherapy techniques including hydrocollator packs, paraffin, or eventually warm whirlpool may be safely used. The purpose of thermotherapy is to increase circulation to the injured area to promote healing. These modalities can also produce some degree of analgesia.

Intermittent compression can once again be used to facilitate removal of injury by-products from the area. Electrical stimulating currents can be used to assist this process by eliciting a muscle contraction and thus inducing a muscle pumping action.

This aids in facilitating lymphatic flow. Electrical currents can once again be used for pain modulation, as can stimulation of trigger points with the low-powered laser.

The sports therapist must continue to stress the importance of range-of-motion and strengthening exercises and progress with them appropriately during this phase.

Maturation-Remodeling Phase

The maturation-remodeling phase is the longest of the four phases and may last for several years, depending on the severity of the injury. The ultimate goal during this maturation stage of the healing process is a return to activity. The injury is no longer painful to the touch, although some progressively decreasing pain may still be felt with movement. The collagen fibers must be realigned according to the tensile stresses and strains placed upon them. Virtually all modalities may be safely used during this stage; thus decisions should be based on what seems to work most effectively in a given situation.

At this point, some type of heating modality contributes to the healing process. The deep-heating modalities, ultrasound, or shortwave and microwave diathermy should be used to increase circulation to the deeper tissues. Ultrasound is particularly useful during this period, since collagen absorbs a high percentage of the available acoustic energy. Increased blood flow delivers the essential nutrients to the injured area to promote healing, and increased lymphatic flow assists in the breakdown and removal of waste products. The superficial heating modalities are certainly less effective at this point.

Electrical stimulating currents can be used for a number of purposes. As before, they may be used in pain modulation. They may also be used to stimulate muscle contractions to increase both range of motion and muscular strength.

Low-power laser can also assist in modulating pain. If pain is reduced, therapeutic exercises may be progressed more quickly.

THE ROLE OF PROGRESSIVE CONTROLLED MOBILITY IN THE MATURATION-REMODELING PHASE. Wolff's Law states that both bone and soft tissue will respond to the physical demands placed upon them, causing them to remodel or realign along lines of tensile force.[15] Therefore it is critical that injured structures be exposed to progressively increasing loads, particularly during the maturation-remodeling phase. Controlled mobilization is superior to immobilization for scar formation, revascularization, muscle regeneration, and reorientation of muscle fibers and tensile properties in animal models.[17] However, immobilization of the injured tissue during the inflammatory response phase will likely facilitate the process of healing by controlling inflammation, thus reducing clinical symptoms. As healing progresses to the fibroblastic-repair phase, controlled activity directed toward return to normal flexibility and strength should be combined with protective support or bracing. Generally, clinical signs and symptoms disappear at the end of this phase.

As the maturation-remodeling phase begins, aggressive range of motion and strengthening exercises should be incorporated to facilitate tissue remodeling and realignment. To a great extent, pain will dictate rate of progression. Pain is intense with initial injury and tends to decrease and eventually subside altogether as healing progresses. Any exacerbation of either pain, swelling, or other clinical symptoms during or after a particular exercise or activity indicates that the load is too great for the level

TABLE 2-2   **Indications and Contraindications for Therapeutic Modalities**

Therapeutic Modality	Physiologic Resources (Indications for Use)	Contraindications and Precautions
Electrical stimulating currents—high voltage	Pain modulation Muscle reeducation Muscle pumping contractions Retard atrophy Muscle strengthening Increase range of motion Fracture healing Acute injury	Pacemakers Thrombophlebitis Superficial skin lesions
Electrical stimulating currents—low voltage	Wound healing Fracture healing Iontophoresis	Malignancy Skin hypersensitivities Allergies to certain drugs
Electrical stimulating currents—interferential	Pain modulation Muscle reeducation Muscle pumping contractions Fracture healing Increase range of motion	Same as high-voltage
Electrical stimulating currents—Russian	Muscle strengthening	Pacemakers
Electrical stimulating currents—MENS	Fracture healing Wound healing	Malignancy Infections
Shortwave and microwave diathermy	Increase deep circulation Increase metabolic activity Reduce muscle guarding/spasm Reduce inflammation Facilitate wound healing Analgesia Increase tissue temperatures over a large area	Metal implants Pacemakers Malignancy Wet dressings Anesthetized areas Pregnancy Acute injury and inflammation Eyes Areas of reduced blood flow Anesthetized areas
Cryotherapy—cold packs, ice massage	Acute injury Vasoconstriction—decreased blood flow Analgesia Reduce inflammation Reduce muscle guarding/spasm	Allergy to cold Circulatory impairments Wound healing Hypertension
Thermotherapy—hot whirlpool, paraffin, hydrocollator, infrared lamps	Vasodilation—increased blood flow Analgesia Reduce muscle guarding/spasm Reduce inflammation Increase metabolic activity Facilitate tissue healing	Acute and postacute trauma Poor circulation Circulatory impairments Malignancy
Low-power laser	Pain modulation (trigger points) Facilitate wound healing	Pregnancy Eyes

Continued.

TABLE 2-2   Indications and Contraindications for Therapeutic
Modalities — cont'd

Therapeutic Modality	Physiologic Resources (Indications for Use)	Contraindications and Precautions
Ultraviolet	Acne Aseptic wounds Folliculitis Pityriasis rosea Tinea Septic wounds Sinusitis Increase calcium metabolism	Psoriasis Eczema Herpes Diabetes Pellagra Lupus erythematosus Hyperthyroidism Renal and hepatic insufficiency Generalized dermatitis Advanced atherosclerosis
Ultrasound	Increase connective tissue extensibility Deep heat Increased circulation Treatment of most soft tissue injuries Reduce inflammation Reduce muscle spasm	Infection Acute and postacute injury Epiphyseal areas Pregnancy Thrombophlebitis Impaired sensation Eyes
Intermittent compression	Decrease acute bleeding Decrease edema	Circulatory impairment

of tissue repair or remodeling. The sports therapist must be aware of the timelines required for the healing process and realize that being overly aggressive can interfere with that process.

Other Considerations in Treating Injury

During the rehabilitation period after injury, athletes must alter their training and conditioning habits to allow the injury to heal sufficiently. The sports therapist must not neglect fitness training in designing a rehabilitation program. Consideration must be given to maintaining levels of strength, flexibility, and cardiorespiratory endurance. Modality use should be combined with antiinflammatory medication, particularly during the initial acute and acute inflammatory phases of rehabilitation.

INDICATIONS AND CONTRAINDICATIONS

Table 2-2 is a summary list of indications, contraindications, and precautions in using the various modalities. This list should aid the sports therapist in making decisions regarding the appropriate use of a therapeutic modality in a given clinical situation.

SUMMARY

1. Clinical decisions on how and when therapeutic modalities may best be used should be based on recognition of signs and symptoms, as well as some

awareness of the time frames associated with the various phases of the healing process.

2. Once an acute injury has occurred, the healing process consists of the inflammatory response phase, the fibroblastic-repair phase, and the maturation-remodeling phase.

3. There are a number of pathologic factors that can impede the healing process.

4. Modality use in the initial treatment phase should be directed toward limiting the amount of swelling and reducing pain.

5. It is critical to use logic and common sense based on sound theoretical knowledge when selecting the appropriate modalities to use during the different phases of healing.

6. During the rehabilitation period after injury, athletes must alter their training and conditioning habits to allow the injury to heal sufficiently.

GLOSSARY

acute injury An injury in which active inflammation is present that includes the classic symptoms of tenderness, swelling, redness, and so on.

chronic injury An injury in which the normal cellular response in the inflammatory process is altered, replacing leukocytes with macrophages and plasma cells, along with degeneration of the injured structure.

fibroplasia The period of scar formation that occurs during the fibroblastic-repair phase.

macrotears Significant damage to soft tissues caused by acute trauma that result in clinical symptoms and functional alterations.

microtears Minor damage to soft tissue most often associated with overuse.

REFERENCES

1 Arnheim D, Prentice W: *Principles of athletic training,* ed 8, St Louis, 1993, Mosby.

2 Bryant MW: Wound healing, *CIBA Clinical Symposia* 29(3): 2-36, 1977.

3 Carrico TJ, Mehrhof AI, Cohen IK: Biology and wound healing, *Surg Clin North Am* 64(4): 721-734, 1984.

4 Cheng N: The effects of electrocurrents on ATP generation, protein synthesis and membrane transport, *J Orth Rel Res* 171: 264-272, 1982.

5 Fantone J: *Basic concepts in inflammation.* In Leadbetter W, Buckwalter J, Gordon S, editors: *Sports-induced inflammation,* Park Ridge, Ill, 1990, American Academy of Orthopaedic Surgeons.

6 Fernandez A, Finlew JM: Wound healing: helping a natural process, *Postgrad Med* 74(4): 311-318, 1983.

7 Hettinga DL: *Inflammatory response of synovial joint structures.* In Gould JA, Davies GJ, editors: *Orthopaedic and sports physical therapy,* St Louis, 1990, Mosby.

8 Leadbetter W: *Introduction to sports-induced soft-tissue inflammation.* In Leadbetter W, Buckwalter J, Gordon S, editors: *Sports-induced inflammation,* Park Ridge, Ill, 1990, American Academy of Orthopaedic Surgeons.

9 Leadbetter W, Buckwalter J, Gordon S: *Sports-induced inflammation,* Park Ridge, Ill, 1990, American Academy of Orthopaedic Surgeons.

10 Marchesi VT: *Inflammation and healing.* In Kissane JM, editor: *Anderson's pathology,* ed 8, St Louis, 1985, Mosby.

11 Riley WB: Wound healing, *Am Fam Physician* 24: 5, 1981.

12 Robbins SL, Cotran RS, Kumar V: *Pathologic basis of disease,* ed 3, Philadelphia, 1984, WB Saunders.

13 Rywlin AM: *Hemopoietic system.* In Kissane JM, editor: *Anderson's pathology,* ed 8, St Louis, 1985, Mosby.

14 Wahl S, Renstrom P: *Fibrosis in soft-tissue injuries.* In Leadbetter W, Buckwalter J, Gordon S, editors: *Sports-induced inflammation,* Park Ridge, Ill, 1990, American Academy of Orthopaedic Surgeons.

15 Wolff J: *Gesetz der transformation der knochen,* Berlin, 1892, Aug. Hirschwald.

16 Woo SL-Y, Buckwalter J, editors: *Injury and repair of musculoskeletal soft tissues,* Park Ridge, Ill, 1988, American Academy of Orthopaedic Surgeons.

17 Zachezewski J: *Flexibility for sports.* In Sanders B, editor: *Sports physical therapy,* Norwalk, Conn, 1990, Appleton & Lange.

Managing Pain with Therapeutic Modalities

3

Phillip B. Donley and Craig R. Denegar

OBJECTIVES

After completion of this chapter, the student will be able to do the following:

- Define pain, its types, and its positive and negative effects.

- Describe the characteristics of sensory receptors.

- Describe how the nervous system relays information about painful stimulation.

- Describe an appropriate neurophysiologic mechanism for pain control for the therapeutic modalities used by the sports therapist.

- Describe how pain perception can be modified by cognitive factors.

UNDERSTANDING PAIN

The International Association for the Study of Pain defines **pain** as "an unpleasant sensory and emotional experience associated with actual or potential tissue damage, or described in terms of such damage."[22] Pain is a subjective sensation with more than one dimension and an abundance of descriptors of its characteristics. In spite of its universality, pain is composed of a variety of human discomforts, rather than being a single entity.[20] The perception of pain can be subjectively modified by past experiences and expectations. Much of what we do to treat athletes' pain is to change their perception of pain.[4]

Pain does have a purpose. It warns us that there is something wrong and can provoke a withdrawal response to avoid further injury. It also results in muscle spasm and guarding or protection of the injured part. Pain, however, can persist after its usefulness. It can enhance disability and inhibit efforts to rehabilitate the injury. Prolonged spasm, which leads to circulatory deficiency, muscle atrophy, disuse habits, and conscious or unconscious guarding, may lead to a severe loss of athletic ability.[17] Chronic pain may become a disease state in itself. Often lacking an identifiable cause, chronic pain can totally disable a patient.

Research in recent years has led to a better understanding of pain and pain relief. This research also has raised new questions while leaving many unanswered. We now have better explanations for the analgesic properties of the physical agents we use, as well as a better understanding of the psychology of pain. However, new physical agents, such as the laser and microamperage electrical simulators, and new approaches to older agents, such as transcutaneous electrical nerve simulators (TENS), challenge our understanding of injury and pain. Not even the mechanisms for the analgesic response to heat and cold have been fully described.

Pain control is an essential aspect of caring for the injured athlete. The sports therapist has several therapeutic agents with analgesic properties from which to choose. The selection of a therapeutic agent should be based on a sound understanding of its physical properties and physiologic effects. This chapter will not provide a complete explanation of neurophysiology, pain, and pain relief. Instead, it presents an overview of some theories of pain control, intended to provide a stimulus for the sports therapist to develop his or her own rationale for using modalities in the treatment of injured athletes. Ideally, it also will interest some therapists through research to establish the physiologic and psychologic soundness of the use of agents for pain relief and to expand our understanding of pain. Several physiology textbooks provide extensive discussions of human neurophysiology and neurobiology to supplement this chapter.

Many of the modalities discussed in later chapters have analgesic properties. Often, they are used to reduce pain and permit the athlete to perform therapeutic exercises. Some understanding of what pain is, how it affects us, and how it is perceived is essential for the sports therapist who uses these modalities.

TYPES OF PAIN

Pain has been categorized as either acute or chronic. Pain lasting for more than 6 months is generally classified as chronic.[5] There is more research devoted to chronic pain and its treatment, but acute pain, or pain of sudden onset, is a more likely problem for the sports therapist.

Referred pain, which also may be either acute or chronic, is pain that is perceived to be in an area that seems to have little relation to the existing pathology. For example, injury to the spleen often results in pain in the left shoulder. This pattern, known as Kehr's sign, is useful for identifying this serious injury and arranging prompt emergency care. Referred pain can outlast the causative events because of altered reflex patterns, continuing mechanical stress on muscles, learned habits of guarding, or the development of hypersensitive areas, called **trigger points.**

Irritation of nerves and nerve roots can cause radiating pain. Pressure on the lumbar nerve roots associated with a herniated disc or a contusion of the sciatic nerve can result in pain radiating down the lower extremity to the foot.

Deep somatic pain seems to be sclerotomic (associated with a **sclerotome,** a segment of bone innervated by a spinal segment). There is often a discrepancy between the site of the disorder and the site of the pain.

PAIN ASSESSMENT

Pain is a complex phenomenon that is difficult to evaluate and quantify because it is subjective and is influenced by attitudes and beliefs of the sports therapist and the athlete. Quantification is hindered since pain is a very difficult concept to verbalize.

Obtaining an accurate and standardized assessment of pain is problematic, but several tools have been developed. These pain profiles identify the type of pain, quantify the intensity of pain, evaluate the effect of the pain experience on the athlete's level of function, or assess the psychosocial impact of pain.

The pain profiles compel the athlete to verbalize the pain and thereby create an outlet for the athlete and provide the sports therapist with a better understanding of the pain experience. Pain profiles can assist with the evaluation process by improving communication and directing the sports therapist toward appropriate diagnostic tests. These assessments also assist the sports therapist in identifying which therapeutic agents may be effective and when they should be applied. Finally, these profiles provide a standard measure to monitor treatment progress.[12]

Pain Assessment Scales

The following profiles are used in the evaluation of acute and chronic pain associated with sports injuries.

Visual analogue scales are quick and simple tests completed by the athlete (Figure 3-1). These scales consist of a line, usually 10 cm in length, the extremes of which are taken to represent the limits of the pain experience. One end is labeled "None" to show no pain; the other is labeled "Severe" to indicate severe pain. The athlete is asked to mark the line at a point corresponding to the severity of the pain. The distance between None and the mark represents pain severity. A similar scale can be used to assess treatment effectiveness by placing "No pain relief" at one end of the scale and "Complete pain relief" at the other. These scales can be completed daily or more often as pre-treatment and post-treatment assessments.[15]

Pain charts can be used to establish spatial properties of pain. These two-dimensional graphic portrayals are completed by the athlete to assess the location of pain and a number of subjective components. Simple line drawings of the body in several postural positions are presented to the athlete (Figure 3-2). The athlete draws

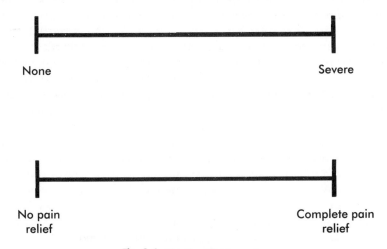

None   Severe

No pain   Complete pain
relief   relief

Fig. 3-1. Visual analogue scales.

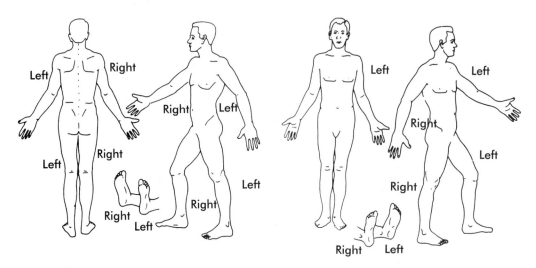

Fig. 3-2. The pain chart. Use the following instructions: "Please use all of the figures to show me exactly where all your pains are and where they radiate to. Shade or draw with *blue marker*. Only the patient is to fill out this sheet. Please be as precise and detailed as possible. Use *yellow marker* for numbness and tingling. Use *red marker* for burning or hot areas and *green marker* for cramping. Please remember: blue = pain; yellow = numbness and tingling; red = burning or hot areas; green = cramping."
From Melzack R: *Pain measurement and assessment,* New York, 1983, Raven Press.)

or colors the pictures in areas that correspond to his or her pain experience. Different colors are used for different sensations. For example, blue is used for aching pain, yellow for numbness or tingling, red for burning pain, and green for cramping pain. Descriptions can be added to the form to enhance the communication value. The form can be completed daily.[18]

The McGill Pain Questionnaire (MPQ) is a tool with 78 words that describe pain (Figure 3-3). These words are grouped into 20 sets that are divided into 4 categories representing dimensions of the pain experience. Completion of the MPQ may take 20 minutes and is often frustrating for athletes who do not speak English well. It is commonly administered to athletes and other patients with low back pain. When administered every 2 to 4 weeks, it demonstrated changes in status very clearly.[20]

The Activity Pattern Indicators Pain Profile measures patient activity. It is a 64 question, self-report tool that may be used to assess functional impairment associated with pain. The instrument measures the frequency of certain behaviors such as housework, recreation, and social activities.[13]

The most common acute pain profile used in sports medicine clinics today is a numeric pain scale. The athlete is asked to rate his or her pain on a scale from 1 to 10 with 10 representing the worst pain they have experienced or could imagine. The question is asked before and after treatment. When treatments provide pain relief, athletes are asked about the extent and duration of the relief. In addition, athletes may be asked to estimate the portion of the day that they experience pain and about specific activities that increase or decrease their pain. When pain affects sleep, athletes may be asked to estimate how long they slept in the previous 24 hours. In addition, the amount of medication required for pain relief can be noted.

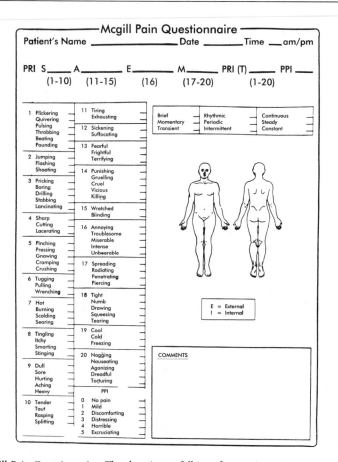

Fig. 3-3. McGill Pain Questionnaire. The descriptors fall into four major groups: sensory, 1 to 10: affective, 11 to 15; evaluative, 16; and miscellaneous, 17 to 20. The rank value for each descriptor is based on its position in the word set. The sum of the rank values is the pain rating index (PRI). The present pain intensity (PPI) is based on a scale of 0 to 5.
From Melzack R: *Pain measurement and assessment,* New York, 1983, Raven Press.)

This information helps the sports therapist assess changes in pain, select appropriate treatments, and communicate more clearly with the athlete about the course of recovery from injury or surgery.

All of these scales help athletes communicate the severity and duration of their pain and appreciate changes that occur. Often in a long recovery, athletes lose sight of how much progress has been made in terms of the pain experience and return to functional activities. A review of these pain scales often can serve to reassure the athlete; foster a brighter, more positive outlook; and reinforce the commitment to the treatment plan.

The efficacy of many of the treatments used in athletic training has not been fully substantiated. These scales are one source of data that can help sports therapists identify the most effective approaches to managing common injuries. These assessment tools can also be useful when reviewing an athlete's progress with physicians, coaches, parents and, in the sports medicine clinical setting, third-party payors.

TISSUE SENSITIVITY

The structures most sensitive to damaging (noxious) stimuli are, first, the **periosteum** and **joint capsule;** second, subchondral bone, tendons, and ligament; third, muscle and cortical bone; and finally, the synovium and articular cartilage. A variety of "silent" fractures produce little or no pain. Different anatomic tissues exhibit varying degrees of sensitivity to pain. **Avulsion fractures** tend to be quite painful because they tear away the periosteum. Musculoskeletal pain is usually spread over a large area unless it is close to the surface. For example, a hamstring strain usually results in pain over the posterior thigh, whereas an acromioclavicular sprain usually localizes over the joint.

GOALS IN MANAGING PAIN

Regardless of the cause of pain, its reduction is an essential part of treatment. Medical or surgical treatment or immobilization is necessary to treat some conditions, but physical therapy and an early return to activity are appropriate after many athletic injuries. The sports therapist's objectives are to encourage the body to heal through exercise designed to progressively increase the capacity for athletic work and to return the athlete to competition as swiftly and safely as possible. Pain will inhibit therapeutic exercise. The challenge for the sports therapist is to control acute pain and protect the athlete from further injury, while encouraging progressive exercise in a supervised environment.

PAIN PERCEPTION AND NEURAL TRANSMISSION
Sensory Receptors

There are several types of sensory receptors in the body, and the sports therapist should be aware of their existence and the types of stimuli that activate them (Table 3-1).[31] Activation of some of these sense organs with therapeutic agents will decrease the athlete's perception of pain.

Six different types of receptor nerve endings are commonly described:
1. Meissner's corpuscles are activated by light touch.
2. Pacinian corpuscles respond to deep pressure.
3. Merkel's corpuscles respond to deep pressure but more slowly than pacinian corpuscles and also are activated by hair follicle deflection.
4. Ruffini corpuscles in the skin are sensitive to touch, tension, and possibly heat; those in the joint capsules and ligaments are sensitive to change in position.
5. Krause's end bulbs are thermoreceptors that react to a decrease in temperature and touch.[26]
6. Pain receptors, called **nociceptors** or **free nerve endings,** are sensitive to extreme mechanical, thermal, or chemical energy.[3] They respond to noxious stimuli, such as cuts, burns, and sprains. The term *nociceptive* is from the Latin *nocere,* to damage, and is used to imply pain information.

These organs respond to superficial forms of heat and cold, analgesic balms, and massage.

TABLE 3-1	Some Characteristics of Selected Sensory Receptors			
	Stimulus		Receptor	
Type of Sensory Receptors	General Term	Specific Nature	Term	Location
Mechanoreceptors	Pressure	Movement of hair in a hair follicle	Afferent nerve fiber	Base of hair follicles
		Light pressure	Meissner's corpuscle	Skin
		Deep pressure	Pacinian corpuscle	Skin
		Touch	Merkel's touch corpuscle	Skin
Nociceptors	Pain	Distension (stretch)	Free nerve endings	Wall of gastrointestinal tract, pharynx, skin
Proprioceptors	Tension	Distension	Corpuscles of Ruffini	Skin and capsules in joints and ligaments
		Length changes	Muscle spindles	Skeletal muscle
		Tension changes	Golgi tendon organs	Between muscles and tendons
Thermoreceptors	Temperature change	Cold	Krause's end bulbs	Skin
		Heat	Corpuscles of Ruffini	Skin and capsules in joints and ligaments

From Previte JJ: *Human physiology*, New York, 1983, McGraw-Hill.

Proprioceptors found in muscles, joint capsules, ligaments, and tendons provide information regarding joint position and muscle tone. The muscle spindles react to changes in length and tension when the muscle is stretched or contracted. The Golgi tendon organs also react to changes in length and tension within the muscle. See Table 3-1 for a more complete listing of sensory receptors.

Some sensory receptors respond to phasic activity and produce an impulse when the stimulus is increasing or decreasing but not during a sustained stimulus. They adapt to a constant stimulus. Meissner's corpuscles and pacinian corpuscles are examples of such receptors.

Tonic receptors produce impulses as long as the stimulus is present. Examples of tonic receptors are muscle spindles, free nerve endings, and Krause's end bulbs. The initial impulse is at a higher frequency than later impulses that occur during sustained stimulation.

Accommodation is the decline in generator potential and the reduction of frequency that occurs with a prolonged stimulus or with frequently repeated stimuli. If some physical agents are used too often or for too long, the receptors may adapt to or accommodate the stimulus and reduce their impulses. The accommodation phenomenon can be observed with the use of superficial hot and cold agents, such as ice packs and hydrocollator packs.

As a stimulus becomes stronger, the number of receptors excited and the frequency of the impulses increase. This provides more electrical activity at the spinal cord level, which may facilitate the effects of some physical agents.

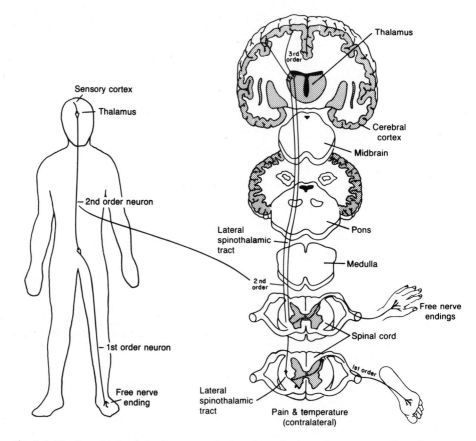

Fig. 3-4. The lateral spinothalamic tract carries impulses of pain and temperature from the sensory receptors to the cortex.

NEURAL TRANSMISSION

Afferent nerve fibers transmit impulses from the sensory receptors toward the brain, while **efferent** fibers, such as motor neurons, transmit impulses from the brain toward the periphery. First-order or primary afferent fibers transmit the impulses from the sensory receptor to the dorsal horn of the spinal cord (Figure 3-4). There are four different types of first-order neurons (Table 3-2). Note that A-alpha and A-beta fibers are characterized as being large-diameter afferents and A-delta and C fibers as small-diameter afferents.

Second-order afferent fibers carry sensory messages from the dorsal horn to the brain. Second-order afferent fibers are categorized as wide dynamic range or nociceptive specific. The wide dynamic range second-order afferents receive input from A-beta, A-delta, and C fibers. These second-order afferents serve relatively large, overlapping receptor fields. The nociceptive specific second-order afferents respond exclusively to noxious stimulation. They receive input only from A-delta and C fibers. These afferents serve smaller receptor fields that do not overlap. All of these neurons

TABLE 3-2   Classification of Afferent Neurons

Size	Type	Group	Subgroup	Diameter (Micrometers)	Conduction Velocity	Receptor	Stimulus
Large	A α	I	1a	12-20 (22)	70-120	Proprioceptive mechanoreceptor	Muscle velocity and length change, muscle shortening of rapid speed
	A α	I	1b				
	A β	II	Muscle	6-12	36-72	Proprioceptive mechanoreceptor	Muscle length information from touch and pacinian corpuscles
	A β	II	Skin			Cutaneous receptors	Touch, vibration, hair receptors
	A δ	III	Muscle	1-5 (6)	6(12)-36(80)	75% mechanoreceptors and thermoreceptors	Temperature change
Small	A δ	III	Skin			25% nociceptors, mechanoreceptors and thermoreceptors (hot and cold)	Noxious mechanical and temperature ($>45°$ C, $<10°$ C)
	C	IV	Muscle	0.3-1.0	0.4-1.0	50% mechanoreceptors and thermoreceptors	Touch and temperature
	C	IV	Skin			50% nociceptors, 20% mechanoreceptors, and 30% thermoreceptors (hot and cold)	Noxious mechanical and temperature ($>45°$ C, $<10°$ C)

synapse with third-order neurons that carry information to various brain centers where the input is integrated, interpreted, and acted upon.

Facilitators and Inhibitors of Synaptic Transmission

For information to pass between neurons, a transmitter substance must be released from one neuron terminal (presynaptic membrane), enter the synaptic cleft, and attach to a receptor site on the next neuron (postsynaptic membrane). In the past, all the activity within the synapse was attributed to neurotransmitters, such as acetylcholine. The **neurotransmitters,** when released in sufficient quantities, cause depolarization of the postsynaptic neuron. In the absence of the neurotransmitter, no depolarization occurs.

It is now apparent that several compounds that are not true neurotransmitters can facilitate or inhibit synaptic activity. These compounds are classified as biogenic amine transmitters or neuroactive peptides. Serotonin and norepinephrine are examples of biogenic amine transmitters. About 25 neuroactive peptides have been identified, including **substance P, enkephalins,** and **β-endorphin.**[3]

Serotonin and **enkephalins** are active in descending (efferent) pathways that block the pain message.[7] Enkephalin is an **endogenous** (made by the body) **opioid** that inhibits the depolarization of second-order nociceptive nerve fibers. It is released from **interneurons,** enkephalin neurons with short axons. The enkephalins are stored in nerve-ending vesicles found in the **substantia gelatinosa** and several areas of the brain. When released, enkephalin may bind to presynaptic or postsynaptic membranes.[3]

Norepinephrine is a biogenic amine transmitter that is released by the depolarization of some neurons and binds to the postsynaptic membranes. Norepinephrine is found in several areas of the nervous system, including a tract that descends from the pons, which inhibits synaptic transmission between first- and second-order nociceptive fibers, thus decreasing pain sensation.[16]

Other endogenous opioids, **endorphins,** may be active analgesic agents. These neuroactive peptides are released into the central nervous system and have an action similar to that of morphine, an opiate analgesic. There are specific **opiate receptors** located at strategic sites, called binding sites, to receive these compounds. β-endorphin, a 31-amino acid peptide, and **dynorphin** have potent analgesic effects. These endorphins are released within the central nervous system by mechanisms that are not fully understood at this time.

Nociception

A nociceptive neuron transmits pain signals. Its cell body is in the dorsal root ganglion near the spinal cord. Approximately 25% of the myelinated A-delta and 50% of the unmyelinated C fibers contact nociceptors and are considered nociceptive, afferent neurons (see Table 3-2). Once a nociceptor is stimulated, it releases a neuropeptide (substance P) that initiates the electrical impulses along the afferent fiber toward the spinal cord. Substance P also serves as a transmitter substance between the first- and second-order afferent fibers (see Figure 3-4) at the dorsal horn of the spinal column.

The A-delta and C fibers that transmit sensations of pain and temperature have different diameters (A-delta are larger) and different conduction velocities (A-delta are faster). The C fibers also are connected to more of the nociceptive specific second-order afferents. These differences result in two qualitatively different types of pain, termed fast and slow.[3] Fast pain is brief, well-localized, and well-matched to the stimulus—for example, the initial pain of an unexpected pinprick. Slow pain is an aching, throbbing, or burning sensation that is poorly localized and less specifically related to the stimulus. There is a delay in the perception of slow pain after injury, but the pain will continue long after the noxious stimulus is removed. Fast pain is transmitted over the larger, faster-conducting A-delta afferent neurons and originates from receptors located in the skin. Slow pain is transmitted by the C afferent neurons and originates from both superficial (skin) and deeper (ligaments and muscle) tissue.[3]

The various types of afferent fibers follow different courses as they ascend toward the brain. Some A-delta and most C afferent neurons enter the spinal cord through the dorsolateral tract of Lissauer and synapse in marginal zone (lamina 1) or the substantia gelatinosa (lamina 2) with a second-order neuron.[16] Most nociceptive second-order neurons ascend to higher centers along one of three tracts: (1) lateral spinothalamic tract, (2) spinoreticular tract, and (3) spinoencephalic tract, with the remainder ascending along the spinocervical tract or as projections to the cuneate and gracile nuclei of the medulla.[16] Approximately 90% of the wide dynamic range second-order afferents terminate in the thalamus.[16] Third-order neurons project to the sensory cortex and numerous other centers in the central nervous system. These projections allow us to perceive pain. They also permit the integration of past experiences and emotions that form our response to the pain experience. These connections are also believed to be parts of complex circuits that the sports therapist may stimulate to manage pain. Most analgesic physical agents used in sports medicine are believed to slow or block the impulses ascending along the A-delta and C afferent neuron pathways through direct input into the dorsal horn or through descending mechanisms. These pathways are discussed in more detail in the following section.

NEUROPHYSIOLOGIC EXPLANATIONS OF PAIN CONTROL

The neurophysiologic mechanisms of pain control through stimulation of cutaneous receptors have not been fully explained. Much of what is known and current theory result from work involving electroacupuncture and TENS.[32] However, this information often provides an explanation for the analgesic response to other modalities, such as massage, analgesic balms, and moist heat.

The concepts of the analgesic response to cutaneous receptor stimulation presented here were first proposed by Melzack and Wall[21] and Castel.[7] These models essentially present three analgesic mechanisms:

1. Stimulation from ascending A-beta afferents results in the blocking of impulses (pain messages) carried along A-delta and C afferent fibers.
2. Stimulation of descending pathways in the dorsolateral tract of the spinal cord by A-delta and C fiber afferent input results in a blocking of the impulses carried along the A-delta and C afferent fibers.
3. The stimulation of A-delta and C afferent fibers causes the release of endogenous opioids (β-endorphin), resulting in a prolonged activation of descending analgesic pathways.

These theories or models are not necessarily mutually exclusive. Recent evidence suggests that pain relief may result from combinations of dorsal horn and central nervous system activity.[2,9]

A decrease in input along nociceptive afferents also results in pain relief. Cooling afferent fibers decreases the rate at which they conduct impulses. Thus a 20-minute application of cold is effective in relieving pain because of the decrease in activity rather than an increase in activity along afferent pathways.

Blocking the Pain Impulses with Ascending A-Beta Input

Pain modulation caused by sensory stimulation and the resultant increase in the impulses in the large diameter (A-beta) afferent fibers was proposed by the gate control theory of pain[21] (Figure 3-5). Impulses ascending on these fibers stimulate the substantia gelatinosa as they enter the dorsal horn of the spinal cord. Stimulation of the substantia gelatinosa inhibits synaptic transmission in the large- and small- (A-delta

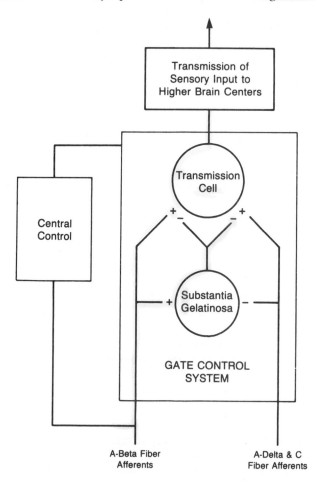

Fig. 3-5. The gate control system. Increases A-beta input and stimulates the substantia gelatinosa, which inhibits the flow of afferent input to sensory centers.

and C) fiber afferent pathways. The "pain message" carried along the small-diameter fibers is not transmitted to the second-order neurons and never reaches sensory centers. The balance between the input from the small- and large-diameter afferents determines how much of the pain message is blocked or gated.

The concept of sensory stimulation for pain relief, as proposed by the gate control theory, has empiric support. Rubbing a contusion, applying moist heat, or massaging sore muscles decreases the perception of pain. The analgesic response to these treatments is attributed to the increased stimulation of large-diameter afferent fibers.

The gate control theory also proposes that A-delta and C fiber impulses inhibit the substantia gelatinosa, facilitating the perception of pain. The sensation of pain does not diminish rapidly because free nerve endings do not accommodate and the afferent impulses from them "open the gate" to further pain message transmission.

The discovery and isolation of endogenous opioids in the 1970s led to new theories of pain relief. Castel[7] introduced an endogenous opioid analogue to the gate control theory (Figure 3-6). This theory proposes that A-beta impulses trigger a release of enkephalin from **enkephalinergic interneurons** found in the dorsal horn. These neuroactive amines inhibit synaptic transmission in the A-delta and C fiber afferent pathways. The end result, as in the gate control theory, is that the pain message is blocked before it reaches sensory levels.

Descending Pain Control Mechanisms

The gate control theory[21] proposed a second analgesic mechanism that involves descending efferent fibers. The central control, originating in higher centers of the central nervous system, could affect the dorsal horn gating process.[6] Impulses from the thalamus and brain stem **(central biasing)** are carried into the dorsal horn on efferent fibers in the dorsal or dorsal lateral paths (or tracts). Impulses from the higher centers act to close the gate and block transmission of the pain message at the dorsal horn

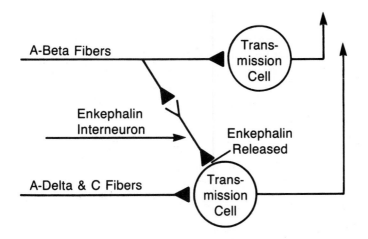

Fig. 3-6. Presynaptic inhibition of dorsal horn synapse transmission caused by A-beta fiber stimulation at enkephalin interneurons.

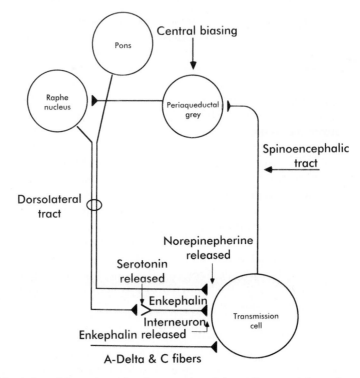

Fig. 3-7. Stimulation of the periaqueductal grey region of the midbrain and the raphe nucleus in the pons and medulla by ascending neural input, especially from A-delta and C fiber afferents, and possibly central biasing, activates the descending mechanism.

synapse. Through this system, it was theorized, previous experiences, emotional influences, sensory perception, and other factors could influence the transmission of the pain message and the perception of pain.

Castel[7] offers an endogenous opioid model of descending influence over dorsal horn synapse activity (Figure 3-7). Stimulation of the **periaqueductal grey** region of the midbrain and the **raphe nucleus** in the pons and medulla by ascending neural input, especially from A-delta and C fiber afferents, and possibly central biasing, activate the descending mechanism. The periaqueductal grey stimulates the raphe nucleus, which sends impulses along serotonergic efferent fibers in the dorsal lateral tract, which synapse with enkephalinergic interneurons. The interneurons release enkephalin into the dorsal horn, inhibiting the synaptic transmission of impulses to the second-order afferent neurons.

More recently, a second descending, norandrenergic pathway projecting from the pons to the dorsal horn has been identified.[16] The significance of these parallel pathways is not fully understood. It is also not known if these norandrenergic fibers directly inhibit dorsal horn synapses or stimulate the enkephalinergic interneurons.

This model provides a physiologic explanation for the analgesic response to brief, intense stimulation. The analgesia after accupressure and the use of some TENS, such as point simulators, is attributed to this descending pain control mechanism.

β-Endorphin and Dynorphin

There is evidence that stimulation of the small-diameter afferents (A-delta and C) can stimulate the release of other endogenous opioids.* β-endorphin and dynorphin are neuroactive peptides with potent analgesic affects. The term endorphin refers to an opiate-like substance produced by the body. The mechanisms regulating the release of β-endorphin and dynorphin have not been fully elucidated. However, these large endogenous substances play a role in the analgesic response to some forms of stimuli used to treat patients in pain.

One of the sources of β-endorphin is the anterior pituitary gland. Here it shares the prohormone propiomelanocortin (POMC) with adrenocorticotropin **(ACTH).** Prolonged (20 to 40 minutes) small-diameter afferent fiber stimulation has been thought to trigger the release of β-endorphin from the anterior pituitary gland. Electroacupuncture and possibly TENS with long phase durations and low pulse rates (1 to 5 pulses/second), will cause small-diameter afferent fiber depolarization necessary for β-endorphin release. Recent findings do not support the anterior pituitary gland as a source of β-endorphin in low pulse rate, long pulse width TENS-induced analgesia.[11] These results and the recognition that β-endorphin does not readily cross the blood-brain barrier[3] suggest that if β-endorphin or other endogenous opioids are active and analgesic agents within the central nervous system, they are released from areas within the brain.

The neurons in the hypothalamus that send projections to the periaqueductal grey and noradrenergic nuclei in the brain stem contain β-endorphin. It is possible that β-endorphin released from these neurons by stimulation of the hypothalamus is responsible for the analgesic response to the treatments[6] (Figure 3-8).

Dynorphin, a more recently isolated endogenous opioid, is found in the periaqueductal grey, rostroventral medulla, and the dorsal horn.[16] It has been demonstrated that dynorphin is released during electroacupuncture.[14] Dynorphin may be responsible for suppressing the response to noxious mechanical stimulation.[16]

Summary of Pain Control Mechanisms

The body's pain control mechanisms are probably not mutually exclusive. Rather, analgesia results from overlapping processes. It is also important to realize that the theories presented are only models. They are useful in conceptualizing the perception of pain and pain relief. These models will help the sports therapist understand the effects of therapeutic modalities and form a sound rationale for modality application. As more research is conducted and as the mysteries of pain and neurophysiology are solved, new models will emerge. The sports therapist should adapt these models to fit new developments.

COGNITIVE INFLUENCES

Pain perception and the response to a painful experience may be influenced by a variety of cognitive processes, including anxiety, attention, depression, past pain experiences, and cultural influences. These individual aspects of pain expression are mediated by

---

* References 8, 10, 19, 23, 24, 25, 27-30.

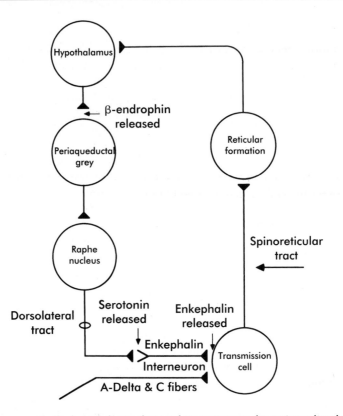

Fig. 3-8. The neurons in the hypothalamus that send projections to the periaqueductal grey and noradrenergic nuclei in the brain stem contain β-endorphin. It is possible that β-endorphin released from these neurons by stimulation of the hypothalamus is responsible for the analgesic response to the treatments.

higher centers in the cortex in ways that are not clearly understood.[6] Pain perception may influence both the sensory discriminative and motivational affective dimensions of pain.

Many mental processes modulate the perception of pain through descending systems. Behavior modification, the excitement of the moment, happiness, positive feelings, **focusing** (directed attention toward specific stimuli), hypnosis, and suggestion may modulate pain perception. Past experiences, cultural background, personality, motivation to play, aggression, anger, and fear are all factors that could facilitate or inhibit pain perception. Strong central inhibition may mask severe injury for a period of time. At such times, evaluation of the injury is quite difficult.

Athletes with chronic pain may become very depressed and experience a severe loss of fitness. They tend to be less active and may have altered appetites and sleep habits. They have a decreased will to perform and often develop a reduced sex drive. They may turn to self-abusive patterns of behavior. Tricyclic drugs are often used to inhibit serotonin depletion for the athlete with chronic pain.

Just as pain may be inhibited by central modulation, it may also arise from central origins. Phobias, fear, depression, anger, grief, and hostility can all produce pain in the absence of local pathologic processes. In addition, pain memory, which is associated with old injuries, may result in pain perception and pain response that are out of proportion to a new, often minor, injury. Substance abuse can also alter and confound the perception of pain. Substance abuse may lead to depression and psychosomatic pain.

PAIN MANAGEMENT

How should the sports therapist approach pain? First, the source of the pain must be identified. Unidentified pain may hide a serious disorder, and treatment of such pain may delay the appropriate treatment of the disorder. Once a diagnosis has been made, many physical agents can provide pain relief. The therapist should match the therapeutic agent to each athlete's situation. Casts and braces may prevent the application of ice or moist heat. However, TENS electrodes often can be positioned under a cast or brace for pain relief. After acute injuries, ice may be the therapeutic agent of choice because of the effect of cold on the inflammatory process. There is not one "best" therapeutic agent for pain control. The sports therapist must select the therapeutic agent that is most appropriate for each athlete, based on the knowledge of the modalities and professional judgment. In no situation should the therapist apply a therapeutic agent without first developing a clear rationale for the treatment.

In general, physical agents can be used to do the following:
1. Stimulate large-diameter afferent fibers. This can be done with TENS, massage, and analgesic balms.
2. Decrease pain fiber transmission velocity with cold or ultrasound.
3. Stimulate small-diameter afferent fibers and descending pain control mechanisms with accupressure, deep massage, or TENS over acupuncture points or trigger points.
4. Stimulate a release of β-endorphin or other endogenous opioids through prolonged small-diameter fiber stimulation with TENS.

Other useful pain control strategies include the following:
1. Encourage central biasing through cognitive processes, such as motivation, tension diversion, focusing, relaxation techniques, positive thinking, thought stopping, and self-control.
2. Minimize the tissue damage through the application of proper first aid and immobilization.
3. Maintain a line of communication with the athlete. Let the athlete know what to expect after an injury. Pain, swelling, dysfunction, and atrophy will occur after injury. The athlete's anxiety about these events will increase his or her perception of pain. Often, an athlete who has been told what to expect by someone he or she trusts will be less anxious and suffer less pain.
4. Recognize that all pain, even psychosomatic pain, is very real to the athlete.
5. If the activity will not cause further harm to the athlete, encourage supervised exercise to encourage blood flow, promote nutrition, increase metabolic activity, and reduce stiffness and guarding.

The physician may choose to prescribe oral or injectable medications in the treatment of the injured athlete. The most commonly used medications are classified as analgesics, antiinflammatory agents, or both. The sports therapist should become familiar with these drugs and note if the athlete is taking any medications. It is also important to work with the team physician to ensure that the athlete takes the medications appropriately.

The sports therapist's approach to the athlete has a great impact on the success of the treatment. The athlete will not be convinced of the efficacy and importance of the treatment unless the therapist appears confident about it. The sports therapist must make the athlete a participant rather than a passive spectator in the treatment and rehabilitation process.

The goal of most treatment programs is to encourage early pain-free exercise. The physical agents used to control pain do little to promote tissue healing. They should be used to relieve acute pain after injury or surgery or to control pain and other symptoms, such as swelling, to promote progressive exercise. The sports therapist should not lose sight of the effects of the physical agents or the importance of progressive exercise in restoring the athlete's athletic ability.

Reducing the perception of pain is as much an art as a science. Selection of the proper physical agent, proper application, and marketing are all important and will continue to be so even as we increase our understanding of the neurophysiology of pain. There is still the need for a good empirical rationale for the use of a physical agent. The sports therapist is encouraged to keep abreast of the neurophysiology of pain and the physiology of tissue healing to maintain a current scientific basis for selecting modalities and managing the injured athlete.

SUMMARY

1. Pain is a response to a noxious stimulus and is subjectively modified by past experiences and expectations.
2. Pain is classified as either acute or chronic and can exhibit many different patterns.
3. Early reduction of pain in a treatment program will facilitate therapeutic exercise.
4. Stimulation of sensory receptors via the therapeutic modalities can modify the athlete's perception of pain.
5. Four mechanisms of pain control may explain the analgesic affects of physical agents:
   a. Decreased transmission of input along nociceptive pathways.
   b. Dorsal horn modulation caused by input from large-diameter afferents through a gate control system, the release of enkephalins, or both.
   c. Descending efferent fiber activation caused by effects of small-fiber afferent input on higher centers including the thalamus, raphe nucleus, and periaqueductal grey region.
   d. The central release of endogenous opioids, including β-endorphin, through prolonged small-diameter afferent stimulation.
6. Pain perception may be influenced by a variety of cognitive processes mediated by the higher brain centers.

7. The selection of a therapeutic modality for controlling pain should be based on current knowledge of neurophysiology and the psychology of pain.
8. The application of physical agents to control pain should not occur until the diagnosis of the injury has been established.
9. The selection of a therapeutic modality for managing pain should be based on establishing the primary cause of pain.

GLOSSARY

accommodation Adaption by the sensory receptors to various stimuli over an extended period of time.

ACTH Adrenocorticotropic hormone. This hormone stimulates the release of glucocorticoids (cortisol) from the adrenal glands.

acute Pain of sudden onset often associated with physical trauma.

afferent Conduction of a nerve impulse toward an organ.

avulsion fracture A fracture in which a small piece of bone is torn away by an attached tendon or ligament.

β-Endorphin A neurohormone derived from proopiomelanocortin (POMC). It is similar in structure and properties to morphine. β-endorphin has a half-life of 4 hours.

central biasing A theory of pain modulation where higher centers such as the cerebral cortex influence the perception of and response to pain.

chronic pain Pain lasting more than 6 months.

dynorphin An endogenous opioid derived from the prohormone prodynorphin.

efferent Conduction of a nerve impulse away from an organ.

endogenous opioids Opiate-like substances made by the body.

endorphins Endogenous opioids whose actions have analgesic properties (i.e., β-endorphin).

enkephalin Neurotransmitter proteins that block the passage of noxious stimuli from first-order to second-order afferents. These proteins inhibit the release of substance P and are produced by enkephalinergic neurons.

enkephalinergic interneurons Neurons with short axons that release enkephalin. They are widespread in the central nervous system and are found in the substantia gelatinosa, raphe nucleus, and periaqueductal grey matter.

free nerve endings Receptors that are sensitive to extreme mechanical, chemical, or thermal energy.

focusing Narrowing attention to the appropriate stimuli in the environment.

interneurons Neurons contained entirely in the central nervous system. They have no projections outside the spinal cord. Their function is to serve as relay stations within the central nervous system.

joint capsule Ligamentous structure that surrounds and encapsulates a joint.

Kehr's sign Referred pain pattern involving pain in the left jaw, shoulder, and arm.

neurotransmitter Substance that passes information between neurons. It is released from one neuron terminal (presynaptic membrane), enters the synaptic cleft, and attaches (binds) to a receptor on the next neuron (postsynaptic membrane). Substance P, enkephalins, serotonin, methionine, and leucine enkephalin are neurotransmitters.

nociceptors Pain information or signals of pain stimuli.

norepinephrine A neurotransmitter.

opiate receptors Neurons that have receptors that bind to opiate substances.

pain An unpleasant sensory and emotional experience associated with actual or potential tissue damage.

periaqueductal grey A midbrain structure that plays an important role in descending tracts that inhibit synaptic transmission of noxious input in the dorsal horn.

periosteum A highly vascularized and innervated membrane lining the surface of bone.

radiating pain Pain that moves away from the site of a lesion, usually associated with some pressure in the area of injury.

raphe nucleus Part of the brain that is known to inhibit pain impulses being transmitted through the ascending system.

referred pain (referred myofascial pain) When nociceptive impulses reach the dorsal grey matter, they converge and their summation can depolarize internuncial neurons over several spinal segments, causing the individual to feel pain in distal areas innervated by these segments.

sclerotome A segment of bone innervated by a spinal segment.

sensitization Prolonged depolarization of nociceptive neurons that results in continuous stimulation. Most sensory receptors are rendered less sensitive after prolonged stimulation. This is not the case with nociceptive neurons.

serotonin A neurotransmitter found in neurons descending in the dorsolateral tract. The dorsolateral tract is thought to play a significant role in pain control. Serotonin is found in the vesicles in nerve endings that bind when released to postsynaptic membranes. Its action is terminated by reuptake into presynaptic membranes. It is probably involved in both endogenous pain

control and opiate analgesia. Increased levels of serotonin in the central nervous system are generally associated
with increased analgesia.

substance P A peptide believed to be the neurotransmitter
of small-diameter primary afferent. It is released from
both ends of the neuron.

substantia gelatinosa Lamina 2 of the dorsal horn of the
gray matter. Melzack and Wall[21] proposed that it is
responsible for closing the gate to painful stimuli.

trigger point Localized deep tenderness in a palpable firm
band of muscle. When stretched, a palpating finger can
snap the band like a taut string, which produces local
pain, a local twitch of that portion of the muscle, and a
jump by the patient. Sustained pressure on a trigger point
reproduces the pattern of referred pain for that site.

REFERENCES

1 Addison RG: Chronic pain syndrome, *Am J Med* 77: 54, 1985.
2 Anderson S, Ericson T, Holmgren E, et al.: Electroacupuncture
affects pain threshold measured with electrical stimulation of
teeth, *Brain* 63: 393-396, 1973.
3 Berne RM, Levy MN: *Physiology,* St Louis, 1988, Mosby.
4 Bishop B: Pain: its physiology and rationale for management, *Phys
Ther* 60: 13-37, 1980.
5 Bonica JJ: *The management of pain,* Philadelphia, 1990, Lea &
Febiger.
6 Bowsher D: *Central pain mechanisms.* In Wells PE, Frampton V,
Bowsher D, editors: *Pain management in physical therapy,*
Norwalk Conn., 1988, Appleton & Lange.
7 Castel JC: *Pain management: acupuncture and transcutaneous
electrical nerve stimulation techniques,* Lake Bluff, Ill, 1979, Pain
Control Services.
8 Chapman CR, Benedetti C: Analgesia following electrical
stimulation: partial reversal by a narcotic antagonist, *Life Sci* 26:
44-48, 1979.
9 Cheng R, Pomeranz B: Electroacupuncture analgesia could be
mediated by at least two pain relieving mechanisms: endorphin
and non-endorphin systems, *Life Sci* 25: 1957-1962, 1979.
10 Clement-Jones V, McLaughlin L, Tomlin S, et al.: Increased
beta-endorphin but not net-enkephalin levels in human cerebrospinal fluid after electroacupuncture for recurrent pain,
Lancet 2: 946-948, 1980.
11 Denegar GR, Perrin DH, Rogol AD, et al.: Influence of transcutaneous electrical nerve stimulation on pain, range of motion
and serum cortisol concentration in females with induced
delayed onset muscle soreness, *J Orthop Sports Phys Ther* 11:
101-103, 1989.
12 Dickerman Joel: The use of pain profiles in clinical practice, *Fam
Pract* 14(3): 21-39, 1992.
13 Gatchel RJ: Million behavioral health inventory: its utility in
predicting physical functioning patients with low back pain *Arch
Phys Med Rehabil* 67: 878, 1986.
14 Ho WKK, Wen HL: Opioid-like activity in the cerebrospinal fluid
of pain patients treated by electroacupuncture, *Neuropharma-
cology* 28: 961-966, 1989.
15 Huskisson EC: *Visual analogue scales.* In Melzack R, editor:
Pain measurement and assessment, New York, Raven Press,
1983.
16 Jessell TM, Kelly DD: *Pain and analgesia.* In Kandel ER,

Schwartz JH, Jessell TM, editors *Principles of neural science,*
Norwalk, Conn., 1991, Appleton & Lange.
17 Kuland DN: The injured athletes' pain. *Curr Concepts Pain* 1:
3-10, 1983.
18 Margoles MS: *The pain chart: spatial properties of pain.* In
Melzack R, editor: *Pain measurement and assessment,* New
York, Raven Press, 1983.
19 Mayer DJ, Price DD, Rafii A: Antagonism of acupuncture
analgesia in man by the narcotic antagonist naloxone, *Brain Res*
121: 368-372, 1977.
20 Melzack R: *Concepts of pain measurement.* In Melzack R, editor:
Pain measurement and assessment, New York, 1983, Raven
Press.
21 Melzack R, Wall P: Pain mechanisms: a new theory, *Science* 150:
971-979, 1965.
22 Merskey H, Albe Fessard DG, Bonica JJ, et al.: Pain terms: a list
with definitions and notes on usage, *Pain* 6: 249-252, 1979.
23 Pomeranz B, Chiu D: Naloxone blockade of acupuncture
analgesia: enkephalin implicated, *Life Sci* 19: 1757-1762, 1976.
24 Pomeranz B, Paley D: Brain opiates at work in acupuncture, *New
Scientist* 73: 12-13, 1975.
25 Pomeranz B, Paley D: Electro-acupuncture hypoalgesia is mediated by afferent impulses: an electrophysiological study in mice,
Exp Neurol 66: 398-402, 1979.
26 Previte JJ: *Human physiology,* New York, 1983, McGraw-Hill.
27 Salar G, Job I, Mingringo S, et al.: Effects of transcutaneous
electrotherapy on CSF beta-endorphin content in patients
without pain problems, *Pain* 10: 169-172, 1981.
28 Sjolund B, Eriksson M: Electroacupuncture and endogenous
morphines, *Lancet* 2: 1085, 1976.
29 Sjoland B, Eriksson M: Increased cerebrospinal fluid levels of
endorphins after electro-acupuncture, *Acta Physiol Scand* 100:
382-384, 1977.
30 Wen HL, Ho WKK, Ling N, et al.: The influence of electroacupuncture on naloxone: induces morphine withdrawal: elevation
of immunoassayable beta-endorphin activity in the brain but not
in the blood, *Am J Clin Med* 7: 237-240, 1979.
31 Willis WD, Grossman RC: *Medical neurobiology,* ed 3, St Louis,
1981, Mosby.
32 Wolf SL: *Neurophysiologic mechanisms in pain modulation:
relevance to TENS.* In Manheimer JS, Lampe GN, editors:
Clinical applications of TENS, Philadelphia, 1984, FA Davis.

Basic Principles of Electricity

4

William E. Prentice

OBJECTIVES

After completion of this chapter, the student will be able to do the following:

- Define potential difference, ampere, volt, ohm, and watt.
- Give Ohm's law and its mathematical expression.
- Differentiate between alternating, direct, and pulsed currents.
- Discuss various waveforms and pulse characteristics.
- Discuss current modulation.
- Differentiate between series and parallel circuit arrangement.
- Discuss current flow through various types of biologic tissue.
- Discuss safety in the use of electrical equipment by the sports therapist.

Many of the modalities discussed in this text may be classified as electrical modalities. These pieces of equipment can take the electrical current flowing from a wall outlet and modify it to produce a specific, desired physiologic effect in human biologic tissue.

Understanding the basic principles of electricity is usually difficult even for the sports therapist who is accustomed to using electrical modalities on a daily basis. To understand how current flow affects biologic tissue, it is first necessary to become famliar with some of the principles that describe how electricity is produced and how it behaves in an electrical circuit.

These principles and concepts presented in this chapter can be applied to the use of all of the electrical modalities to be discussed in this text, including iontophoresis (Chapter 6), biofeedback (Chapter 7), the diathermies (Chapter 8), low power laser (Chapter 10), ultraviolet (Chapter 11), and even ultrasound (Chapter 12), but they are particularly applicable to electrical stimulating currents (Chapter 5).

COMPONENTS OF ELECTRICAL CURRENTS

All matter is composed of atoms that contain positively and negatively charged particles called **ions.** These charged particles possess electrical energy and thus are able to move about. They tend to move from an area of higher concentration toward an area of lower concentration. An electrical force is capable of propelling these particles from higher to lower energy levels, thus establishing **electrical potentials.** The more ions an object has, the higher its potential electrical energy. Particles with a positive charge tend to move toward negatively charged particles, and those particles that are negatively charged tend to move toward the positively charged particles (Figure 4-1).[10]

Electrons are particles of matter possessing a negative charge and very small mass. The net movement of electrons is referred to as an **electrical current.** The movement or flow of these electrons will always go from a higher potential to a lower potential.[17] An electrical force is oriented only in the direction of the applied force. This flow of electrons may be likened to a domino reaction.

The unit of measurement that indicates the rate at which electrical current flows is the **ampere** (amp); 1 amp is defined as the movement of 1 **coulomb** or 6.25×10^{18} electrons per second. Amperes indicate the rate of electron flow, while coulombs indicate the number of electrons. In the case of therapeutic modalities, current flow is generally described in milliamperes ($\frac{1}{1000}$ of an amp, denoted as mA) or in microamperes ($\frac{1}{1,000,000}$ of an amp, denoted as μA).

The electrons will not move unless an electrical potential difference in the concentration of these charged particles exists between two points. The electromotive force, which must be applied to produce a flow of electrons, is called a **volt** (V) and is defined as the difference in electron population (potential difference) between two points.[3]

Voltage is the force resulting from an accumulation of electrons at one point in an electrical circuit, usually corresponding to a deficit of electrons at another point in the circuit. If the two points are connected by a suitable conductor, the potential difference (difference in electron population) will cause electrons to move from the area of higher population to the area of lower population.

Commercial current flowing from wall outlets produces an electromotive force of either 115 V or 220 V. The electrotherapeutic devices used in injury rehabilitation modify voltages. Electrical generators are sometimes referred to as being either **low-voltage current** or **high-voltage current.** These terms are somewhat useless in meaning, although some older texts have referred to generators that produce less than 150 V as low-volt and those that produce several hundred volts as high-volt.[3]

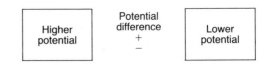

Fig. 4-1. The difference between high potential and low potential is potential difference. Electrons tend to flow from areas of higher concentration to areas of lower concentration. A potential difference must exist if there is to be any movement of electrons.

TABLE 4-1   Electron Flow as Analogous to Water Flow

Electron Flow		Water Flow
Volt	=	Pump
Amperes	=	Gallons
Ohm (properties of conductor)	=	Resistance (length and distance of pipe)

Electrons can move in a current only if there is a relatively easy pathway to move along. Materials that permit this free movement of electrons are referred to as **conductors. Conductance** is a term that defines the ease with which current flows along a conducting medium. Metals (copper, gold, silver, aluminum) and electrolyte solutions are good conductors of electricity because both are composed of large numbers of free electrons that are given up readily. Thus materials that offer little opposition to current flow are good conductors. Materials that resist current flow are called **insulators.** Insulators contain relatively few free electrons and thus offer greater resistance to electron flow. Air, wood, and glass are all considered insulators. The number of amps flowing in a given conductor depends both on the voltage applied and on the conduction characteristics of the material.[16]

The opposition to electron flow in a conducting material is referred to as **resistance** or **electrical impedance** and is measured in a unit known as an **ohm.** Thus an electrical circuit that has high resistance (ohms) will have less flow (amps) than a circuit with less resistance and the same voltage.[2]

The mathematical relationship between current flow, voltage, and resistance is demonstrated in the formula:

$$\text{Current flow} = \frac{\text{Voltage}}{\text{Resistance}}$$

This formula is the mathematical expression of **Ohm's law,** which states that the current in an electrical circuit is directly proportional to the voltage and inversely proportional to the resistance.

An analogy comparing the movement of water with the movement of electricity may help to clarify this relationship between current flow, voltage, and resistance (Table 4-1).

For water to flow, some type of pump must create a force to produce movement. Likewise, the volt is the pump that produces the electron flow. The resistance to water flow is dependent on the length, diameter, and smoothness of the water pipe. The resistance to electrical flow depends on the characteristics of the conductor. The amount of water flowing is measured in gallons, while the amount of electricity flowing is measured in amps.

The amount of energy produced by flowing water is determined by two factors: (1) the number of gallons flowing per unit of time and (2) the pressure created in the pipe. Electrical energy, or power, is a product of the voltage or electromotive force and the amount of current flowing. Electrical power is measured in a unit called a **watt.**

$$\text{Watts} = \text{Volts} \times \text{Amperes}$$

Simply, the watt indicates the rate at which electrical power is being used. A watt is defined as the electrical power needed to produce a current flow of 1 amp at a pressure of 1 volt.

ELECTROTHERAPEUTIC CURRENTS

Electrotherapeutic devices generate three different types of current, which, when introduced into biologic tissue, are capable of producing specific physiologic changes. These three types of current are referred to as **alternating (AC), direct (DC),** or **pulsed.** The therapeutic effects of these various types of electrical stimulating currents will be discussed in detail in Chapter 5.

Direct current, also referred to in some texts as galvanic current, has a unidirectional flow of electrons toward the positive pole (Figure 4-2, A). On most modern direct current devices the polarity, and thus the direction of current flow, can be reversed.[17] Some generators have the capability of automatically reversing polarity, in which case the physiologic effects will be similar to AC current.[15]

In an alternating current, the flow of electrons constantly changes direction, or stated differently, reverses its polarity. Electrons flowing in an alternating current always move from the negative to positive pole, reversing direction when polarity is reversed (Figure 4-2, B).

Pulsed currents usually contain three or more pulses grouped together (Figure 4-2, C). These groups of pulses are interrupted for short periods of time and repeat themselves at regular intervals. Pulsed currents are used in interferential and so-called ''Russian'' currents, which will be discussed in Chapter 5.[1,7]

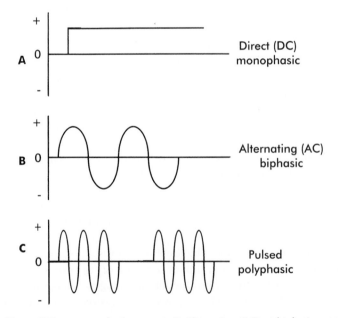

Fig. 4-2. A, Direct (DC) or monophasic current. **B,** Alternating (AC) or biphasic current. **C,** Pulsed or polyphasic current.

Generators of Electrotherapeutic Currents

A great deal of confusion has developed relative to the terminology used to describe electrotherapeutic currents. Basically, all therapeutic electrical generators regardless of whether they deliver AC, DC, or pulsed currents through electrodes attached to the skin are **transcutaneous electrical stimulators.** The majority of these are used to stimulate peripheral nerves and are correctly called **transcutaneous electrical nerve stimulators (TENS).** Occasionally the terms **neuromuscular electrical stimulator (NMES)** or electrical muscle stimulator (EMS) are used, however these terms are only appropriate when the electrical current is being used to stimulate muscle directly, as would be the case with denervated muscle where peripheral nerves are not functioning. In recent years, a new type of transcutaneous electrical stimulator has gained popularity that uses current intensities too small to excite peripheral nerves. The most common term used to describe these generators is **microcurrent electrical nerve stimulators (MENS).**[1,12,14]

There is no relationship between the type of current being delivered to the patient by the generator and the type of current being used as a power source to drive the generator (i.e., a wall outlet or battery). Generators that produce electrotherapeutic currents may be driven by either alternating or direct currents. Devices that plug into the standard electrical wall outlet use alternating current. The commercially produced alternating current changes its direction of flow 120 times per second. In other words, there are 60 complete cycles per second. The number of cycles occurring in 1 second is called frequency and is indicated in Hertz (Hz), pulses per second (PPS), or cycles per second (CPS). The voltage of electromotive force producing this alternating directional flow of electrons is set at a standard 115 V or 220 V. Thus commercial alternating current is produced at 60 Hz with a corresponding voltage of either 115 V or 220 V.

Other electrotherapeutic devices are driven by batteries that always produce direct current, ranging between 1.5 and 9 V, although the devices driven by batteries may in turn produce modified types of current.

A series of electrical components within the stimulating unit converts current coming from an AC power source to a DC current delivered to the patient: a **transformer,** a **rectifier,** a **filter,** a **regulator,** an **amplifier,** and an **oscillator.**[5,6] A transformer "steps down" or reduces the amount of voltage from the power supply. The rectifier converts AC current to pulsating DC current. The filter changes the pulsating DC current to smooth DC current. The regulator produces a specific controlled voltage output. An **output amplifier** within the stimulating unit is used to magnify or increase the amplitude of the voltage output of the generator and control it at a specific level, regardless of the electrical impedance of the remainder of the circuit (including the electrodes and patient). The oscillator is used to produce and output a specific waveform, which again may be different from that used to power or drive the stimulating unit.

WAVEFORMS

The term **waveform** indicates a graphic representation of the shape, direction, amplitude, duration, and pulse frequency of the electrical current being produced by

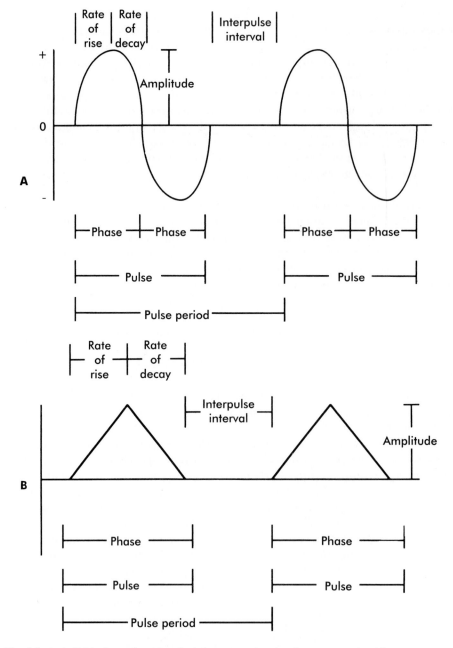

Fig. 4-3. An individual waveform is referred to as a pulse. A pulse may contain either one or two phases, that portion of the pulse that rises above or below the baseline for some period of time. **A,** Biphasic pulse. **B,** Monophasic pulse.

the electrotherapeutic device, as displayed by an instrument called an oscilloscope (Figure 4-3).

Waveform Shape

Electrical currents may take on *sine, rectangular,* or *triangular* waveform configurations depending on the capabilities of the generator producing the current. (Figure 4-4, *A-I*). Alternating, direct, and pulsed currents may take on any of the waveform shapes.

Pulses Versus Phases and Direction of Current Flow

On an oscilloscope, an individual waveform is referred to as a pulse. A pulse may contain either one or two **phases,** the portion of the pulse that rises above or below the baseline for some period of time. Direct current, also referred to as **monophasic current,** produces waveforms that have only a single phase in each pulse. Current flow is unidirectional, always flowing in the same direction toward either the positive or negative pole (see Figure 4-2, *A.*) Conversely, alternating current, also referred to as

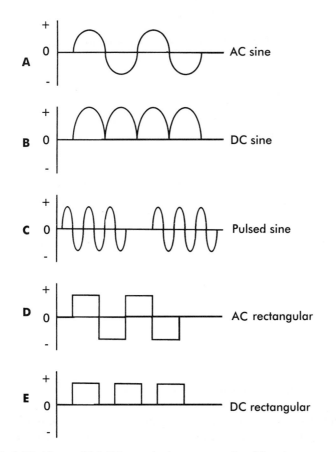

Fig. 4-4, A to I. Waveforms of AC, DC, or pulsed current may be either sine, rectangular, or triangular in shape.   *Continued*

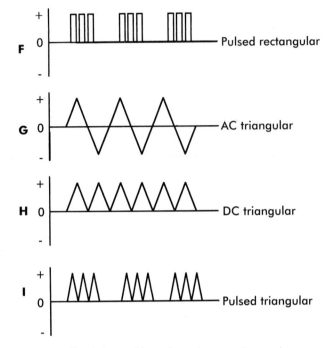

Fig. 4-4, cont'd. For legend see previous page.

biphasic current, produces waveforms that have two separate phases during each individual pulse. Current flow is bidirectional, reversing direction or polarity once during each pulse. Biphasic waveforms may be symmetrical or asymmetrical. If both phases of the waveform are symmetrical, the shape and size of each phase is identical (see Figure 4-2, *B*). Pulsed current waveforms are called **polyphasic** currents and are representative of electrical current that is conducted as a series of pulses of short duration (μsec) followed by a short period of time when current is not flowing called the **interpulse interval** (msec). Single pulses may be inturrupted by an **intrapulse interval** (see Figure 4-2, *C*). Pulsed current may flow in one direction as in DC current or may reverse direction of flow as in AC current. With pulsed currents, there is always some interruption of current flow.

Pulse Amplitude

The **amplitude** of each pulse reflects the intensity of the current, the maximum amplitude being the tip or highest point of each phase (see Figure 4-3). The term amplitude is synonymous with the terms voltage and current intensity. The higher the amplitude, the greater the peak voltage or intensity. However, the peak amplitude should not be confused with the total amount of current being delivered to the tissues.

On electrical generators that produce short duration pulses, the total current produced (columbs/sec) is low compared to peak current amplitudes due to long interpulse intervals that have current amplitudes of zero. Thus the **average current** or the amount of current flowing per unit of time is relatively low, ranging from as low as 2 mA to as high as 100 mA on some interferential generators. Average current can

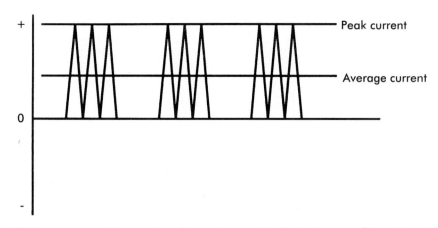
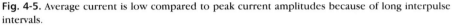

Fig. 4-5. Average current is low compared to peak current amplitudes because of long interpulse intervals.

be increased by either increasing pulse duration, increasing pulse frequency, or by some combination of the two (Figure 4-5).

Pulse Charge

The term **pulse charge** refers to the total amount of electricity being delivered to the patient during each pulse. With monophasic current, the phase charge and the pulse charge are the same and are always greater than zero. With biphasic current the pulse charge is equal to the sum of the phase charges. If the pulse is symmetrical the net pulse charge will be zero. In asymmetrical pulses the net pulse charge is greater than zero, which by definition is a DC current.[1]

Pulse Rate of Rise and Decay Times

The **rate of rise** in amplitude or the rise time refers to how quickly the pulse reaches its maximum amplitude in each phase. Conversely, **decay time** refers to the time in which a pulse goes from peak amplitude to 0 V. The rate of rise is important physiologically because of the **accommodation** phenomenon, in which a fiber that has been subjected to a constant level of depolarization will become unexcitable at that same intensity or amplitude. Rate of rise and decay times are generally short, ranging from nanoseconds (billionths of a second) to milliseconds (thousandths of a second) (see Figure 4-3).

By observing the three different waveforms, it is apparent that the sine wave has a gradual increase and decrease in amplitude for both alternating and direct currents (see Figure 4-4, A-C). The rectangular wave has an almost instantaneous increase in amplitude, which plateaus for a period of time and then abruptly falls off (see Figure 4-4, D-F). The triangular wave has a rapid increase and decrease in amplitude (see Figure 4-4, G-I). The shape of these waveforms as they reach their maximum amplitude or intensity is directly related to the excitability of the nervous tissue. The more rapid the increase in amplitude or the rate of rise, the greater the current's ability to excite nervous tissue.

Most modern DC generators make use of a twin-peak triangular pulse of very short duration (1 to 70 microseconds) and peak amplitudes as high as 500 V (Figure 4-6).

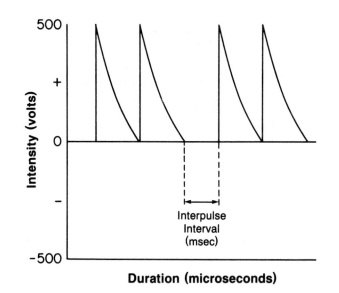

Duration (microseconds)

Fig. 4-6. Most DC generators produce a twin-peak triangular pulse of short duration and high amplitude.

Combining high-peak intensity with a short-phase duration produces a very comfortable type of current as well as an effective means of stimulating sensory, motor, and pain fibers.[18]

The effects of the various waveforms on biologic tissue will be discussed in Chapter 5.

ASYMMETRIC WAVEFORMS. Asymmetric biphasic waveforms have been used in the past but are seldom available on generators used by sports therapists. Occasionally, manufacturers will indicate that their equipment is producing **faradic current.** However, the true faradic waveform is no longer used. The so-called faradic current is most likely a high-frequency (greater than 400 Hz) pulsed wave. The original faradic waveform (Figure 4-7, A) could only have used alternating current because there was always a reversal of direction of current flow. The amplitude of the portion of the wave in the negative direction was not great enough to produce any physiologic response. Thus the effects of this faradic wave would be similar to those of a DC pulsed wave.[8]

In the monophasic sawtooth or exponential waveform (Figure 4-7, B) the amplitude rises very gradually and then falls abruptly. Current that uses this waveform stimulates denervated muscle without affecting normally innervated muscle, since the gradual rise in amplitude allows for accommodation of the normal muscle.[8]

Pulse Duration

The **duration** of each pulse indicates the length of time that current is flowing in one cycle. With monophasic current the phase duration is the same as the pulse duration and is the time from initiation of the phase to its end. With biphasic current the pulse duration is determined by the combined phase durations. In some electrotherapeutic devices the duration is preset by the manufacturer. Other devices can change duration. The phase duration may be as short as a few microseconds or may be a long-duration direct current that flows for several minutes.

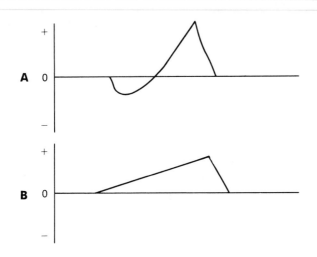

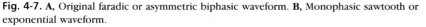

Fig. 4-7. A, Original faradic or asymmetric biphasic waveform. **B,** Monophasic sawtooth or exponential waveform.

With pulsed currents, and in some instances with alternating and direct currents, the current flow is off for a period of time. The combined time of the pulse duration and the interpulse interval is referred to as the **pulse period** (see Figure 4-3).

Pulse Frequency

Pulse **frequency** indicates the number of pulses per second. Each individual pulse represents a rise and fall in amplitude. As the frequency of any waveform is increased, the amplitude tends to increase and decrease more rapidly. The muscular and nervous system responses depend on the length of time between pulses and on how the pulses or waveforms are modulated.[16] Muscle will respond with individual twitch contractions to pulse rates of less than 50 pulses per second. At 50 pulses per second or greater, a **tetany** will result, regardless of whether the current is biphasic, monophasic, or polyphasic.

Stimulators have been clinically labeled as either low-, medium-, or high-frequency generators, and a great deal of misunderstanding exists over how these frequency ranges are classified.[1] Generally, all stimulating units are low-frequency electrical generators that deliver between one and several hundred pulses per second. Recently a number of so-called medium-frequency generators have been developed that are claimed to have frequencies of 2500 to as high as 10,000 pulses per second. However, these high-frequency pulses are in reality groups of pulses combined as **bursts** that range in frequency from 1 to 200 pulses per second. These modulated bursts can produce a physiologically effective frequency of stimulation only in this 1 to 200 pulse per second range owing to the limitations of the absolute refractory period of nerve cell membranes. Therefore many of the claims of equipment manufacturers relative to medium-frequency generators are inaccurate.[1]

Current Modulation

The physiologic responses to the various waveforms depend to a large extent on current **modulation.** Modulation refers to any alteration in the magnitude or any

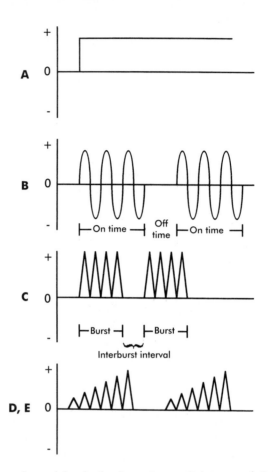

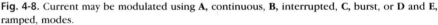

Fig. 4-8. Current may be modulated using **A,** continuous, **B,** interrupted, **C,** burst, or **D** and **E,** ramped, modes.

variation in duration of these pulses. Modulation may be continuous, interrupted, burst, or ramped.[1,9] The parameters of this modulation must be established according to various treatment goals.

CONTINUOUS MODULATION. Continuous modulation means that the amplitude of current flow remains the same for several seconds or perhaps minutes. Continuous modulation is usually associated with long-pulse duration direct current (Figure 4-8, *A*). With direct current, flow is always in a uniform direction. In the discussion of physiologic responses to electrical currents, it was indicated that positive and negative ions are attracted toward poles or, in this case, electrodes of opposite polarity. This accumulation of charged ions over a period of time creates either an acidic or alkaline environment that may be of therapeutic value. This therapeutic technique has been referred to as **medical galvanism.** The technique of **iontophoresis** (see Chapter 6) also uses continuous direct current to drive ions into the tissues. If the amplitude is great enough to produce a muscle contraction, the contraction will occur only when the current flow is turned on or off. Thus with direct current continuous modulation, there will be a muscle contraction both when the current is turned on and when it is turned off. Continuous modulation is also used with alternating current primarily to elicit muscle contractions.

INTERRUPTED MODULATION. With interrupted modulation, current flows for some period of time called the *on-time*, and is then periodically turned off during the *off-time*. On most units, on-time may be set between 1 and 60 seconds, while off-time may be set between 1 and 120 seconds. Interrupted modulation is used with monophasic or biphasic currents. Currents with sine, rectangular, or triangular shaped waveforms may be interrupted. Interrupted modulation is used clinically for muscle reeducation and strengthening and for improving range of motion (Figure 4-8, *B*).

BURST MODULATION. Burst modulation occurs when pulsed current flows for a short duration (milliseconds) and then is turned off for a short time (milliseconds) in a repetitive cycle. With polyphasic currents, sets of pulses are combined. These combined pulses are most commonly referred to in the literature as bursts but have also been called *packets, envelopes, pulse trains,* or *beats* (as is the case with interferential currents). The interruptions between individual bursts are called interburst intervals (Figure 4-8, *C*). The interburst interval is much too short to have any effect on a muscle contraction. Thus the physiologic effects of a burst of pulses will be the same as with a single pulse.[1] Bursts may be used with monophasic and biphasic currents as well.

RAMPING MODULATION. In **ramping** modulation, also called surging modulation, current amplitude will increase or ramp up gradually to some preset maximum and may also decrease or ramp down in intensity (Figure 4-8, *D* and *E*). Ramp-up time is usually preset at about one third of the on-time. The ramp-down option is not available on all machines. Most modern stimulators allow the sports therapist to set the on-time and the off-time between 1 and 10 seconds. Ramping modulation is used clinically to elicit muscle contraction and is generally considered to be a very comfortable type of current, since it allows for a gradual increase in the intensity of a muscle contraction.

ELECTRICAL CIRCUITS

The path of current from a generating power source through various components back to the generating source is called an electrical **circuit.** A closed circuit is one in which electrons are flowing, and in an open circuit the current flow ceases. Electronic circuits are not ordinarily composed of single elements; they often encompass several branches or components with different resistances. The current in each branch may be easily calculated if the individual resistances are known and if the amount of voltage applied to the circuit is also known.[4]

With the development of the microelectronics industry, we all know that electrical circuits can be extremely complex. However, all electrical circuits have several basic components: (1) There is a power source that is capable of producing voltage. (2) There is some type of conducting medium or pathway, along which current travels, carrying the flowing electrons. (3) There is some component or group of components that are driven by this flowing current. These driven elements provide resistance to electrical flow.[4]

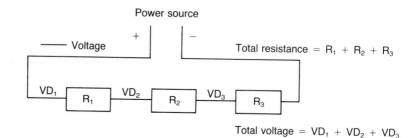

Fig. 4-9. In a series circuit the component resistors are placed end to end. The total resistance to current flow is equal to the resistance of all the components added together. There is a voltage decrease at each component such that the sum of the voltage decreases is equal to the total voltage.

Series and Parallel Circuits

The components that provide resistance to current flow may be connected to one another in one of two different patterns: (1) a **series circuit** or (2) a **parallel circuit.** The main difference between these patterns is that in a series circuit there is only one path for current to get from one terminal to another. In a parallel circuit, two or more routes exist for current to pass between the two terminals.

In a series circuit the components are placed end to end (Figure 4-9). The number of amps of an electrical current flowing through a series circuit is exactly the same at any point in that circuit. The resistance to current flow in this total circuit is equal to the resistance of all the components in the circuit added together.

$$R_T = R_1 + R_2 + R_3$$

Electrical energy is required to force the current through the resistor, and this energy is dissipated in the form of heat. Consequently, there is a decrease in voltage at each component such that the total voltage at the beginning of the circuit is equal to the sum of the voltage decreases at each component.

$$V_T = VD_1 + VD_2 + VD_3$$

In a parallel circuit, the component resistors are placed side by side and the ends are connected (Figure 4-10). Each of the resistors in a parallel circuit receives the same voltage. The current passing through each component depends on its resistance, so the total voltage will be exactly the same as the voltage at each component.

$$V_T = V_1 = V_2 = V_3$$

Each additional resistance added to a parallel circuit in effect decreases the total resistance. Adding an alternative pathway regardless of its resistance to current flow improves the ability of the current to get from one point to another. The current will, in general, choose the pathway that offers the least resistance. The formula for determining total resistance in a parallel circuit according to Ohm's law is

$$\frac{1}{R_T} = \frac{1}{R_1} + \frac{1}{R_2} + \frac{1}{R_3}$$

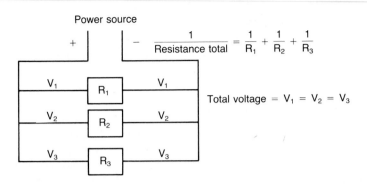

Fig. 4-10. In a parallel circuit the component resistors are placed side by side and the ends are connected. The current flow in each of the pathways is inversely proportional to the resistance of the pathway. The total voltage is the sum of the voltages at each component.

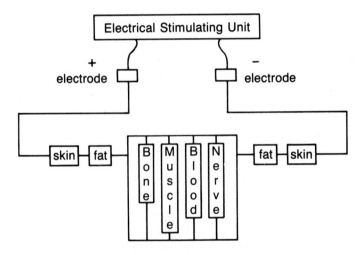

Fig. 4-11. The electrical circuit that exists when electrons flow through human tissue is in reality a combination of a series and parallel circuit.

Thus component resistors connected in a series circuit have a higher resistance and lower current flow, and resistors in a parallel circuit have a lower resistance and a higher current flow.

The electrical modalities in general make use of some combination of both series and parallel circuits.[8] For example, to elicit a muscle contraction, the electrodes from an electrical stimulating unit are placed on the skin (Figure 4-11). The current from those electrodes must pass directly through the skin and fat. The total resistance to current flow seen by the electrical stimulating unit is equal to the combined resistances at each electrode. This passage of current through the skin is basically a series circuit.

After the current passes through the skin and fat, it comes in contact with a number of different types of biologic tissue (i.e., bone, connective tissue, blood, muscle). The current has several different pathways through which it may reach the muscle to be stimulated. The total current travelling through these tissues is the sum of the currents in each different type of tissue, and since there are additional tissues through which current may travel, the total resistance is effectively reduced. Thus in this typical application of a therapeutic modality, both parallel and series circuits are used to produce the desired physiologic effect.

CURRENT FLOW THROUGH BIOLOGIC TISSUES

As stated previously, electrical current tends to choose the path that offers the least resistance to flow or, stated differently, the material that is the best conductor.[18] The conductivity of the different types of tissue in the body is variable. Typically tissue that is highest in water content and consequently highest in ion content is the best conductor of electricity.

The skin has different layers that vary in water content, but generally the skin offers the primary resistance to current flow and is considered an insulator. Skin preparation to reduce electrical impedance is of primary concern with electrodiagnostic apparatus (see Chapter 7), but it is also important with electrotherapeutic devices. The greater the impedance of the skin, the higher the voltage of the electrical current must be to stimulate underlying nerve and muscle. Chemical changes in the skin can make it more resistant to certain types of current. Thus skin impedance is generally higher with direct current than with alternating current.

Blood is a biologic tissue that is composed largely of water and ions and is consequently the best electrical conductor of all of the tissues. Muscle is composed of about 75% water and depends on the movement of ions for contraction. Muscle tends to propagate an electrical impulse much more effectively longitudinally than transversely. Muscle tendons are considerably more dense than muscle, contain relatively little water, and are considered poor conductors. Fat contains only about 14% water and is thought to be a poor conductor. Peripheral nerve conductivity is approximately 6 times that of muscle. However, the nerve is generally surrounded by fat and a fibrous sheath, both of which are considered to be poor conductors. Bone is extremely dense, contains only about 5% water, and is considered to be the poorest biologic conductor of electrical current. It is essential for the sports therapist to understand that many biologic tissues will be stimulated by an electrical current. Selecting the appropriate treatment parameters is critical if the desired tissue response is to be attained.

Physiologic Responses to Electrical Current

The effects of electrical current passing through the various tissues of the body may be thermal, chemical, or physiologic.[15]

All electrical currents cause a rise in temperature in a conducting tissue. The tissues of the body possess varying degrees of resistance, and those of higher resistance should heat up more when electrical current passes through. As indicated in previous chapters, the diathermies generate a continuous high frequency electrical current that is designed to produce a tissue temperature increase. The electrical currents used for nerve and muscle stimulation have a relatively low average current flow that produces minimal thermal effects.

Basically, electrical currents are used to produce either muscle contractions or modification of pain impulses through effects on the motor and sensory nerves. This function is dependent to a great extent on selecting the appropriate treatment parameters based on the principles identified in this chapter.

Electrical currents are also used to produce chemical effects. Most biologic tissue contains negatively and positively charged ions. A direct current flow will cause migration of these charged particles toward the pole of opposite polarity. At the positive pole the negatively charged particles cause an acidic reaction in which there is coagulation of protein and hardening of the tissues. At the negative pole the positively charged particles produce an alkaline reaction, liquefying protein and causing softening of the tissues.

SAFETY IN THE USE OF ELECTRICAL EQUIPMENT

Electrical safety in the sports-medicine setting should be of maximal concern to the professional sports therapist. Too often there are reports of athletes being electrocuted as a result of faulty electrical circuits in whirlpools. This type of accident can be avoided by taking some basic precautions and acquiring some understanding of the power distribution system and electrical grounds.

The typical electrical circuit consists of a source producing electrical power, a conductor that carries the power to a resistor or series of driven elements, and a conductor that carries the power back to the power source.

Electrical power is carried from generating plants through high-tension power-lines carrying 2200 V. The power is decreased by a transformer and is supplied in the wall outlet at 220 V or 120 V with a frequency of 60 Hz. The voltage at the outlet is alternating current, which means that one of the poles, the "hot" or "live" wire, is either positive or negative with respect to other neutral lines. Theoretically the voltage of the neutral pole should be zero. Actually the voltage of the neutral line is about 10 V. Thus both hot and neutral lines carry some voltage with respect to the earth, which has zero voltage. The voltage from either of these two leads may be sufficient to cause physiologic damage.

The two-pronged plug has only two leads, both of which carry some voltage. Consequently the electrical device has no true ground. The term true **ground** means the electrical circuit is connected to the earth or the ground, which can accept large electrical charges without becoming charged itself. The ground will continually accept these charges until the electrical potential has been neutralized. Therefore any electrical charge that may be potentially hazardous (i.e., any electricity escaping from the circuit) is almost immediately neutralized by the ground. If an individual were to come in contact with a short-circuited instrument that was not grounded, the electrical current would flow through that individual to reach the ground.

Electrical devices that have two-pronged plugs generally rely on the chassis or casing of the power source to act as a ground. The danger with the two-pronged plug devices is that there is no true ground. So if an individual were to touch the casing of the instrument while in contact with some object or instrument that has a true ground, an electrical shock may result. With three-pronged plugs, the third prong is grounded directly to the earth and all excess electrical energy should theoretically be neutralized through this prong.

By far the most common mechanism of injury from therapeutic devices results

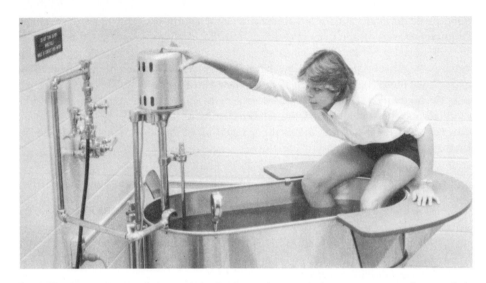

Fig. 4-12. There is danger of electrical shock when a therapeutic device is not properly grounded. This is a major problem in a whirlpool.

TABLE 4-2   **Physiologic Effects of Electrical Shock at Varying Magnitudes**

Intensity	Physiologic Effects
0-1 mA	Imperceptible
1-15 mA	Tingling sensation and muscle contraction
15-100 mA	Painful electrical shock
100-200 mA	Cardiac or respiratory arrest
> 200 mA	Instant tissue burning and destruction

when there is some damage, breakdown, or short circuit to the power cord. When this happens, the casing of the machine becomes electrically charged. In other words, there is a voltage leak and in a device that is not properly grounded, electrical shock may occur (Figure 4-12).

The magnitude of the electrical shock is a critical factor in terms of potential health danger (Table 4-2). Shock from electrical currents flowing at one or less mA will not be felt and is referred to as **microshock.** Shock from a current flow greater than 1 mA is called **macroshock.** Currents that range between 1 and 15 mA produce a tingling sensation or perhaps some muscle contraction. Currents flowing at 15 to 100 mA cause a painful electrical shock. Currents between 100 and 200 mA may result in fibrillation of cardiac muscle or respiratory arrest. When current flow is above 200 mA, there is rapid burning and destruction of tissue.[11]

Most electrotherapeutic devices (e.g., muscle stimulators, ultrasound, and the diathermies) are generally used in dry environments. All new electrotherapeutic equipment being produced has three-pronged plugs and is thus grounded to the earth.

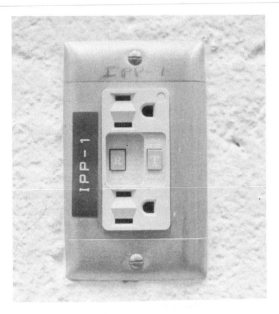

Fig. 4-13. A typical ground-fault interruptor.

However, in a wet or damp area the three-pronged plug may not provide sufficient protection from electrical shock.

We know that the body will readily conduct electricity because of its high water content. If the body is wet or if an individual is standing in water, the resistance to electrical flow is reduced even more. Thus if a short should occur, the shock could be as much as five times greater in this damp or wet environment. The potential danger that exists with whirlpools or tubs is obvious. The ground on the whirlpool will supposedly conduct all current leakage from a faulty motor or power cord to the earth. However, an individual in a whirlpool is actually a part of that circuit and is subject to the same current levels as any other component of the circuit. Small amounts of current can therefore be potentially harmful, no matter how well the apparatus is grounded. For this reason in 1981 the National Electrical Code required that all health-care facilities using whirlpools and tubs install **ground-fault interruptors (GFI)** (Figure 4-13). These devices constantly compare the amount of electricity flowing from the wall outlet to the whirlpool turbine with the amount returning to the outlet. If there is any leakage in current flow detected, the ground-fault circuit breaker will automatically interrupt current flow in as little as one fortieth of a second, thus shutting off current flow and reducing the chances of electrical shock.[13] These devices may be installed either in the electrical outlet or in the circuit-breaker box.

Regardless of the type of electrotherapeutic device being used and the type of environment, the following safety practices should be considered:

1. The entire electrical system of the building or training room should be designed or evaluated by a qualified electrician. Problems with the electrical system may exist in older buildings or in situations where rooms have been

modified to accommodate therapeutic devices (e.g., putting a whirlpool in a locker room where the concrete floor is always wet or damp).

2. It should not be assumed that all three-pronged wall outlets are automatically grounded to the earth. The ground must be checked.

3. The sports therapist should become very familiar with the equipment being used and with any potential problems that may exist or develop. Any defective equipment should be immediately removed from the clinic.

4. The plug should not be jerked out of the wall by pulling on the cable.

5. Extension cords or multiple adaptors should never be used.

6. Equipment should be reevaluated on a yearly basis and should conform to National Electrical Code guidelines. If a clinic or training room is not in compliance with this code, then there is no legal protection in a lawsuit.

7. Common sense should always be exercised when using electrotherapeutic devices. A situation that appears to be potentially dangerous may result in injury or death.

SUMMARY

1. Electrons move along a conducting medium as an electrical current.

2. A volt is the electromotive force that produces a movement of electrons; an ampere is a unit of measurement that indicates the rate at which electrical current is flowing.

3. Ohm's law expresses the relationship between current flow voltage and resistance. The current flow is directly proportional to the voltage and inversely proportional to the resistance.

4. Electrotherapeutic devices generate three different types of current, alternating (AC) or biphasic, direct (DC) or monophasic, or pulsed or polyphasic, which when introduced into biologic tissue are capable of producing specific physiologic changes.

5. Confusion exists relative to the terminology used to describe electrotherapeutic currents, but all therapeutic electrical generators regardless of whether they deliver AC, DC, or pulsed currents through electrodes attached to the skin are transcutaneous electrical stimulators.

6. The term pulse is synonomous with waveform, which indicates a graphic representation of the shape, direction, amplitude, duration, and pulse frequency of the electrical current being produced by the electrotherapeutic device, as displayed by an instrument called an oscilloscope.

7. Modulation refers to any alteration in the magnitude or any variation in duration of a pulse (or pulses) and may be continuous, interrupted, burst, or ramped.

8. The main difference between a series and a parallel circuit is that in a series circuit there is a single pathway for current to get from one terminal to another and in a parallel circuit two or more routes exist for current to pass.

9. The electrical circuit that exists when electron flow is through human tissue is a combination of both a series and a parallel circuit.

10. The effects of electrical current moving through biologic tissue may be chemical, thermal, or physiologic.

11. Electrical safety is critical when using electrotherapeutic devices. It is the responsibility of the sports therapist to make sure that all electrical modalities conform to the National Electrical Code.

GLOSSARY

accommodation Adaptation by the sensory receptors to various stimuli over an extended period of time.

alternating current Current that periodically changes its polarity or direction of flow.

ampere Unit of measure that indicates the rate at which electrical current is flowing.

amplifier A device using electrical components to increase electrical power.

amplitude The intensity of current flow as indicated by the height of the waveform from baseline.

average current The amount of current flowing per unit of time.

biphasic current Another name for alternating current, in which the direction of current flow reverses direction.

bursts A combined set of three or more pulses; also referred to as packets or envelopes.

circuit The path of current from a generating source through the various components back to the generating source.

conductance The ease with which a current flows along a conducting medium.

conductors Materials that permit the free movement of electrons.

coulomb Measurement indicating the number of electrons flowing in a current.

decay time The time required for a waveform to go from peak amplitude to 0 V.

direct current Galvanic current that always flows in the same direction and may flow in either a positive or a negative direction.

duration Sometimes referred to as pulse width. Indicates the length of time the current is flowing.

electrical current The net movement of electrons along a conducting medium.

electrical impedance The opposition to electron flow in a conducting material.

electrical potential The difference between charged particles at a higher and lower potential.

electron Fundamental particles of matter possessing a negative electrical charge and very small mass.

faradic current An asymmetric biphasic waveform seldom used on modern electrical generators.

filter Changes pulsating DC current to smooth DC.

frequency The number of cycles or pulses per second.

ground A wire that makes an electrical connection with the earth.

ground-fault interruptor (GFI) A safety device that automatically shuts off current flow and reduces the chances of electrical shock.

high-voltage current Current in which the waveform has an amplitude of greater than 150 V with a relatively short pulse duration.

insulators Materials that resist current flow.

interpulse interval The interruptions between individual pulses or groups of pulses.

intrapulse interval The period of time between individual pulses.

ion A positively or negatively charged particle.

iontophoresis Use of continuous direct current to drive ions into the tissues.

low-voltage current Current in which the waveform has an amplitude of less than 150 V.

macroshock An electrical shock that can be felt and has a leakage of electrical current of greater than 1 mA.

medical galvanism Creation of either an acidic or alkaline environment that may be of therapeutic value.

microcurrent electrical nerve stimulator (MENS) Used primarily in tissue healing, the current intensities are too small to excite peripheral nerves.

microshock An electrical shock that is imperceptible because of a leakage of current of less than 1 mA.

modulation Refers to any alteration in the magnitude or any variation in the duration of an electrical current.

monophasic current Another name for direct current, in which the direction of current flow remains the same.

neuromuscular electrical stimulator (NMES) Also called an electrical muscle stimulator (EMS), it is used to stimulate muscle directly as would be the case with denervated muscle where peripheral nerves are not functioning.

ohm A unit of measure that indicates resistance to current flow.

Ohm's law The current in an electrical circuit is directly proportional to the voltage and inversely proportional to the resistance.

oscillator Used to produce and output a specific waveform, which may be different from that used to power or drive the stimulating unit.

output amplifier Used to magnify or increase the amplitude of the voltage output of the generator and control it at a specific level.

parallel circuit A circuit in which two or more routes exist for current to pass between the two terminals.

phases That portion of the pulse that rises above or below the baseline for some period of time.

polyphasic current Current that contains three or more grouped phases in a single pulse and that is used in interferential and ''Russian'' currents.

pulse An individual waveform.

pulse charge The total amount of electricity being delivered to the athlete during each pulse.

pulse period The combined time of the pulse duration and the interpulse interval.

ramping Another name for surging modulation, in which the current builds gradually to some maximum amplitude.

rate of rise How quickly a waveform reaches its maximum amplitude.

rectifier Converts AC current to pulsating DC current.

regulator Produces a specific controlled voltage output.

resistance The opposition to electron flow in a conducting material.

series circuit A circuit in which there is only one path for current to get from one terminal to another.

tetany Muscle condition that is caused by hyperexcitation and results in cramps and spasms.

transcutaneous electrical nerve stimulator (TENS) A transcutaneous electrical stimulator used to stimulate peripheral nerves.

transcutaneous electrical stimulator All therapeutic electrical generators regardless of whether they deliver AC, DC, or pulsed currents through electrodes attached to the skin.

transformer Reduces the amount of voltage from the power supply.

volt The electromotive force that must be applied to produce a movement of electrons.

voltage The force resulting from an accumulation of electrons at one point in an electrical circuit, usually corresponding to a deficit of electrons at another point in the circuit.

watt A measure of electrical power. Mathematically, Watts = Volts × Amperes.

waveform The shape of an electrical current as displayed on an oscilloscope.

REFERENCES

1 Alon G: *Principles of electrical stimulation.* In Nelson R, Currier D, editors: *Clinical electrotherapy,* Norwalk, Conn, 1991, Appleton & Lange.

2 Bergueld P: *Electromedical instrumentation: a guide for medical personnel,* Cambridge, 1980, Cambridge University Press.

3 Chamishion R: *Basic medical electronics,* Boston, 1964, Little, Brown.

4 Cohen HL, and Brunilik J: *Manual of electroneuromyography,* ed 2, New York, Harper & Row, 1925.

5 Cook T, Barr JO: *Instrumentation.* In Nelson R, and Currier D, editors: *Clinical electrotherapy,* Norwalk, Conn, 1991, Appleton & Lange.

6 Cromwell L, Arditti M, Weibell F: *Medical instrumentation for health care,* Englewood Cliffs, NJ, 1976, Prentice-Hall.

7 DeDomenico G: *Basic guidelines for interferential therapy,* Sydney, Australia, 1981, Theramed.

8 Griffin J, Karselis T: *Physical agents for physical therapists,* Springfield, Ill, 1988, Charles C. Thomas.

9 Kloth L, Cummings JP: *Electrotherapeutic terminology in physical therapy.* Alexandria, Virginia, 1990, Section on Clinical Electrophysiology and the American Physical Therapy Association.

10 Licht S: *Therapeutic electricity and ultraviolet radiation,* vol IV, ed 2, Baltimore, 1969, Waverly.

11 Myklebust B, Kloth L: *Electrodiagnostic and electrotherapeutic instrumentation: characteristics of recording and stimulation systems and principles of safety.* In Gersh MR: *Electrotherapy in rehabilitation,* Philadelphia, 1992, FA Davis.

12 Myklebust B, Robinson AJ: *Instrumentation.* In Snyder-Mackler L, Robinson AJ, editors: *Clinical electrophysiology, electrotherapy and electrophysiologic testing.* Baltimore, 1989, Williams & Wilkins.

13 Porter M, Porter J: Electrical safety in the training room, *Ath Train* 16(4): 263-264, 1981.

14 Robinson AJ: *Basic concepts and terminology in electricity.* In Snyder-Mackler L, Robinson AJ, editors: *Clinical electrophysiology, electrotherapy and electrophysiologic testing,* Baltimore, 1989, Williams & Wilkins.

15 Shriber W: *A manual of electrotherapy,* ed 4, Philadelphia, 1975, Lea & Febiger.

16 Stillwell GK: *Therapeutic electricity and ultraviolet radiation,* ed 3, Baltimore, 1983, Williams & Wilkins.

17 Watkins AL: *A manual of electrotherapy,* ed 3, Philadelphia, 1968, Lea & Febiger.

18 Wolf SL: *Electrotherapy: clinics in physical therapy,* vol 2, New York, 1981, Churchill Livingstone.

SUGGESTED READINGS

Alon G: *High voltage stimulation: a monograph,* Chattanooga, Tenn, 1984, Chattanooga Corporation.

Alon G: *Electrical stimulators,* Chattanooga, Tenn. 1985, Chattanooga Corporation (Video presentation).

Alon G, Allin J, Inbar G: Optimization of pulse duration and pulse charge during TENS, *Aust J Physiother* 29: 195, 1983.

Benton L, Baker L, Bowman B, et al.: *Functional electrical stimulation: a practical clinical guide*, Downey, Calif, 1980, Rancho Los Amigos Hospital.

Binder S: *Electrical stimulating currents.* In Wolf S, editor: *Electrotherapy*, New York, 1981, Churchill Livingstone.

Brown I: *Fundamentals of electrotherapy course guide*, Madison, Wis, 1963, University of Wisconsin Press.

Campbell J: A critical appraisal of the electrical output characteristics of ten TENS units, *Clin Phys Physiol Meas* 3: 141, 1982.

Geddes L: A short history of electrical stimulation of excitable tissue, *Physiologist* 27: 1, 1984.

Geddes L, Baler L: *Applied biomedical instrumentation*, New York, 1975, John Wiley.

Kottke F: *Handbook of physical medicine and rehabilitation*, ed 3, Philadelphia, 1982, WB Saunders.

Lane J: Electrical impedances of superficial limb tissues, epidermis, dermis, and muscle sheath, *Ann NY Acad Sci* 238: 812, 1974.

Licht S: *Electrodiagnosis and electromyography*, vol 1, ed 3, Baltimore, 1971, Waverly.

Mannheimer J, Lampe G: *Clinical transcutaneous electrical nerve stimulation*, Philadelphia, 1984, FA Davis.

Nelson R, Currier D: *Clinical electrotherapy*, Norwalk, Conn, 1987, Appleton & Lange.

Newton RA: *Electrotherapy: selecting wave form parameters*, paper presented at the American Physical Therapy Association Conference, Washington, DC, 1981.

Newton RA: *Electrotherapeutic treatment: selecting appropriate wave form characteristics*, Clinton, NJ, 1984, Preston.

Reismann M: A comparison of electrical stimulators eliciting muscle contraction, *Phys Ther* 64: 751, 1984.

Scott P: *Clayton's electrotherapy and actinotherapy*, eds 5 and 7, Baltimore, 1965 and 1975, Williams & Wilkins.

Sunderland S: *Nerves and nerve injuries*, Baltimore, 1968, Williams & Wilkins.

Wadsworth H, and Chanmugan A: *Electrophysical agents in physical therapy*, Marickville, Australia, 1983, Science Press.

Ward A: *Electricity waves and fields in therapy*, Marickville, Australia, 1980, Science Press.

Electrical Stimulating Currents

5

Daniel N. Hooker

OBJECTIVES

After completion of this chapter, the student will be able to do the following:

- Describe muscle and nerve responses to electrical stimulation.

- Describe nonexcitatory cell and tissue responses to electrical stimulation.

- Describe the uses of electrically stimulated muscle contractions.

- Describe the various treatment parameters that must be considered with electrical stimulating currents.

- Describe the effect of non-contractable stimulation on edema.

- Describe the modulation of pain through the use of electrical stimulating currents.

- Discuss specialized electrical current generators in relation to physiologic changes and benefits.

- Identify problems that might respond to electrical stimulation.

Often the sports therapist uses electrical currents for treatment in an effort to create a quick cure for the physical problems suffered by his or her patients or athletes. Although electrical treatments can provide dramatic results at times, this is the exception rather than the rule. The use of electricity in treating an injury can be beneficial, but the sports therapist must base the use of electricity on facts about the effects of electricity on biologic tissues. The treatment program must be tailored toward influencing the problems identified in the evaluation. Electrical therapy should not be used in a "shotgun" approach if we are to maximize the effectiveness of this modality.

There has been considerable activity in the last 10 years in the commercial development of new therapeutic electrical generators. The clinical use of electrotherapy has changed as the changing technology has enabled the equipment manufacturers to design and promote their latest product lines. Modern electronics have opened the doors to electronic equipment that could conceivably generate any electrical output desired. Wave shapes, amplitudes, and frequencies can all be manipulated so that any combination might be possible.

The research is, as usual, lagging behind commercial development. Of the research that has been and will be conducted, experts will continue to disagree with or challenge the interpretations of the results. Researchers in the biologic responses find it difficult to isolate one variable for experimentation and maintain control of all the other variables that could affect their results. Deciding whether the results of a study are significant for cause and effect or merely a chance happening or significant but not directly caused by the manipulation of the experimental variable is very difficult for the clinician. There are still more questions than answers in this field of research.

Electrotherapy of the future is moving toward attempts at controlling cellular and tissue function with externally generated electrical currents. The sports therapist will need the concepts of **bioelectromagnetics,** the study of biologic tissues' electrical and magnetic properties, to apply and understand the therapeutic outcomes of the next generation of electrical modalities. Knowledge of the electric properties of cells, intercellular and intracellular communication, bioelectric potentials, tissue currents, strain generated electric potentials, and the biologic effects of other nonionizing energy will be essential for the expert clinician to use present and future electrical modalities for maximum therapeutic benefit.[17,18]

PHYSIOLOGIC RESPONSE TO ELECTRICAL CURRENTS

Electricity will have an effect on each cell and tissue that it passes through.[17,18,87] The type and extent of this response are dependent on (1) the type of tissue and its response characteristics (for example, how it normally functions and how it grows or changes under normal stress) and (2) the nature of the current applied (that is, direct or alternating, intensity, duration, voltage, and density). The tissue should respond to electrical energy in a manner similar to that in which it normally functions or grows. These statements are true within a certain range of current parameters, but current density above critical levels can cause coagulation and tissue destruction.[1] Clinically, sports therapists use electrical currents for the following:

1. Creating muscle contraction through nerve or muscle stimulation.
2. Stimulating sensory nerves to help in treating pain.
3. Creating an electrical field in biologic tissues to stimulate or alter the healing process.
4. Creating an electrical field on the skin surface to drive ions beneficial to the healing process into or through the skin.

As electricity moves through the body's conductive medium, changes in the physiologic functioning can occur at various levels of the total system. Four levels can be readily identified from the functional standpoint:

I. Cellular
II. Tissue
III. Segmental
IV. Systematic

As in all classification systems, there is some overlap and assignment to one level may be a bit arbitrary. The effects can be defined as follows:

Cellular Level: can be broken down into five major effects
1. Excitation of nerve cells
2. Changes in cell membrane permeability
3. Protein synthesis
4. Stimulation of fibrobloast, osteoblast
5. Modification of microcirculation

Tissue Level: this requires multiple cellular events
1. Skeletal muscle contraction
2. Smooth muscle contraction
3. Tissue regeneration

Segmental Level: involves a regional effect of the previous two level activities
1. Modification of joint mobility
2. Muscle pumping action to change circulation and lymphatic activity
3. Alteration of the microvascular system not associated with muscle pumping

Systematic Effects:
1. Analgesic effects as endongenous pain suppressors are released and act at different levels to control pain
2. Analgesic effects from the stimulation of certain neurotransmitters to control neural activity in the presence of pain stimuli[2]

These responses can be broken into direct and indirect effects. There is always a direct effect along the lines of current flow and under the electrodes. Indirect effects occur remote to the area of current flow and are usually the result of stimulating a natural physiologic event to occur.[2,21]

If a certain effect is desired from stimulation, goals must be established to achieve a specific physiologic response from treatment. These responses can be grouped into two basic physiologic responses: nonexcitatory and excitatory.

The excitatory response is the most obvious and most used in treating athletes. In sports medicine, most time is spent trying to get the excitatory response from the nerve cells and muscle tissue. Athletes perceive excitatory responses as electric sensation, muscle contraction, and electric pain. Physiologically, the nerves that affect these perceptions fire in that order as the stimulus is gradually increased. Nerves have very little discriminatory ability. They can tell only if there is electricity in sufficient magnitude to cause a depolarization of the nerve membrane. They have very little regard for the different shape and polarities of waveforms. To the nerve cell, electricity is electricity. As in all things dealing with higher level organisms, there is a large range of responses to the same stimulus depending on the environmental and systemic factors.

All perception is a product of the brain receiving the signal that a nerve has been stimulated electrically. This further enlarges the broad range of systemic effects that occur in response to the electric stimulation.

Stimulation events will change the body's perception. As the strength or duration of the current increases, more nerve cells will fire. As the strength of the stimulus increases and these events occur, certain quality judgments about the electric stimuli are made. Is the current pleasant or unpleasant? Is the intensity of the stimulus weak or strong? The broad range of individual responses to these quality judgments has a significant impact on the beneficial effects of this therapy.[28,29]

Muscle and Nerve Responses to Electrical Currents

Presently, the major therapeutic uses of electricity center on muscle contraction, sensory stimulation, or both. Let us look in a general way at the physiologic effects of electricity on nerve and muscle tissue. Specific currents or frequencies will be discussed later in the chapter.

Nerves and muscles are both excitable tissues. This excitability is dependent on the cell membrane's **voltage sensitive permeability.** The nerve or muscle cell membrane regulates the interchange of substances between the inside of the cell and the environment outside the cell. This voltage sensitive permeability produces an unequal distribution of charged ions on each side of the membrane, which in turn creates a potential difference between the charge of the interior of the cell and the exterior of the cell. The membrane then is considered to be polarized. The potential difference between the inside and outside is known as the **resting potential**[1] because the cell tries to maintain this electrochemical gradient as its normal homeostatic environment.[17]

Both electrical and chemical gradients are established along the cell membrane, with a greater concentration of diffusible positive ions on the outside of the membrane than on the inside. Using its active transport mechanism, the cell continually moves Na^+ from inside the cell to outside and balances this positive charge movement by moving K^+ to the inside. K^+ will have a larger concentration on the inside of the cell, but the overall charge difference produces an electrical gradient with positive charges outside and negative charges inside (Figure 5-1). As explained by Guyton, "The potential is proportional to the difference in tendency of the ions to diffuse in one direction versus the other direction. Two conditions are necessary for the membrane potential to develop: (1) The membrane must be semipermeable, allowing ions of one charge to diffuse through the pores more readily than ions of the opposite charge. (2) The concentration of the diffusable ions must be greater on one side of the membrane than on the other side."[17,42]

The resting membrane potential is generated because the cell is an ionic battery whose concentration of ions inside and outside the cell is maintained by regulatory NA^+/K^+ pumps within the cell wall. In addition to the ability of the nerve and muscle cell membranes to develop and maintain the resting potential, the membranes are excitable.[17,42]

To create transmission of an impulse in the nerve tissue, resting membrane

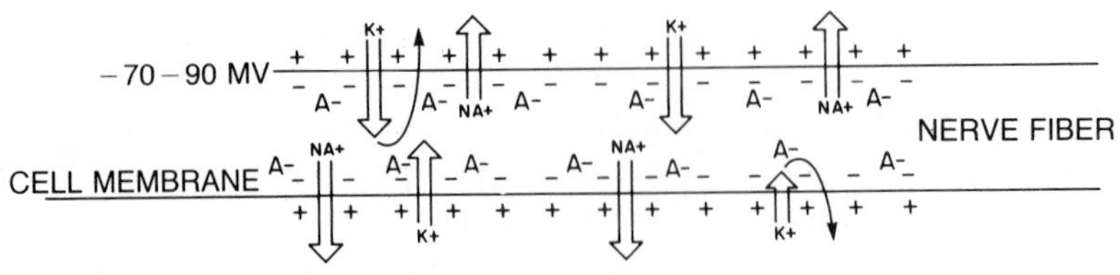

Fig. 5-1 Nerve cell membrane with active transport mechanisms maintaining the resting membrane potential.

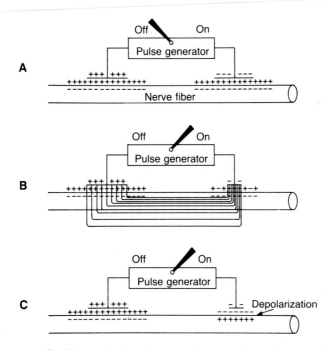

Fig. 5-2 A to **C,** Depolarization of nerve cell membrane.

potential must be reduced below a threshold level. Changes in the membrane's permeability may then occur. These changes create an **action potential** that will propagate the impulse along the nerve in both directions from the location of the stimulus. An action potential created by a stimulus from chemical, electrical, thermal, or mechanical means always creates the same result, membrane **depolarization.**

Not all stimuli are effective in causing an action potential and depolarization. To be an effective agent, the stimulus must have an adequate intensity and last long enough to equal or exceed the membrane's basic threshold for excitation. The stimulus must alter the membrane so that a number of ions are pushed across the membrane, exceeding the ability of the active transport pumps to maintain the resting potentials. A stimulus of this magnitude forces the membrane to depolarize and results in an action potential.[42,95]

DEPOLARIZATION. As the charged ions move across the nerve fiber membranes beneath the **anode** and **cathode,** membrane depolarization occurs. The cathode is usually the site of depolarization (Figure 5-2, *A*). As the concentration of negatively charged ions increases, the membrane's voltage potential becomes low and is brought toward its threshold for depolarization (Figure 5-2, *B*). The anode makes the nerve cell membrane potential more positive, increasing the threshold necessary for depolarization (Figure 5-2, *C*). The cathode in this example becomes the active electrode; the anode becomes the **indifferent electrode.** The anode and cathode may switch active and indifferent roles under other circumstances.[2,9,95] The number of ions needed to exceed the membrane pump's ability to maintain the normal membrane resting potential is tissue dependent.

Depolarization propagation. After excitement and propagation of the impulse

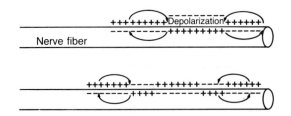

Fig. 5-3 Propagation of the nerve impulse.

along the nerve fiber, there is a brief period during which the nerve fiber is incapable of reacting to a second stimulus. This is the **absolute refractory period,** which lasts about 0.5 μsec. Excitability is restored gradually as the nerve cell membrane repolarizes itself. The nerve then is capable of being stimulated again. The maximum number of possible discharges of a nerve may reach 1000 per second, depending on fiber type.[8,9,42,95]

The difference in electrical potential between the depolarized region and the neighboring inactive regions causes the current to flow from the depolarized region through the intercellular material to the inactive membrane. The current also flows through the extracellular materials, back to the depolarized area, and finally into the cell again. This forms a complete local circuit and makes the depolarization self-propagating as the process is repeated all along the fiber in each direction from the depolarization site. Energy released by the cell keeps the intensity of the impulse uniform as it travels down the cell.[8,9,42,95] This process is illustrated in Figure 5-3.

Depolarization effects. As the nerve impulse reaches its effector organ or another nerve cell, the impulse is transferred between the two at a motor end plate or a synapse. At this junction, a transmitter substance is released from the nerve, rather than the impulse jumping from one nerve to another. This transmitter substance causes the other excitable tissue to discharge (Figure 5-4).[9,95]

In terms of muscle excitation, a **twitch muscle contraction** results. This contraction, initiated by an electrical stimulus, is the same as a twitch contraction coming from voluntary activity. Voluntary muscular activity is different only in the rate and synchrony (simultaneous response) of the muscle fiber contractions.[9,70] A graphic illustration of this threshold and propagation and contraction is the **strength-duration curve** (Figure 5-5).

As illustrated, there is a nonlinear relationship between current duration and current intensity, in which shorter duration stimuli require increasing intensities to reach the threshold of the nerve or muscle. Nerve and muscle membrane thresholds differ significantly. Different sizes and types of nerve fibers also have different thresholds. The strength-duration curves for different classes of nerve and muscle tissue illustrate the different thresholds of excitability of these tissues. The curves are basically symmetric, but the intensity of current necessary to reach the membrane's threshold for excitation differs for each tissue (Figure 5-6).[42,69,95,100]

STRENGTH-DURATION CURVE. Three important concepts are represented in the strength-duration curve. These terms and ideas are used frequently in discussions on the effects of electrical currents on the nerve cellular level.[44,95]

1. The shape of the curve relates the intensity of the electrical stimulus and the length of time (duration) necessary to cause the tissue to depolarize.

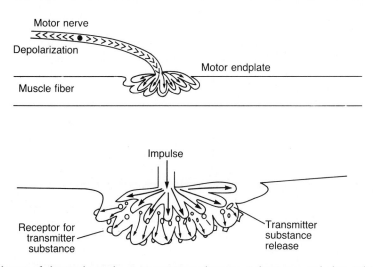

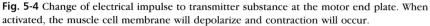

Fig. 5-4 Change of electrical impulse to transmitter substance at the motor end plate. When activated, the muscle cell membrane will depolarize and contraction will occur.

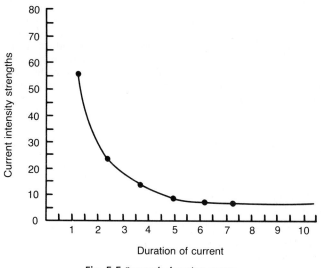

Duration of current

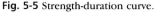

Fig. 5-5 Strength-duration curve.

2. The **rheobase** describes the minimum intensity of current necessary to cause tissue excitation when applied for a maximum duration (Figure 5-7).

3. **Chronaxie** describes the length of time (duration) required for a current of twice the intensity of the rheobase current to produce tissue excitation (see Figure 5-7).

If you look at the strength-duration curve and wish to obtain maximum sensory or motor response, use a stimulus with a high intensity and short duration. Electrical engineers have designed some units to maximize this effect. As the charge increases and

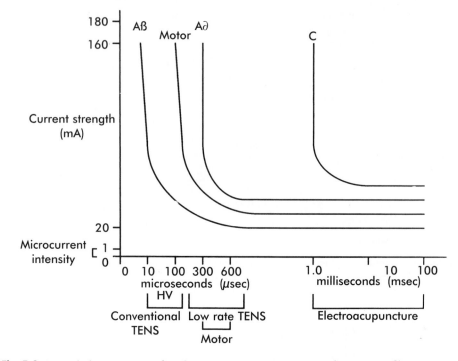

Fig. 5-6. Strength duration curves for Aβ sensory, motor, A∂ sensory, and pain nerve fibers. Durations of several electrical stimulators are indicated along the lower axis. Corresponding intensities would be necessary to create a depolarizing stimulus for any of the nerve fibers. Microcurrent intensity is so low that the nerve fibers will not depolarize. This current travels through other body tissues to create effects.

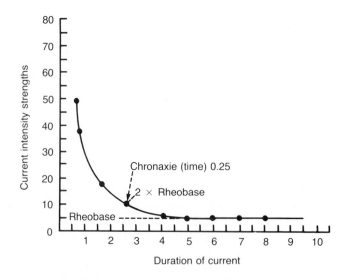

Fig. 5-7. Excitation time of nerve cell membrane.

more and more nerve fibers fire, the brain becomes more and more involved in the perceptual part of the experience.

MUSCULAR RESPONSES TO ELECTRICAL CURRENT. Stimulation of the motor nerve is the method used in most clinical applications of electrical muscular contractions. In the absence of innervation, muscle contraction can be stimulated by an electrical current that causes the muscle membrane to depolarize. This will create the same muscle contraction as a natural stimulus.

The **all-or-none response** is another important concept in applying electrical current to nerve or muscle tissue. Once a stimulus reaches a depolarizing threshold, the nerve or muscle membrane depolarizes, and propagation of the impulse or muscle contraction occurs. This reaction remains the same regardless of increases in the strength of the stimulus used. Either the stimulus causes depolarization—the all—or it does not cause depolarization—the none. There is no gradation of response; the response of the single nerve or muscle fiber is maximal or nonexistant.[9,70,95]

This all-or-none phenomenon does not mean that muscle fiber shortening and overall muscle activity cannot be influenced by changing the intensity, pulses per second, or duration of the stimulating current. Adjustments in current parameters can cause changes in the shortening of the muscle fiber and in the overall muscle activity.

THE EFFECTS OF ELECTRICAL STIMULATION ON NONEXCITABLE TISSUES AND CELLS

The nonexcitatory cells respond to electric current in a variety of ways consistent with the cell type and tissue function. To understand the theory of stimulating these nonexcitatory cells, a good understanding of the cell as a part of the body's bioelectric system is needed.

CELLULAR ELECTRICAL CIRCUITS

The cell membrane. The basic cell with cell membrane, nucleus, organelles, and so on acts like an ionic battery with the inside of the cell electrically negative and the outside electrically positive. The cell's plasma membrane is responsible for maintaining this electrochemical gradient as well as sending and receiving messages. The membrane is made up of phospholipid molecules studded with several types of proteins that project into or through the phospholipid layers. These proteins support, transport things in and out, receive specific molecules that alter cell functions, and promote reactions on the cell surface (Figure 5-8, A).

General cell electrical gradients are similar to those described for nerve cells but contain four electrical zones. The central cytoplasm area is negative and is surrounded by a narrow band of positively charged potassium ions along the inside of the cell membrane. The outer wall of the cell membrane is positively charged with sodium and potassium ions and is surrounded by a negative zone composed of sialic acid molecules (see Figure 5-8).

The difference in potential across the membrane is maintained as described previously for nerve cell membranes with the sodium and potassium pumps in the cell membrane doing the work. Any ionic fluctuations in the cytoplasm cause the ion pumps in the membrane to activate and return the equilibrium of the cell. There are also

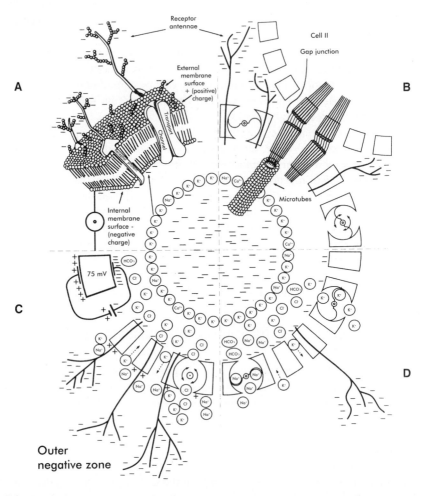

Fig. 5-8. The electric cell with central negative zone, inner positive zone, cell membrane, outer positive zone, and outer negative zone. **A,** Three-dimensional model of the cell membrane with transmembrane receptor proteins, receptor antennae, the outer positive surface charge, and inner negative surface charge. **B,** Gap junctions connect one cell to another and allow direct communication between cells. Receptors connect to microtubes within the cell. **C,** Total electrochemical equilibrium acts as an ion battery, creating a resting potential across the cell membrane. **D,** Cell membrane pumps and passive ion channels act as ion balancers to preserve cell equilibrium.

passive ionic channels in the wall that allow passive ion movement along the electrochemical gradients (Figure 5-8, *D*).

The only difference between excitable and nonexcitable cell membranes is the presence of voltage gated sodium ion channels. In the excitatory cells, these ion channels generate the action potentials once a depolarizing stimulus causes the membrane to become more permeable to the outside NA^+. The NA^+ channels are triggered to open, and NA^+ ions move into the cell, causing a brief reversal of charge. The charge reversal causes these ion channels to close, and the normal membrane potential returns.

The cell membrane is not just an outside covering but is also intimately involved with internal cell structures as an intercellular membrane, surrounds organelles, and supports the internal structure of the cell. This intercellular membrane can then exercise control of the movement of substances out from or into the cytoplasm from the organelles. This movement is controlled by the same type of electrochemical gradients and selective ion channels as are used in maintaining the cell wall[17,18] (see Figure 5-8).

Intercellular structures. The internal cell structure is also made up of a dense network of hollow microtubules. These microtubules can be built and dismantled by the cell relatively rapidly and are **dipoles** with the negatively charged end directed centrally and the positive end directed peripherally. The microtubules are very active in cell function, moving materials like neurotransmitters along the surface of the cell, making cilia move, moving organelles around within the cell, and acting as sensors of the extracellular environment. The microtubules also form the mitotic spindle in the cell division process (Figure 5-8, *B*). Because of its ability to change rapidly and help in cell and intercellular movement, the microtubules are probably significant actors in cell organization during wound healing and regeneration.

Normal cells are signaled and respond to changes when messages contact the outer projections of the cell wall. Likewise, messages from within the cell can be sent outside the cell. The message can be chemical like hormones or possibly an electromagnetic energy coded message. Once the message is received, the signal is conveyed across the membrane to the cell's interior. The message is then transferred to another message system or switchboard, which activates the cell's response to the message. The message may speed the cell up, make it move, stimulate production of extracellular proteins, or increase the secretions of that cell (see Figure 5-8)[17]

Electrical circuits in tissues. Many cells are physically united with neighboring cells of like structure and collectively perform as one tissue. The cell membranes are bound together by junctions between the outer projections of each cell membrane. These specialized junctions allow direct communication between adjacent cells. These specialized junction areas are called **gap junctions** and contain channels for ionic, electrical, and small-molecule signaling. The cells connected by gap junctions can then act together when one cell receives an extracellular message; the tissue can be coordinated in its response by the gap junction's internal message system. Embryonic and regenerating tissues are particularly rich in gap junctions, and they probably play a significant role in tissue growth and differentiation (see Figure 5-8, *B*).

Cells are surrounded by a bonding medium of collagen, elastin, and hyaluronic acid gel. This extracellular matrix can also interact with the adjacent cell surface receptors to modify cell function, orientation and alignment, shape, movement, metabolic rate, and differentiation.[17]

Strain related potentials. The previous discussion on cell structure points out that every cell surface carries a charge. Every support structure within the cell, membranes, or microtubules is a dipole. In effect, cell structures have similar properties to **electrets** (insulators carrying a permanent charge, similar to a permanent magnet). Electrets are capable of **piezoelectric activity,** in which mechanical deformation of the structure causes a change in the surface electrical charge of the structure. They are also capable of **electropiezo activity,** in which changing an electric surface charge would force the electret to change shape. This becomes important when considering the piezoelectric effect of bone and connective tissue and how this change in electrical surface activity may guide or stimulate growth or healing.

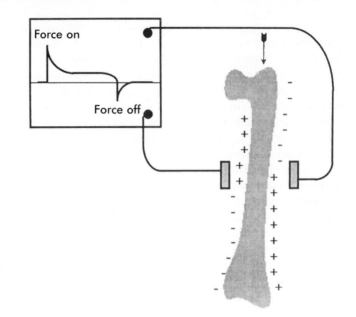

Fig. 5-9. Electrical response of bone tissue to the momentary deforming stress of weight bearing.

Most connective tissues also generate a tissue based electrical potential in response to tissue strain. Tension on surfaces or distraction on the surface creates these **strain related potentials.** Where there is compression, the strain related potentials are negative. Where there is tension, they are positive. Functionally, these strain related potentials have helped provide an electromechanical explanation for Wolff's law governing bone's growth in response to mechanical stress. The controlling mechanism for these events is most likely some form of the intrinsic electrochemical responses discussed earlier in this chapter, since no specific hormonal or neurologic controls have been discovered. The stress generated potential must signal the membranes of the osteoblast, osteocytes, and osteoclasts to add or take away bone in areas of compression or tension. The cells have the necessary mechanisms to receive and decode the strain information, and intrinsically the cells can respond appropriately to maintain the integrity of the tissue[5,13,17] (Figure 5-9).

Cells are grouped together into tissues, creating segmental units that combine into a whole system. Each cell, considered an ionic battery when added together with other cells, can collectively summate the influence and generate potential differences across the surface of the body or between different areas of the same tissue. These endogenous currents with their polarity gradients seem to play a key role in guiding the development, growth, regeneration, and repair of the cells, tissues, and segments of the body.[17]

NORMAL BIOELECTRIC FIELDS. Becker demonstrated a direct current bioelectric field that could be measured in salamanders and other animals. The spatial configuration of this field coincided with the arrangement of their central nervous systems, with the positive areas being located near the major nerve cell accumulations, that is the brain and brachial and lumbar plexus areas. The negative areas were near the major peripheral nerve outflows from these areas.[6,7,8,17,18]

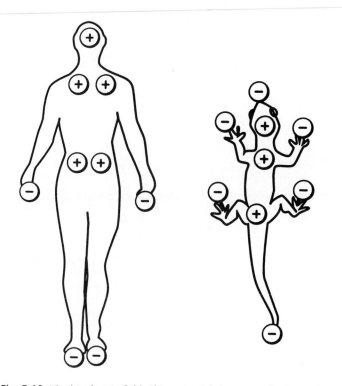

Fig. 5-10. The bioelectric field. Skin potentials in man and salamander.

This bioelectric field has been measured in other animals and has also been recorded for humans. The skin surface also is always negative relative to the dermis, so there is a permanent electrical gradient through the skin tissue.[7,8,17] Potential difference gradients also exist on long bones with the midpoints more positive than the ends and areas of increased cellular activity (i.e., epiphyseal plate area) more negative than other areas. This direct current seems to be in a continuous circuit along the length of the bone and will vary in strength according to local differences in metabolism[17] (Figure 5-10).

Bioelectric activity in skin wounds. When skin is damaged, a steady current will move from the relatively positively charged dermis into the wound area and reenter the skin just below the stratum corneum. The wound currents also generate a lateral potential difference from the outside normal area to the wound edge, forming a lateral electrical gradient. This lateral gradient appears to stimulate epithelial cells in the wound edge to regenerate and begin to grow across the wound. Once the wound edges approximate, the surface integrity is reestablished and the lateral gradient disappears. If the wound dries out, these currents will also drop because of increased resistance to electrical flow. The skin thickness is reestablished as cell layering and the increased electric potentials return to normal[17,36] (Figure 5-11).

Bioelectric field changes in response to injury. Becker's experiments with salamander limb injury showed that the bioelectric field gradient reversed immediately when a salamander limb was amputated. The normal current was -10 mV, and at amputation it jumped to a + 20 mV current. Gradually as healing started to take place,

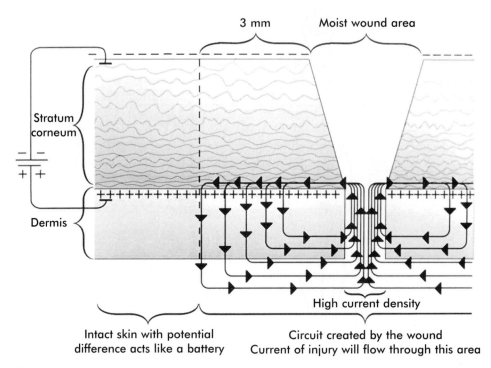

Fig. 5-11. Normal intact skin with electric field (*left side*) and the electric reaction to injury with the current of injury path through the skin wound (*right side*).

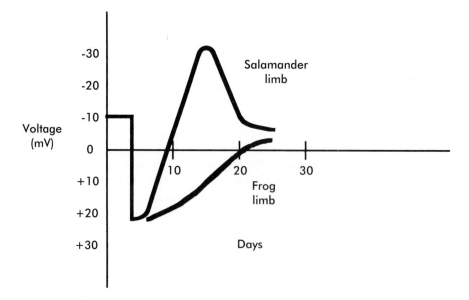

Fig. 5-12. Voltage changes in amputed salamander and frog limbs during regeneration and healing.

this current returned to a highly negative -30 mV current and then gradually returned to baseline values as limb regeneration occurred[6,7,8] (Figure 5-12).

In the frog, a nonregenerating cousin of the salamander, this bioelectric current behaved similarly upon amputation but never jumped back to a negative current. Instead, it gradually moved back to the normal negative baseline values as the stump scarred over and healing became complete. Becker found this **current of injury** was produced by any type of cellular trauma and suggested that it plays a key role in stimulating healing and regeneration of tissue.[6,7,8]

Regeneration is more and more limited as we move up the phylogenetic ladder. Regeneration is also greatest in younger animals. Regeneration in humans is certainly limited, but certain tissues have some capacity to respond (muscle, nerve, bone, skin, connective tissue). Becker felt there were three essential ingredients for regeneration. The first was a powerful initial current of injury, initially a positive current and then becoming strongly negative as the wound blastema formed and gradually returned to baseline value as the limb regenerated. The second was that a high tissue versus innervation density was a critical factor, if innervation density is below a critical level, regeneration will not occur. The third ingredient needed is the presence of peripheral nerves in the wound area and the growth of these nerves to reinnervate the epithelial ingrowth at the amputation site. These neuroepidermal junctions form at about 7 to 8 days in the wound blastema. This event seems to play a significant role in the sudden reversal of the current of injury from positive to negative[6,8,17] (see Figure 5-12).

Becker and others have stimulated regeneration in nonregenerating species (frogs, rats) by applying a direct current to the amputation site that mimics the high negative current found in salamander regeneration during the blastema stage of growth, approximately 7 to 10 days after injury. The electrode must also stay at the growing tip throughout regeneration.[6,7,8,17,45]

This artificial current of injury apparently caused the proliferating cells in the injured area to differentiate to a more primitive cell type and then to differentiate into the appropriate cell types needed to continue the regeneration of the limb. The overall progression of the limb orientation and alignment is also probably guided by the bioelectric field with the distal electrode being negative (see Figure 5-12).

Becker, after several subsequent experiments, concluded that the bioelectric field of animals was a function of DC circuits that originated in and returned to the central nervous system. This conclusion indicates there is a constant flow of direct current present in neural tissue and that the amplitude and direction of current flow are dependent upon central nervous system activity.[8,17]

ELECTRICAL STIMULATION INFLUENCE ON CELLULAR AND TISSUE ACTIVITY. Cell behavior can be influenced by having extracellular molecules lock into receptor sites on the cell membrane, which activate the message relay and action system within the cell (see Figure 5-8, *A*). The recognition of receptor sites and the guiding of the extracellular molecule to that destination is caused by an interaction of the electric fields from the receptor site and the extracellular molecule. Electrical stimulation of the appropriate frequency and amplitude may also be able to activate the cellular receptor sites and stimulate the same cellular changes as the naturally occurring chemical molecular stimulation.

The cell functions by incorporating a multitude of chemical reactions into a living process. Enzymatic activity accelerates these reactions, and each cell contains approximately 3000 enzymes. The enzymatic activity of the cell depends on the availability of specific charged sites on the intracellular membrane surfaces. These sites may be made more or less available for enzymatic reactions by changes in shape or configuration of the surface. These changes usually occur in response to a messenger molecule, but it is conceivable that the appropriate electrical signal could also create more specific sites for enzymatic activity, thereby changing or stimulating cell function[17] (see Figure 5-8).

The microtubule system may selectively receive and transmit electromagnetic signals through the cell. As the energy travels along the microtubule, the signal may stimulate organelles to activate their routine functions. The microtubule system could transmit this energy wave from cell to cell through the tight cell-to-cell contact areas at the gap junctions. This transmission could create cells working together to respond as a tissue and also allow a very small amperage current to move quickly over the length of the tissue (see Figure 5-8).

Cells seem responsive to steady direct current gradients. The cells either move or grow toward one pole and away from the other. The electric field created by the direct current may help guide the healing process or guide the regenerative capabilities of injured or developing tissues.[17]

Cells may also respond to a particular frequency of current. The cell may be selectively responsive to certain frequencies and unresponsive to other frequencies. Some researchers claim that specific genes for protein manufacture can be activated by certain shaped electrical impulses. This frequency could change in certain ways according to the cellular state. This phenomena has been termed the **frequency window selectivity** of the cell.[17]

Overall, we see that small amplitude direct currents are intrinsic to the ways the body works to grow and repair. Clinically if we can duplicate some of these same signals, we may be successful in using electrotherapy in the most effective and efficient manner. The secrets to this type of use are only beginning to be uncovered.

Hopefully after reading this review of cell biology slanted toward the electrical components, the magnitude of the cellular electrical activity and its potential to influence cell function become apparent. Many of the unexplained phenomena surrounding electrotherapy may become more understandable as more research promotes better understanding of the normal electrical activity at the cellular and tissue levels.

In this discussion of how electrical current influences nonexcitatory cells and tissue, we must start to rely on theory more than well proven researched ideas. The student must understand that theories are projections on what might take place to explain observed behavior and the authors expect changes in these theories to occur. So beware and believe cautiously as you incorporate these theories into your clinical practice.[43]

ELECTRICAL CONCEPTS: EFFECTS OF CHANGES IN CURRENT PARAMETERS AND THEIR EFFECT ON TREATMENT PROTOCOLS

When using any of the treatment protocols aimed at the electrical stimulation of muscle or nerve tissue, several concepts must be understood for sports therapists to accomplish their goals:

1. Alternating versus direct current
2. Tissue impedance
3. Current density
4. Frequency of wave or pulse
5. Intensity of wave or pulse
6. Duration of wave or pulse
7. Polarity of electrodes
8. Electrode placement

Changes in these parameters affect how the electrical current changes the physiology of the body part being treated. The wave form used gives us a graphic way to measure and quantify these parameters.[101]

Alternating Versus Direct Current

To further understand electrically stimulated muscle contractions, we must think in terms of multiple stimuli rather than a simple direct current response. The motor nerves are not stimulated by a steady flow of direct current. The nerve repolarizes under the influence of the current and will not depolarize again until a sudden change in current intensity occurs.

If continuous direct current were the only current mode available, we would get a muscle contraction only when the current intensity rose to a stimulus threshold. Once the membrane repolarized, another change in the current intensity would be needed to force another depolarization and contraction (Figure 5-13).

The biggest difference in the effects of alternating and direct currents is the ability of direct current to cause chemical changes. Chemical effects from using direct current usually occur only when the stimulus is continuous and is applied over a period of time. These chemical changes become measurable when the duration of the stimulus reaches the 1-minute mark, but the effect is cumulative over the total treatment time. This type of current is available in most low-voltage equipment. The duration of the current in

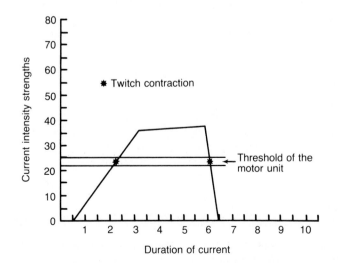

Fig. 5-13 Direct current influence on a motor unit.

most high-voltage stimulators is nonadjustable and is too short to create any chemical effect, unless treatment times in excess of 1 hour are used.[72,95]

Tissue Impedance

Impedance is the resistance of the tissue to the passage of electrical current. Bone and fat are high-impedance tissues; nerve and muscle are low-impedance tissues. If a low-impedance tissue is located under a large amount of high-impedance tissue, the current will never become high enough to cause a depolarization.[9,95]

Current Density

The **current density** (amount of current flow per cubic volume) at the nerve or muscle must be high enough to cause depolarization. The current density is highest where the electrodes meet the skin and diminishes as the electricity penetrates into the deeper tissues (Fig. 5-14).[9,95] If there is a large fat layer between the electrodes and the nerve, the electrical energy may not have a high enough density to cause depolarization (Figure 5-15).

If the electrodes are spaced closely together, the area of highest current density is relatively superficial (Figure 5-16, *A*). If the electrodes are spaced farther apart, the current density will be higher in the deeper tissues, including nerve and muscle (Figure 5-16, *B*).

Electrode size will also change current density. As the size of one electrode relative to another is decreased, the current density beneath the smaller electrode is

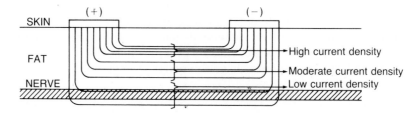

Fig. 5-14 Current density using equal size electrodes spaced close together.

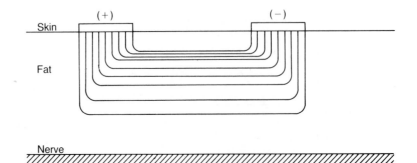

Fig. 5-15 Equal size electrodes spaced close together on body part with thick fat layers. Thus the electrical current does not reach the nerve.

increased. The larger the electrode, the larger the area over which the current is spread, decreasing the current density (Figure 5-17).[1,2,9,70,95]

Using a large **(dispersive) electrode** remote from the treatment area while placing a smaller **(active) electrode** as close as possible to the nerve or muscle motor point will give the greatest effect at the small electrode. The large electrode disperses the current over a large area; the small electrode concentrates the current in the area of the motor point (see Figure 5-17).

Electrode size and placement are key elements that the sports therapist controls that will influence results. High current density close to the neural structure you want to stimulate makes it more certain that you will be successful with the least amount of current. Electrode placement is probably one of the biggest causes of poor results from electrical therapy.[43]

Frequency

The amount of shortening of the muscle fiber and the amount of recovery allowed the muscle fiber is a function of the frequency. The mechanical shortening of the single muscle fiber response can be influenced by stimulating again as soon as the tissue membrane repolarizes. Only the membrane has the absolute refractory period; the contractile mechanism operates on a different timing sequence and is just beginning to contract. When the second stimulus is received by the muscle membrane, the myofilaments are already overlapping and the second stimulus causes an increased mechanical shortening of the muscle fiber. This process of superimposing one twitch

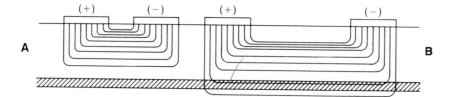

Fig. 5-16 A, Electrodes are very close together, producing a high-density current in the superficial tissues. **B,** Increasing the distance between the electrodes increases the current density in the deeper tissues.

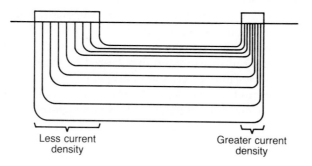

Fig. 5-17 Excitation time of nerve cell membrane.

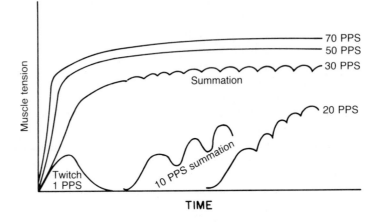

Fig. 5-18 Summation of contractions and tetanization.

contraction on another is called **summation of contractions.** As the number of twitch contractions per second increases, single twitch responses cannot be distinguished and **tetanization** of the muscle fiber is reached (Figure 5-18). The tension developed by a muscle fiber in tetany is much greater than the tension from a twitch contraction. This muscle fiber tetany is strictly a function of the frequency of the stimulating current; it is not dependent on the intensity of the current.[9,70]

The primary difference between electrically induced muscle contraction and voluntary muscle contraction is the asynchrony of firing of motor units under voluntary control versus the synchronous firing of electrically stimulated motor units. Each time the electrical stimulus is applied, the same motor units respond. This may lead to greater fatigue in the electrically stimulated muscles. Normal firing in voluntary muscle contraction varies from one movement to the next because some motor units are contracting while others are inactive. Voluntary contractions do not lead to muscular fatigue as early in the exercise period as do electrical contractions. This synchrony of contraction may also be important in training the muscle to use more synchronous contractions to improve muscular strength.[9,70]

Intensity

Increasing the intensity of the electrical stimulus in Figure 5-19, *A* to that in Figure 5-19, *B* causes the current to reach deeper into the tissue. Depolarization of more fibers is accomplished by two methods: (1) higher threshold fibers within the range of the first stimulus are depolarized by the higher intensity stimulus; and (2) fibers with the same threshold but deeper in the structure are depolarized by the deeper spread of the current. High-voltage stimulators are capable of deeper penetration into the tissue than low-voltage stimulators and may be desirable when stimulating deep muscle tissue. This is one of the most significant differences between high-voltage and low-voltage generators.[2,70]

Duration

We also can stimulate more nerve fibers with the same intensity current by increasing the duration that an adequate stimulus is available to depolarize the membranes

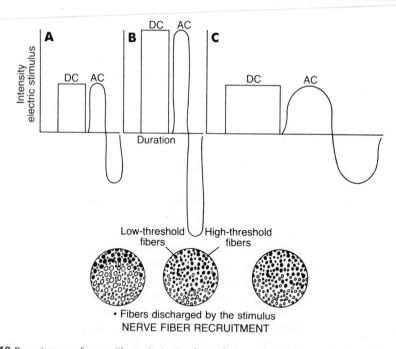

• Fibers discharged by the stimulus
NERVE FIBER RECRUITMENT

Fig. 5-19 Recruitment of nerve fibers. **A,** A stimulus pulse at a duration-intensity just above threshold will excite the closest and largest fibers. Each electrical pulse of the same intensity at the same location will cause the same fibers to contract. **B,** Increasing the intensity will excite smaller fibers and fibers farther away. **C,** Increasing the duration will also excite smaller fibers and fibers farther away.

(Figure 5-19, C). Greater numbers of nerve fibers would react to the same intensity stimulus because the current would be available for a longer period of time.[9,44,95] This method requires the use of a stimulator with an adjustable duration. The low-voltage stimulators usually are available with this parameter, whereas the high-voltage stimulators usually have a preset pulse duration.

Polarity

During the use of any stimulator, an electrode that has a greater level of electrons is called the negative electrode or the cathode. The other electrode in this system has a lower level of electrons and is called the positive electrode or the anode. The cathode attracts positive ions and the anode attracts negative ions and electrons. With AC waves, these electrodes change polarity with each current cycle.

With a direct current generator, the sports therapist can designate one electrode as the cathode and one as the anode and for the duration of the treatment the electrodes will provide that polar effect. The polar effect can be thought of in terms of three characteristics: (1) chemical effects, (2) ease of excitation, and (3) direction of current flow.*

---

*References 8, 9, 60, 70, 77, 95.

CHEMICAL EFFECTS. Changes in pH under each electrode, a reflex vasodilation, and the ability to drive oppositely charged ions through the skin into the tissue (iontophoresis) are all thought of as chemical effects. A tissue stimulating effect is ascribed to the cathode. To create these effects, longer pulse durations (greater than 1 minute) are required.[8,35,72,77] The **bacteriostatic** effect was achieved at either the anode or cathode with intensities in the 5 to 10 mA range. While at 1 mA or below, the greatest bacteriostatic effect was found at the cathode.[4,41] Another study using treatment times exceeding 30 minutes found some bacteriostatic effect of high-voltage pulsed currents.[51]

EASE OF EXCITATION OF EXCITABLE TISSUE. The polarity of the active electrode usually should be negative when the desired result is a muscle contraction because of the greater facility for membrane depolarization at the cathode. However, current density under the anode can be increased rapidly enough to create a depolarizing effect. Using the positive electrode as the active electrode is not as efficient, since it will require more current intensity to create an action potential. This may cause the patient to be less comfortable with the treatment. In treatment programs requiring muscle contraction or sensory nerve stimulation, patient comfort should dictate the choice of positive or negative polarity. Negative polarity is usually the most comfortable in this instance.[70,95]

DIRECTION OF CURRENT FLOW. In some treatment schemes, the direction of current flow is also considered important. Generally speaking, the cathode is positioned distally and the anode proximally. This arrangement tries to replicate the naturally occurring pattern of electrical flow in the body.[8,62]

The direction of current flow could also influence shifting of the water content of the tissues and movement of colloids (fluid suspension of the intracellular fluid). Neither of these phenomena is well documented or understood, and further study is needed before clinical treatments are designed around these concepts.[67,79,95]

True polar effects can be substantiated when they occur close to the electrodes through which the current is entering the tissue. In laboratory situations in physics and physical therapy, polar effects occur in very close proximity to the electrode. To cause these effects, the current must flow through a medium. If the tissue to be treated is centrally located between the two electrodes, results cannot be assigned to polar effects.[8,43] Clinically, polar effects are an important consideration in iontophoresis, stimulating motor points or peripheral nerves, and in the biostimulative effect on nonexcitatory cells.

Electrode Placement

When using any of the treatment protocols aimed at the electrical stimulation of sensory nerves for pain suppression, there are several guidelines that will help the sports therapist select the appropriate sites for electrode placement. Transcutaneous electrical nerve stimulation (TENS) uses similar-sized electrodes placed according to a pattern and moved in a trial-and-error pattern until pain is decreased. The following patterns may be used:

1. Electrodes may be placed on or around the painful area.

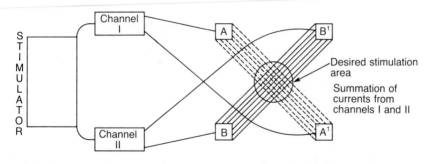

Fig. 5-20 Current flow would be from *A* to *A* and *B* to *B*. As the currents cross the area of stimulation, they summate in intensity.

2. Electrodes may be placed over specific dermatomes, myotomes, or sclerotomes that correspond to the painful area.

3. Electrodes may be placed close to the spinal cord segment that innervates an area that is painful.

4. Peripheral nerves that innervate the painful area may be stimulated by placing electrodes over sites where the nerve becomes superficial and can be stimulated easily.

5. Vascular structures contain neural tissue as well as ionic fluids that would transmit electrical stimulating currents and may be most easily stimulated by electrode placement over superficial vascular structures.

6. Electrode placement over trigger point locations.[93]

7. Both acupuncture and trigger points have been conveniently mapped out and illustrated. A reference on acupuncture and trigger areas is included in Appendix A. The sports therapist should systematically attempt to stimulate the points listed as successful for certain areas and types of pain. If they are effective, the patient will have decreased pain. These points also can be identified using an ohm meter–point locator to determine areas of decreased skin resistance.

8. Combinations of any of the above systems and bilateral electrode placement can also be successful.[53,54,60,100]

9. Crossing patterns, also referred to as an interferential technique, involve electrode application such that the electrical signals from each set of electrodes add together at some point in the body. The electrodes are usually arranged in a criss-cross pattern around the point to be stimulated (Figure 5-20).[89]

The sports therapist should not be limited to any one system but should evaluate electrode placement for each patient. The effectiveness of sensory stimulation is closely tied in with proper electrode placement. As in all trial-and-error treatment approaches, a systematic, organized search is always better than a shotgun, hit-and-miss approach. Numerous articles have identified some of the best locations for common pain problems, and these locations may be used as a starting point for the first approach.[53] If the treatment is not achieving the desired results, the electrode placement should be reconsidered.

THERAPEUTIC USES OF ELECTRICALLY INDUCED MUSCLE CONTRACTION

A variety of therapeutic gains can be made by electrically stimulating a muscle contraction:

1. Muscle reeducation
2. Muscle pump contractions
3. Retardation of atrophy
4. Muscle strengthening
5. Increasing range of motion

Any electrical stimulator—high voltage, low voltage, alternating current, **hybrid current,** or TENS—may be used to cause muscle contraction. The efficiency and effectiveness of treatment can be increased by following the protocols as closely as possible with the available equipment.

Muscle fatigue should be considered when deciding on treatment parameters. The variables that have an influence of muscle fatigue follow:

1. Force of contraction—combination of the pulse stimulus' amplitude intensity and the pulse duration
2. The number of pulses or bursts per second
3. On time
4. Off time

Muscle force is varied by changing the intensity to recruit more or less motor units. Muscle force can also be varied to a certain degree by increasing the summating quality of the contraction with high burst or pulse rates. The greater the force and the greater the demands on the muscle are, the greater the occulsion of muscle blood flow and the greater the fatigue will be. If high muscle forces are not required, the intensity and frequency can be adjusted to desired levels but fatigue can still be a factor. To minimize fatigue associated with forceful contractions, a combination of the lowest frequency and the highest intensity will keep the force constant and the most fatigue resistant.[11]

If high force levels are desired, then higher frequencies and intensities can be used. To keep the muscle fatigue as low as possible, the rest time between contractions should be at least 60 seconds for each 10 seconds of contraction time. A variable frequency train, in which a high frequency then low frequency stimulus are used, will also help minimize fatigue in repetitive functional electric stimulation.[11]

Neuromuscular induced contraction at the higher torques is associated with patient perceptions of pain, either from the current used or the intensity of the contraction. This is often a limiting factor in the success of any of the following protocols. Each patient needs supervision and good therapist-patient confidence for the most effective compliance with the treatment goals.[11,27,43]

When using electrical stimulation for muscle contraction, motor point stimulation can give the best individual muscle contraction. To find the motor point of a muscle, a probe electrode should be used to stimulate the muscle. Stimulation should be started in the approximate location of the desired motor point. (See Appendix A for motor point chart.) The intensity should be increased until contraction is visible, and the current intensity should be maintained at that level. The probe should be moved around until the best visible contraction for that current intensity is found; this is the motor point.[9,94] By choosing this location for stimulation, the current density can be increased in an area where numerous motor nerve fibers can be affected, maximizing the muscular response from the stimulation.

Muscle Reeducation

Muscular inhibition after surgery or injury is the primary indication for muscle reeducation. If the neuromuscular mechanisms of a muscle have not been damaged, then central nervous system inhibition of this muscle usually is a factor in loss of control. The atrophy of synaptic contacts that remain unused for long periods is theorized as a source of this sensorimotor alienation. The addition of electrical stimulation of the motor nerve provides an artificial use of the inactive synapses and helps restore a more normal balance to the system, since the ascending sensory information will be reintegrated into the patient's movement control patterns. A muscle contraction usually can be forced by electrically stimulating the muscle. Forcing the muscle to contract causes an increase in the sensory input from that muscle. The patient feels the muscle contract, sees the muscle contract, and can attempt to duplicate this muscular response.[9,25,31,69]

Protocols for muscle reeducation do not list specific parameters to make this treatment more efficient, but the following criteria are essential for effective electrical stimulation:

1. Current intensity must be adequate for muscle contraction but comfortable for the athlete.
2. Pulse duration must be set as close as possible to the duration needed for chronaxie of the tissue to be stimulated. This is preset on most therapeutic generators.
3. Pulses per second should be high enough to give a tetanic contraction (20 to 40 pulses per second).
4. Interrupted or surged current must be used.
5. On time should be 1 to 2 seconds.
6. Off time should be 4 to 10 seconds.
7. The patient should be instructed to allow just the electricity to make the muscle contract, letting the patient feel and see the response desired. Next, the patient should alternate voluntary muscle contractions with current-induced contractions.
8. Total treatment time should be about 15 minutes, but this can be repeated several times daily.
9. High-voltage pulsed or medium-frequency alternating current may be most effective (Figure 5-21).[9,25,31]

Muscle Pump Contractions

Electrically induced muscle contraction can be used to duplicate the regular muscle contractions that help stimulate circulation by pumping fluid and blood through venous and lymphatic channels back into the heart. A discussion of edema formation is included in Chapter 13. Using sensory level stimulation has also decreased edema in sprain and contusion injuries in animals.[79]

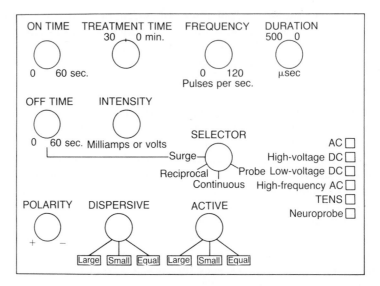

Fig. 5-21 Electrical stimulator control panel.

Electrical stimulation of muscle contractions in the affected extremity can help reestablish the proper circulatory pattern while keeping the injured part protected.

The following criteria must be satisfied for the electrical treatment to be successful in helping to reduce swelling:

1. Current intensity must be high enough to provide a strong, comfortable muscle contraction.
2. Pulse duration is preset on most of the therapeutic generators. If adjustable, it should be set as close as possible to the duration needed for chronaxie of the motor nerve to be stimulated.
3. Pulses per second should be in the beginnings of tetany range (20 pulses per second).
4. Interrupted or surged current must be used.
5. On time should be 5 to 10 seconds.
6. Off time should be 5 to 10 seconds.
7. The part to be treated should be elevated.
8. The patient should be instructed to allow the electricity to make the muscles contract. Active range of motion may be encouraged at the same time if it is not contraindicated.
9. Total treatment time should be between 20 and 30 minutes; treatment should be repeated two to five times daily.
10. High-voltage pulsed or medium-frequency alternating current may be most effective[25,31,73,76,88] (see Figure 5-21).
11. Use this protocol in addition to the normal ICE for best effect.[33,67]

Retardation of Atrophy

Prevention or retardation of atrophy has traditionally been a reason for treating patients with electrically stimulated muscle contraction. The maintenance of muscle tissue after an injury that prevents normal muscular exercise can be accomplished by substituting an electrically stimulated muscle contraction. The electrical stimulation reproduces the physical and chemical events associated with normal voluntary muscle contraction and helps to maintain normal muscle function.

Again, no specific protocols exist. In designing a program, the practitioner should try to duplicate muscle contractions associated with normal exercise routines. The following criteria can be used as guidelines in developing effective treatment protocols:

1. Current intensity should be as high as can be tolerated by the patient. This can be increased during the treatment since some sensory accommodation takes place. The contraction should be capable of moving the limb through the antigravity range or of achieving 25% or more of the normal **maximum voluntary isometric contraction (MVIC)** torque for the muscle. The higher torque readings seem to have the best results.

2. Pulse duration is preset on most of the therapeutic generators. If it is adjustable, it should be set as close as possible to the duration needed for chronaxie of the motor nerve to be stimulated.

3. Pulses per second should be well into the tetany range (65 to 85 pulses per second).

4. Interrupted or surge type current should be used.

5. On time should be between 6 and 15 seconds.

6. Off time should be at least 1 minute or preferably 2 minutes.

7. The muscle should be given some resistance, either gravity or external resistance provided by the addition of weights or by fixing the joint so that the contraction becomes isometric.

8. The athlete can be instructed to work with the electrically induced contraction, but voluntary effort is not necessary for the success of this treatment.

9. Total treatment time should be 15 to 20 minutes or enough time to allow a minimum of 10 contractions; some protocols have been successful with 3 sets of 10 contractions. The treatment can be repeated twice daily. Some protocols using battery powered rather than line powered units have advocated longer bouts with more repetitions probably because of low contraction force.

10. A medium-frequency alternating current stimulator is the machine of choice (see Figure 5-21).*

Muscle Strengthening

Muscle strengthening from electrical muscle stimulation has been used with some good results in patients with weakness or denervation of a muscle group. The protocol is better established for this use, but more research is needed to clarify the procedures and allow us to generalize the results to other electrical stimulators. The following summarizes the protocols used successfully:

1. Current intensity should be high enough to make the muscle develop 60% of the torque developed in an MVIC.

---

*References 11, 25, 26, 27, 31, 69, 81, 83, 84.

2. Pulse duration is preset on most therapeutic generators. If adjustable, it should be set as close as possible to the duration needed for chronaxie of the motor nerve to be stimulated. In general, longer pulse durations should include more nerves in response.

3. Pulses per second should be near the top of the tolerable range (approximately 65 to 85 pulses per second).

4. Surged or interrupted current with a gradual ramp to peak intensity is most effective.

5. On time should be in the 10 to 15 second range.

6. Off time should be in the 50 seconds to 2 minute range.

7. Resistance usually is applied by immobilizing the limb. The muscle is then given an isometric contraction torque equal to or greater than 25% of the MVIC torque. The greater the percentage of torque produced, the better the results.

8. The patient can be instructed to work with the electrically induced contraction, but voluntary effort is not necessary for the success of the treatment.

9. Total treatment time should include a minimum of 10 contractions, but mimicking normal active resistive training protocols of 3 sets of 10 contractions can also be productive. Fatigue is a major factor in this set-up. Electrical stimulation bouts should be scheduled at least three times weekly. Generally, strength gains will continue over the treatment course, but intensities may need to increase to keep pace with the most current maximum voluntary contraction torques.

10. A medium-frequency alternating current stimulator is the machine of choice (see Figure 5-21).*

Increasing Range of Motion

Increasing the range of motion in contracted joints is also a possible and documented use of electrical muscle stimulation. Electrically stimulating a muscle contraction pulls the joint through the limited range. The continued contraction of this muscle group over an extended time appears to make the contracted joint and muscle tissue modify and lengthen. Reduction of contractures in patients with hemiplegia has been reported, although no studies have reported this type of use in contracted joints from athletic injuries or surgery. The protocol needed to affect joint contracture is the following:

1. Current intensity must be of sufficient intensity and duration to make a muscle contract strongly enough to move the body part through its antigravity range. Intensity should be increased gradually during treatment.

2. Pulse duration is preset on most of the therapeutic generators. If it is adjustable, it should be set as close as possible to the duration needed for chronaxie of the motor nerve to be stimulated.

3. Pulses per second should be at the beginning of the tetany range (20 to 30 pulses per second).

4. Interrupted or surged current should be used.

*References 11, 25, 26, 27, 69, 81, 83, 84.

5. On time should be between 15 and 20 seconds.

6. Off time should be equal to or greater than on time; fatigue is a big consideration.

7. The stimulated muscle group should be antagonistic to the joint contracture, and the patient should be positioned so that the joint will be moved to the limits of the available range.

8. The patient is passive in this treatment and does not work with the electrical contraction.

9. Total treatment time should be 90 minutes daily. This can be broken into three 30-minute treatments.

10. High-voltage pulsed or medium-frequency alternating current stimulators are the best choices (see Figure 5-21).

The Effect of Noncontractile Stimulation on Edema

Ion movement within biologic tissues is a basic theory in the electrotherapy literature. This is clearly seen in the action potential model of nerve cell depolarization. The effects of sensory level stimulation on edema have been theorized to work on this principle. Research has not documented the effectiveness of this type of treatment, and sports therapists should continue to use other more proven mechanisms to decrease edema. See Chapter 13 for a discussion of edema formation.

Since 1987, numerous studies using rat and frog models have helped to more clearly define the effects of electrical stimulation on edema formation and reduction. The muscle pumping theory has seemed the most viable way to affect this problem. Most of the recent studies have focused on a sensory level stimulation. Early theory supported the use of sensory level direct current as a driving force to make the charged plasma protein ions in the interstitial spaces move in the direction of the oppositely charged electrode. This theory has not been totally refuted, but it has not been supported by the recent research. If this theory does have any basis, an effective treatment would require the following:

1. Extended treatment times

2. Direct current stimulation with polarity arranged in correct fashion

3. Electrodes arranged to pull or push plasma proteins into the lymphatic system and be moved back into the circulatory system via the thoracic duct

Another proposed mechanism is that a μA stimulation of the local neurovascular components in an injured area may cause a vasoconstriction and reduce the permeability of the capillary walls to limit the migration of plasma proteins into the interstitial spaces. This would retard the accumulation of plasma proteins and the associated fluid dynamics of the edema exudate. In a study on the histamine stimulated leakage of plasma proteins, animals treated with small doses of electrical current produced less leakage. The underlying mechanisms were a reduced pore size in the capillary walls and reduced pooling of blood in the capillaries that could have been initiated by hormonal, neural, mechanical, or electrochemical factors.[79]

Theory on exact mechanisms of action is cloudy, but the research has given us a viable model to use in trying to stimulate and achieve the same edema control mechanisms clinically as have been proven in the laboratory. The following is an edema control sensory stimulation protocol:

1. Current intensity should be 30 to 50 V or 10% less than needed to produce a visible muscle contraction.
2. Preset short duration currents on the high voltage equipment are effective.
3. High pulse frequencies (120 pps) are most effective.
4. Interrupted direct currents are most effective. Biphasic currents showed increases in volume.
5. The animals treated with a negative distal electrode had a significant treatment effect. The animals with a positive distal electrode showed no change.
6. Time of treatment after injury—the best results were reported when treatment began immediately after injury. Treatment started after 24 hours showed an effect on the accumulation of new edema volume but showed no effect on the existing edema volume.
7. A 30 minute treatment showed good control of volume for 4 to 5 hours.
8. The water immersion electrode technique was effective, but using surface electrodes was not effective.
9. High voltage pulsed generators were effective, but low voltage generators were not effective.*

THERAPEUTIC USES OF ELECTRICAL STIMULATION OF SENSORY NERVES

Clinically, efforts are made to stimulate the sensory nerves to change the patient's perception of a painful stimulus coming from an injured area. To understand how to maximally affect the perception of pain through electrical stimulation, it is necessary to understand pain perception. The gate control theory, the **central biasing** theory, and the opiate pain control theory are the theoretical bases for pain reduction phenomena. These theories are covered in depth in Chapter 3.

Gate Control Theory

Electrically stimulating the large sensory fibers when there is pain in a certain area will force the central nervous system to make the brain's recognition area aware of the electrical stimuli. As long as the stimuli are applied, the perception of pain is diminished. Electrical stimulation of sensory nerves will evoke the gate control mechanism and diminish awareness of painful stimuli. As long as the stimulation is causing firing of the sensory nerves, the gate to pain should be closed. If accommodation to the electrical stimulus occurs or if the stimulus stops, the gate is then open and pain is perceived.†

The physical dominance, enkephalin release model is used in treating pain from acute injuries, problems with the musculoskeletal system, or postoperative pain. The following criteria can be used as guidelines in developing effective treatment protocols:

1. Current intensity should be adjusted to tolerance but should not cause a muscular contraction; the higher the better.
2. Pulse duration (pulse width) should be 75 to 150 μsec or maximum possible on the machine.
3. Pulses per second should be 80 to 125 or as high as possible on the machine.

*References 2, 10, 14, 24, 32, 33, 39, 49, 50, 51, 56, 65, 66, 67, 68, 91, 92.
†References 12, 13, 53, 54, 55, 62, 63, 80, 81, 84, 95.

4. A transcutaneous electrical stimulator waveform should be used.

5. On time should be continuous mode.

6. Total treatment time should correspond to fluctuations in pain; the unit should be left on until pain is no longer perceived, turned off, then restarted when pain begins again.

7. If this treatment is successful, the patient will have some pain relief within the first 30 minutes of treatment.

8. If it is not successful but you feel this is the best theoretical or most clinically applicable approach, change the electrode placements and try again. If this is not successful, then using a different theoretical approach may offer more help.

9. Any stimulator that can deliver this current is acceptable. Portable units are better for 24-hour pain control[53,54,59] (see Figure 5-21).

Central Biasing Theory

Intense electrical stimulation of the smaller fibers (C fibers or pain fibers) at peripheral sites (trigger and acupoint) for short time periods causes stimulation of descending neurons, which then affects transmission of pain information by closing the gate at the spinal cord level[16] (see Figure 3-5).

The central biasing set-up is used on sharp chronic pain or severe pathologic pain. Changing the bias of the central nervous system and increasing the descending influences on the transmission of pain are best accomplished with the following protocols:

1. Current intensity should be very high, approaching a noxious level; muscular contraction is not desirable.

2. Pulse duration should be 10 msec.

3. Pulses per second should be 80.

4. On time should be 30 seconds to 1 minute.

5. Stimulation should be applied over trigger or acupuncture points.

6. Selection and number of points used varies according to the part treated.

7. A low-frequency, high-intensity generator is the stimulator of choice for central biasing[16] (see Figure 5-21).

8. If this treatment is successful, pain will be relieved shortly after the treatment.

9. If this treatment is not successful, try different electrode set-ups by expanding the treatment points used.

Opiate Pain Control Theory

Electrical stimulation of sensory nerves may stimulate the release of enkephaline from local sites throughout the central nervous system and the release of β-endorphin from the pituitary gland into the cerebral spinal fluid. The mechanism that causes the release and then the binding of enkephalin and β-endorphin to some nerve cells is still unclear. It is certain that a diminution or elimination of pain perception is caused by applying an electrical current to areas close to the site of pain or to acupuncture or trigger points, both local and distant to the pain area.*

---

*References 16, 22, 58, 63, 64, 81, 86, 99.

To use the influence of hyperstimulation analgesia and B-endorphin release, a point stimulation set-up must be used. A large dispersive pad and a small pad or handheld probe point electrode are used in this approach. The point electrode is applied to the chosen site, and the intensity is increased until it is perceived by the patient. The probe is then moved around the area, and the patient is asked to report relative changes in perception of intensity. When a location of maximum-intensity perception is found, the current intensity is increased to maximum tolerable levels. This is much the same as finding a motor point, as described earlier.[16,74]

β-endorphin stimulation may offer better relief for the deep aching or chronic pain similar to that perceived in overuse injury. β-endorphin production may be stimulated using the following protocols:

1. Current intensity should be high, approaching a noxious level; muscular contraction is acceptable.
2. Pulse duration should be 200 μsec to 10 msec.
3. Pulses per second should be between 1 and 5.
4. High-voltage pulsed current should be used.
5. On time should be 30 to 45 seconds.
6. Stimulation should be applied over trigger or acupuncture points.
7. Selection and number of points used vary according to the part and condition being treated.
8. A high-voltage pulsed current or a low-frequency, high-intensity machine is best for this effect[16,63,64] (see Figure 5-21).
9. If stimulation is successful, you should know at the completion of the treatment. The analgesic effect should last for 6 to 7 hours.
10. If not successful, try expanding the number of stimulation sites. Add the same stimulation points on the opposite side of the body, add auricular acupuncture points, or add more points on the same limb.

A combination of intense point stimulation and TENS may be used. The TENS applications should be used as much as needed to make the patient comfortable, and the intense point stimulation should be used on a periodic basis. Periodic use of intense point stimulation gives maximal pain relief for a period of time and allows some gains in overal pain suppression. Daily intense point stimulation may eventually bias the central nervous system and decrease the effectiveness of this type of stimulation.[43]

Placebo Effect Of Electrical Stimulation

All three of these theories of sensory electrical stimulation produce their effects on the transmission lines of pain by interrupting or slowing the flow of pain information to the brain. The brain is the reception and interpretation center for these pain messages, and incorporating this area into treatment can enhance the treatment's effects. This is crucial to a successful treatment because the sports therapist is trying to alter the athlete's pain perception. This perceptual change is influenced by many factors at the cognitive and affective levels.

There is a big placebo effect in all that sports therapists do in providing any therapy to athletes. This placebo effect is a basic and extremely important tool to help achieve the best results. The attitude toward athletes and presentation of the therapy to them are crucial. When the sports therapist demonstrates a sincere interest in the athlete's problems, the athlete uses that interest to add to his or her own conviction and motivation to get well.

When these factors are active, real physiologic changes occur that assist in the healing process. The sports therapist should not intentionally deceive the athlete with a sham treatment but should use the treatment to have the best impact on the athlete's perception of the problem and the effectiveness of the treatment.

The treatment will work better if patients have a profound belief in their treatment's ability to change their problem. To gain the most from this effect, patients need to be intimately involved with their treatment. We must educate, encourage, and empower athletes to get better. Giving athletes the knowledge and ability to feel some control and to be self-determined in healing reduces the stress of injury and enhances the recover powers of athletes. In stressful situations, any measure of control lessens the extent of the stress and results in the improvement of disease resistance or injury recovery factors that will improve treatment outcomes.[43]

CLINICAL USES OF LOW-VOLTAGE CONTINUOUS DIRECT CURRENT
Medical Galvanism

The application of continuous low-voltage direct current causes several physiologic changes that can be used therapeutically. The therapeutic benefits are related to the polar and vasomotor effects and to the acidic reaction around the anode and the alkaline reaction at the cathode. The sports therapist must be concerned with the damaging effects of this variety of current. Acidic or alkaline changes can cause severe skin reactions.[95] These reactions occur only with low-voltage continuous direct current and are not likely with the high-voltage pulsed generators. The pulse duration of the high voltage pulsed generators is too short to cause these chemical changes.[72]

There is also a vasomotor effect on the skin, increasing blood flow between the electrodes. The benefits from this type of direct current are usually attributed to the increased blood flow through the treatment area.[95]

The following protocols for continuous low-voltage direct current can be used to give the greatest vasomotor effects:

1. Current intensity should be to the patient's tolerance; it should be increased as accommodation takes place. These intensities are in the mA range.
2. Continuous direct current should be used.
3. Pulses per second should be 0.
4. A low-voltage direct current stimulator is the machine of choice.
5. Treatment time should be between a 15-minute minimum and a 50-minute maximum.
6. Equal-sized electrodes are used over gauze that has been soaked in saline solution and lightly squeezed.
7. Skin should be unbroken[48,70,74] (see Figure 5-21).

Iontophoresis

Direct current has been used for many years to drive ions from the heavy metals into and through the skin to treat skin infections or for a counterirritating effect. Iontophoresis is discussed in detail in Chapter 6.

Contraindications to Continuous Direct Currents

Skin burns are the greatest hazard of any continuous direct current technique. These burns result from excessive density in any area, usually from direct metal contact with skin or from setting the intensity too high for the size of the active electrode. Both these problems cause a very high density of current in the area of contact.[70,74]

SPECIALIZED ELECTRICAL CURRENTS
Low Intensity Stimulators

Another type of low-voltage equipment is the low intensity stimulator (LIS). The characteristic that distinguishes this type of generator is that the intensity of the stimulus is limited to 1000 μA or less in LIS, while the intensity of the standard low voltage equipment can be increased into the mA range.

Generators that produce LIS are among the newer electrical therapy units available to today's sports therapist. These units were originally called microcurrent electrical neuromuscular stimulators (MENS). However the stimulation pathway is not the usual neural pathway, and they are not designed to stimulate a muscle contraction. Consequently, this type of generator was subsequently referred to as a microcurrent electrical stimulator (MES). LIS is the most recent and currently used term in an ongoing evolution of terminology relative to this type of stimulator.[3]

Perhaps the most important point to emphasize is that currents generated by these devices are not substantially different from the currents discussed previously. These currents still have a direction, and both AC and DC waveforms are available. The currents also have amplitude (intensity), pulse duration, and frequency.

LIS currents are defined as those currents of less than 1 mA or 1000 μA. The generators can produce a variety of waveforms from modified monophasic to biphasic square waves with frequencies from .3 to 50 Hz. The pulse durations are also variable and may be prolonged at the lower frequencies from 1 to 500 msec. This varies as the frequency changes or is preset when pulsed currents are used. Many of these devices are made with an impedance sensitive voltage that adapts the current to the impedance to keep the current constant as selected.[76]

If the current generator can be adjusted to allow increases of intensity above 1000 μA the current becomes like those previously described in this text. If the current provokes an action potential in a sensory or motor nerve, the results on that tissue will be the same as previously described for other currents' sensation or muscle contraction.

Most of the literature on microcurrents and subsequently on LIS has been generated by researchers interested in stimulating the healing process in fractures and skin wounds. Subsequent research is aimed at identifying why and how microcurrents work. The best-researched areas of application of LIS type currents is in the stimulation of bone formation in delayed union or nonunion of fractures of the long bones. Most of this research was done using implanted rather than surface electrodes, and most have used low intensity direct current with the cathode placed at the fracture site.[2,7,26] We are in danger of generalizing treatments for all problems based on success in this one area. These applications were intended to mimic the normal electrical field created during the injury and healing process.[2,32] At present these electrical changes are poorly understood, and the effects of adding additional electric current to the normal electrical activity created by the injury and healing process are still being investigated.

As can be seen in the previous sections on the bioelectric properties of cells and tissues, there are several possible theories that might explain the biostimulative effects of LIS currents and give the sports therapist some guidance in developing clinical protocols.

The current of injury, stress generated potentials, cell metabolism stimulation, and bioelectric fields guiding growth are all natural events that LIS may augment, stimulate, or artifically replace.[17,18]

LIS has been used for two major effects:
1. Analgesia of the painful area
2. Biostimulation of the healing process either for enhancing the process or for acceleration of its stages

ANALGESIC EFFECTS OF LIS. The mechanism of analgesia created by LIS current does not fit into our present theoretical framework since sensory nerve excitation is a necessary component of all three models of electroanalgesia stimulation. At best, LIS can create or change the constant direct current flow of the neural tissues that may have some way of biasing the transmission of the painful stimulus. LIS may also make the nerve cell membrane more receptive to neurotransmitters that will block transmission. The exact mechanism has not yet been established. The research is also equivocal on the effectiveness of LIS in decreasing pain. This lack of consensus and disagreement in the research gives the sports therapist limited security in devising an effective protocol. Most of the research using delayed onset muscle soreness as a pain model has found no significant difference between LIS and placebo treatments.*

PROMOTION OF WOUND HEALING. Low intensity direct current has been used to treat skin ulcers that have poor blood flow. The treated ulcers show accelerated healing rates when compared with untreated skin ulcers.

The following protocol was used to promote wound healing:
1. Current intensity was 200 to 400 μamp for normal skin and 400 to 800 μamp for denervated skin.
2. Long pulse durations or continuous uninterrupted currents can be used.
3. Maximum pulse frequency.
4. Monophasic direct current is best, but biphasic direct current is acceptable. LIS can be used, but other generators with intensities adjusted to sub-sensory levels can also be effective. A battery powered portable unit is most convenient.
5. Treatment time was 2 hours followed by a 4-hour rest time.
6. 2 to 3 treatment bouts per day.
7. The negative electrode is positioned in the wound area for the first 3 days. The positive electrode should be positioned 25 cm proximal to the wound.
8. After 3 days, the polarity is reversed and the positive electrode is positioned in the wound area.

*References 14, 30, 37, 47, 52, 61, 78, 80, 96, 98, 103.

9. If infection is present, the negative electrode should be left in the wound area until the signs of infection are no longer evident. The negative electrode remains in the wound for 3 days after the infection clears.

10. If the wound size decrease plateaus, then return the negative electrode to the wound area for 3 days.

Other protocols have been successful using the anode in the wound area for the entire time. High-volt stimulation has also been used in a manner similar to the negative-positive model presented. The intensity was adjusted to give a μA current. High-volt has been used in a manner similar to the negative-positive model presented. The intensity was adjusted to give a μA current.

In two separate studies, laboratory animals with sutured and circular skin wounds were treated with LIS, following a manufacturers recommended protocol. The current was a monophasic rectangular waveform with a current intensity of 100 μA at 3 Hz, on a 50% duty cycle. This current was applied for 2 hours per day in Leffmann's et al.[56a] study and for 1 hour per day in a study by Byl et al.[14a] Both studies reported no significant effects from this treatment protocol.

The mechanism by which LIS stimulates healing is elusive, but cells are simulated to increase their normal proliferation, migration, motility, DNA synthesis, and collagen synthesis. Receptor levels for growth factor have also shown a significant increase when wound areas are stimulated.* The naturally occurring electrical potential gradients are enhanced after electrical stimulation.[37]

PROMOTION OF FRACTURE HEALING. The use of low intensity direct current may be an adjunctive modality in the treatment of fractures, especially fractures prone to nonunion. Fracture healing may be accelerated by passing a direct current through the fracture site. Getting the current into the bony area without an invasive technique is difficult.†

Using a standard TENS unit, Kahn reported favorable results in the electrical stimulation of callus formation in fractures that had nonunions after 6 months. This information is based on a case study. Results of a more extensive population of nonunions have not been documented. Kahn used the following protocol:

1. Current intensity was just perceptible to the patient.
2. Pulse duration was the longest duration allowed on the unit (100 to 200 msec).
3. Pulses per second were set at the lowest frequency allowed on the unit (5 to 10 pps).
4. Standard monophasic or biphasic current in the TENS units were used.
5. Treatment time was from 30 minutes to 1 hour, three to four times daily.
6. A negative electrode was placed close but distal to the fracture site. A positive electrode was placed proximal to the immobilizing device.
7. If four pads were used, the interferential placement described earlier was used.
8. Results were reassessed at monthly intervals.[48]

PROMOTION OF HEALING IN TENDON AND LIGAMENT. There are only a few research studies on the biostimulative effect of electrical stimulation on tendon or ligament

---

*References 15, 19, 20, 35, 36, 40, 45, 57, 69, 94, 97, 102.
†References 8, 13, 16, 17, 23, 26, 46, 75, 90.

healing. Both tissues have produced strain generated electric potentials naturally in response to stress. These potentials help signal the tissue to grow in response to the stress, according to Wolff's law.

In an experimental study on partial division of dog patellar tendons treated with 20 μA cathodal stimulation, the stimulated tendons showed 92% recovery of normal breaking strength at 8 weeks.[87]

Tendon stimulated in vitro in a culture medium showed increased fibroblastic cellular activity, tendon cellular proliferation, and collagen synthesis. The rate at which stimulated tendons demonstrated histologic repair at the injury site was also significantly accelerated over the control group.[71]

LIS currents can be a valuable addition to the clinical armamentarium of the sports therapist, but they are untested clinically.

For electricity to produce these effects:

1. Cells must be current sensitive
2. Correct polarity orientation may be necessary
3. Correct amounts of current will cause the cells to be more active in the healing process

If results are not going correctly, then change the current intensity or change polarity. Weak stimuli may increase physiologic activity, while much stronger stimuli abolish or inhibit activity.

Weak stimuli may increase physiologic activity, while much stronger stimuli abolish or inhibit activity. Remember the current in LIS is already in the μA range. Current in the middle of the μA range (200-600 μA) seems to have the best effect.

Most generators in use today are capable of producing low intensity current. Simply turn the machine on, but do not increase the intensity to threshold levels. This can also be a function of current density using electrode size and placement as well as intensity to keep current in the μA range.

The sports therapist is certainly entitled to be very skeptical of the manufacturers' claims until more research is reported. Existing protocols for use are not well established, leaving the sports therapist with an insecure feeling about this modality.

Medium Frequency Current Generators

This class of current generators was developed in Canada and the United States after the Russian scientist Yadou M. Kots presented a seminar on the use of electrical muscular stimulators to augment strength gain. The stimulators developed after this presentation were termed **Russian current** generators. These stimulators have evolved and presently deliver a medium (2000 to 10,000 Hz) frequency polyphasic AC waveform. The pulse can be varied from 50 to 250 μsec; the phase duration will be one half of the pulse duration or 25 to 125 μsec. As the pulse frequency increases, the pulse duration decreases.[18,32,38] There are two basic waveforms: a sine wave and a square wave cycle with a fixed intrapulse interval.

The sine wave is produced in a burst mode that has a 50% duty cycle. According to strength duration curve data, to obtain the same stimulation effect as the duration of the stimulus decreases, the intensity must be increased. The intensity associated with this duration of current could be considered painful.

To make this intensity tolerable, current is generated in 50-burst-per-second envelopes with an interburst interval of 10 msec. This slightly reduces the total current

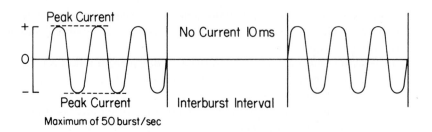

Fig. 5-22 Russian current with polyphasic AC wave form and 10 MS interburst interval.

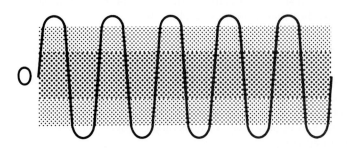

Fig. 5-23 Russian current (without an interburst interval). The light shaded area is equal to the total current.

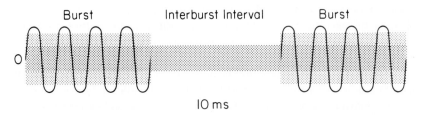

Fig. 5-24 Russian current (with an interburst interval). Dark shaded area represents total current, and light shading indicates total current without the interburst interval.

but allows enough of a peak current intensity to stimulate muscle very well (Figure 5-22). If the current continued without the burst effect, the total current delivered would equal the lightly shaded area in Figure 5-23. When generated with the burst effect, the total current is decreased. Here the total current would equal the darkly shaded area in Figure 5-24. This allows tolerance of greater current intensity by the patient. The other factor affecting patient comfort is the effect that frequency will have on the impedance of the tissue. Higher frequency currents reduce the resistance to the current flow again making this type of wave form comfortable enough that the patient may tolerate higher intensities. As the intensity increases, more motor nerves are stimulated, increasing the magnitude of the contraction. Because it is a fast oscillating alternating current, as soon as the nerve repolarizes it is stimulated again, producing a current that will maximally summate muscle contraction.

The frequency (pulses per second or, in this case, bursts per second) is also a

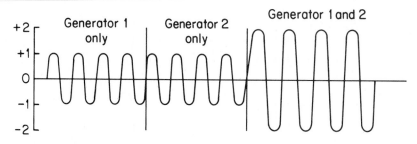

Fig. 5-25 Sine wave from generator 1 and sine wave from generator 2 showing a constructive interference pattern.

variable that can be controlled. This would make the muscle respond with a twitch rather than a gradually increasing mechanical contraction. Gradually increasing the numbers of bursts interrupts the mechanical relaxation cycle of the muscle and causes more shortening to take place[70] (see Figure 5-18).

Interferential Currents

The research and use of interferential currents (IFC) has taken place primarily in Europe. An Austrian scientist, Ho Nemec, introduced the concept and suggested its therapeutic use. Nemec's concept resulted in the creation of a type of electrical generator that is difficult to understand, not because the theory is so complex but because electrical engineers added so many options to the generator that the current can be modified substantially while still maintaining its basic waveform.

The theories and behavior of electrical waves are part of basic physics. This behavior is easiest to understand when continuous sine waves are used as an example.

With only one circuit the current behaves as described earlier; if put on an oscilloscope, it looks like generator 1 in Figure 5-25. If a second generator is brought into the same location, the currents may interfere with each other. This interference can be summative — that is, the amplitudes of the electric wave are combined and increase (see Figure 5-25). Both waves are exactly the same; if they are produced in phase or originate at the same time, they combine. This is called **constructive interference.**

If these waves are generated out of sync Generator 1 starts in a positive direction at the same time that generator 2 starts in a negative direction; the waves then will cancel each other out. This is called **destructive interference;** in the summation the waves end up with an amplitude of 0. (Figure 5-26).

To make this a bit more complex, assume that one generator has a slightly slower or faster frequency and that the generators begin producing current simultaneously. Initially, the electric waves will be constructively summated; however, because the frequencies of the two waves differ, they gradually will get out of phase and become destructively summated. When dealing with sound waves, we hear distinct beats as this phenomenon occurs. We borrow the term **beat** when describing this behavior. When any waveforms are out of phase but are combined in the same location, the waves will cause a beat effect. The blending of the waves is caused by the constructive and destructive interference patterns of the waves and is called **heterodyne** (Figure 5-27).[32,34]

The heterodyne effect is seen on an oscilloscope as a cyclic, rising and falling

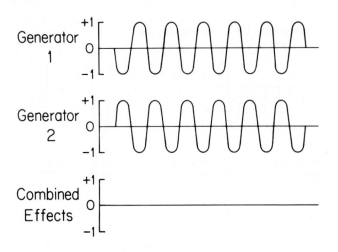

Fig. 5-26 Sine wave from generator 1 and sine wave from generator 2 showing destructive interference pattern.

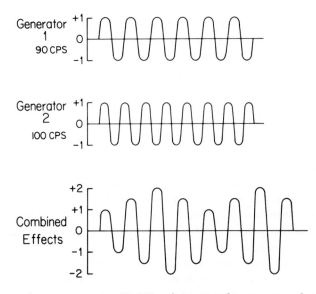

Fig. 5-27 Sine wave from generator 1 at 90 CPS and sine wave from generator 2 at 100 CPS showing the heterodyne, or beating behavior, of wave interference.

waveform. The peaks or beat frequency in this heterodyne wave behavior occur regularly, according to the difference of each current; for example, 100 pps - 90 pps = 10 pps beat frequency. In electric currents, this beat frequency is, in effect, the stimulation frequency of the waveform, because the destructive interference negates the effects of the other part of the wave. The intensity (amplitude) will be set according to sensations created by this peak.[32] When using an interference current for therapy, the sports therapist should select the frequencies to create a beat frequency corresponding to his or her choices of frequency when using other stimulators 20 to

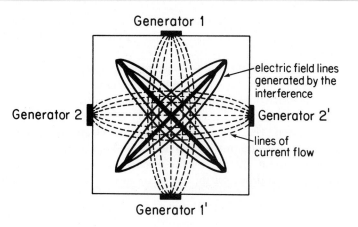

Fig. 5-28 Square electrode alignment and interference pattern of current in a homogeneous medium.

50 pps for muscle contraction, 50 to 120 pps for pain management, or 1 pps for pain relief from stimulation of acupunture points.

When the electrodes are arranged in a square alignment and interferential currents are passed through a homogeneous medium, a predictable pattern of interference will occur. In this pattern, an electric field is created that resembles a four-petaled flower, with the center of the flower located where the two currents cross and the petals falling between the electric current force lines. The maximum interference effect takes place near the center, with the field gradually decreasing in strength as it moves toward the points of the petal (Figure 5-28).[32]

Because the body is not a homogeneous medium, we cannot predict the exact location of this interference pattern; we must rely on the patient's perception. If the patient has a localized structure that is painful, locating the stimulation in the correct location is relatively easy. The therapist moves the electrode placement until the patient centers the feeling of the stimulus in the problem area.[32,34] When a patient has poorly localized pain, the task becomes more difficult. The engineers added features to the generators and created a scanning interferential current that moves the flower petals of force around while the treatment is taking place. This enlarges the effective treatment area. Additional technology and another set of electrodes create a three-dimensional flower effect when one looks at the electrical field. This is called a **stereodynamic** interference current.[32,34]

All these alterations and modifications are designed to spread the heterodyne effect throughout the tissue. Because it is controlled by a cyclic electrical pattern, however, the sports therapist may actually be decreasing the current passed through the structures he or she is trying to treat. The machines seem complex but lack the versatility to do much more than the conventional TENS treatment.[70,86]

Nikolova[73] has used IFC for a variety of clinical problems and found them effective in dealing with pain problems, (e.g., joint sprains with swelling, restricted mobility and pain; neuritis; retarded callus formation after fractures; and pseudarthrosis). These claims are supported by other researchers. Each of these researchers used slightly different protocols in treating the different clinical problems. To be successful in achieving the desired results with interferential currents, the sports therapist must thoroughly review existing protocols and acquire a good working knowledge of the application techniques.

The world of electrical therapy is constantly changing due to the advances in research, engineering, and technology and the competitive pressures of the marketplace. Equipment manufacturers will develop a different machine and try to market it on the basis of a single feature of their product. The old adage "let the buyer beware" is certainly good advice. The more understanding of electrical currents the sports therapist has, the less likely he or she is to be snowed or confused by the salesman's spiel. Even more important, the greater the understanding, the easier it becomes to manipulate the treatment protocols for each patient to optimize the results.[43]

SUMMARY

1. When an electrical system is applied to muscle or nerve tissue, the result will be tissue membrane depolarization, provided that the current has the appropriate intensity, duration, and waveform to reach the tissue's excitability threshold.
2. Nerve function and muscle contraction are the same, regardless of the stimulation mechanism (i.e., natural or electrical).
3. Muscle and nerve tissue respond in an all-or-none fashion; there is no gradation of response.
4. Constant direct current has several major influences. The primary uses involve polar effects (acidic or alkaline), increased blood flow, bacteriostatic effects (negative electrode), and migration and alignment of cellular building blocks in the healing processes.
5. Nonexcitatory cells and tissues respond to electric current and contain continuous direct current circuits.
6. The body responds to injury by producing changes in the local electric circuits that may guide and assist the healing process.
7. Sensory level stimulation may retard edema accumulation in traumatic injuries.
8. Muscle contraction will change according to changes in current. As the frequency of the electrical stimulus increases, the muscle will develop more tension as a result of the summation of the contraction of the muscle fiber through progressive mechanical shortening. Increases in intensity spread the current over a larger area and increase the number of motor units activated by the current. Increases in the duration of the current also will cause more motor units to be activated.
9. Electrically stimulated muscle contractions are used clinically to help with muscle reeducation, muscle contraction for muscle pumping action, reduction of swelling, prevention or retardation of atrophy, muscle strengthening, and increasing range of motion in tight joints.
10. To stimulate a given muscle, location of the muscle's motor point, size and spacing of electrodes, and impedance of the tissue between the electrodes

and the motor points must be selected and adjusted to provide the most effective therapy.

11. Electrically stimulated discharges of sensory nerves help decrease pain perceptions.

12. The pain gating effect of electrical stimulation may occur at different levels in the central nervous system, depending on the type of electrical current used. Types of current similar to that used in transcutaneous electrical nerve stimulation will be gated at the spinal cord level. Hyperstimulation analgesia will stimulate central biasing with inhibitory influences descending from the brain and brain stem levels. Noxious stimuli to acupuncture or trigger areas will cause production of B-endorphin in the spinal cord and brain, with a resultant analgesic effect.

13. Specialized current waveforms all have physiologic responses that can be attributed to the characteristics of their waveforms. The differences in the waveforms and the physiologic response of each have particular effects that can be used therapeutically.

GLOSSARY

absolute refractory period Brief time period (.5 μsec) after membrane depolarization during which the membrane is incapable of depolarizing again.

action potential A recorded change in electrical potential between the inside and outside of a nerve cell, resulting in muscular contraction.

active electrode Electrode at which greatest current density occurs.

all-or-none response The depolarization of nerve or muscle membrane is the same once a depolarizing intensity threshold is reached; further increases in intensity do not increase the response. Stimuli at intensities less than threshold do not create a depolarizing effect.

anode Positively charged electrode in a direct current system.

bacteriostatic A chemical environment in which bacteria is destroyed.

beat Distinct wave pattern created by combining two distinct circuit electrical waves that blend into a gradual rising and falling wave.

bioelectromagnetics The study of biologic tissues' electrical and magnetic properties.

cathode Negatively charged electrode in a direct current system.

central biasing The use of hyperstimulation analgesia to bias the central nervous system against transmitting painful stimuli to the sensory recognition area. This occurs through hormonal influences created by brain stem stimulation.

chronaxie The duration of time necessary to cause observable tissue excitation, given a current intensity of two times rheobasic current.

constructive interference The combined amplitude of two distinct circuits increases the amplitude.

current density Amount of current flow per cubic area.

current of injury A bioelectric current produced by any type of cellular trauma that plays a key role in stimulating healing.

depolarization Process or act of neutralizing the cell membrane's resting potential.

destructive interference Combined amplitude of two distinct circuits decreases the amplitude.

dipoles Molecules whose ends carry opposite charges.

electrets Insulators carrying a permanent charge similar to a permanent magnet.

electropiezo activity Changing electric surface charges of a structure forces the structure to change shape.

frequency window selectivity Cellular responses may be triggered by a certain electrical frequency range.

gap junctions Specialized junction areas connecting cells of like structure, which contain channels for ionic, electrical, and small molecule signaling that pass messages from cell to cell.

heterodyne Cyclic rising and falling waveform of interferential current.

hybrid currents Currents that have waveforms containing parameters that are not classically alternating or direct.

impedance The resistance of the tissue to the passage of electrical current.

indifferent or dispersive electrode Large electrode used to spread out electrical charge and decrease current density at that electrode site.

maximum voluntary isometric contraction Peak torque produced by a muscular contraction.

piezoelectric activity Changing the shape of a structure causes the surfaces of that structure to change electrical charges.

resting potential The potential difference between the inside and outside of a membrane.

rheobase The intensity of current necessary to cause observable tissue excitation given a long current duration.

Russian current A medium frequency (2,000 to 10,000 Hz) polyphasic AC wave generated in 50 burst per second envelopes.

stereodynamic interference current Three distinct circuits blending and creating a distinct electrical wave pattern.

strain related potentials Tissue based electric potentials generated in response to strain of the tissue.

strength-duration curve A graphic illustration of the relationship between current intensity and duration in causing depolarization of a nerve or muscle membrane.

summation of contractions Shortening of muscle myofilaments caused by increasing the frequency of muscle membrane depolarization.

tetanization When individual muscle twitch responses can no longer be distinguished and the responses force maximum shortening of the stimulated muscle fiber.

twitch muscle contraction A single muscle contraction caused by one depolarization phenomenon.

voltage sensitive permeability The quality of some cell membranes that makes them permeable to different ions based on the electric charge of the ions. Nerve and muscle cell membranes allow negatively charged ions into the cell while actively transporting some positively charged ions outside the cell membrane.

REFERENCES

1 Alon G: High voltage stimulation: effects of electrode size on basic excitatory responses, *Phys Ther* 65: 890, 1985.

2 Alon G, DeDomeico G: *High voltage simulation: an integrated approach to clinical electrotherapy,* Chatanooga, Tenn, 1987, Chattanooga Corp.

3 American Physical Therapy Association: *Electrotherapeutic terminology in physical therapy,* Alexandria, VA, 1990, APTA Publications.

4 Barranco SD, Spadero J, Berger T, et al.: In vitro effect of weak direct current on staphylococcus aureus, *Clin Orthop* 100: 250-255, 1974.

5 Basset CAL, Becker RO: Generation of electrical potentials by bone in response to mechanical stress, *Science* 137: 1063-1064, 1962.

6 Becker RO: The bioelectric factors in amphibian-limb regeneration, *J Bone Joint Surg:* 43(A): 643-656, 1961.

7 Becker RO, Bachman CH, and Friedman H: The direct current control system, *NY State J Med* 62: 1169-1176, 1962.

8 Becker RA, Selden G: *The body electric,* New York, 1985, William Morrow.

9 Benton LA, Baker LL, Bowman BR, et al.: *Functional electrical stimulation: a practical clinical guide,* Downey, Calif., 1980, Rancho Los Amigos Hospital.

10 Bettany JA, Fish D, Mendel F, et al.: Influence of high voltage pulsed current on edema formation following impact injury, *Phys Ther* 70: 219-224, 1990.

11 Binder-MacLeod, SA, Snyder-Mackler L: Muscle fatigue: clinical implications for fatigue assessment and neuromuscular electrical stimulation, *Phys Ther* 73: 902-910, 1993.

12 Bishop B: Pain: its physiology and rationale for management, *Phys Ther* 60: 13-37, 1980.

13 Brighton CT: Bioelectric effects on bone and cartilage, *Clin Orthop* 124: 2-4, 1977.

14 Brown SR, Herner A, Birchmeier K, et al.: The effect of microcurrent on edema, range of motion, and pain in treatment of lateral ankle sprains, abstract, *JOSPT* 19: 55, 1994.

14a Byl N, McKenzie A, West J: Pulsed microamperage stimulation: a controlled study of healing of surgically induced wounds in Yucatan pigs, *Phys Ther* 74(3): 201-218, 1994.

15 Carley PJ, Wainapel SF: Electrotherapy for the acceleration of wound healing: low intensity direct current, *Arch Phys Med Rehab* 66: 443-446, 1985.

16 Castel JC: *Pain management with acupuncture and transcutaneous electrical nerve stimulation techniques and photo simulation (laser).* Symposium on Pain Management, Walter Reed Army Medical Center, Nov. 13, 1982.

17 Charman RA: *Bioelectricity and electrotherapy—towards a new paradigm?* 1. The cell, 2. Cellular reception and emission of electromagnetic signals, *Physiotherapy* 76: 502-518. 3. Bioelectric potentials and tissue currents, *Physiotherapy* 76: 643-654. 4. Strain generated potentials in bone and connective tissue, *Physiotherapy* 76: 725-730, 5. Exogenous currents and fields—experimental and clinical applications, *Physiotherapy* 76: 743-750, 1990.

18 Charman RA: *Bioelectricity and Electrotherapy—Towards a New Paradigm.* 6. Environmental current and fields—The natural background, *Physiotherapy* 77: 8-13, 7. Environmental currents and fields—Man Made, *Physiotherapy* 77: 129-149. 8. Grounds for a New Paradigm? *Physiotherapy* 77: 211-221, 1991.

19 Chreng N, Van Houf H, Bockx E, et al.: The effects of electric current on ATP generation, protein synthesis, and membrane transport in rat skin, *Clin Orthop* 171: 264-272, 1982.

20 Chu CS: Weak direct current accelerates split thickness: graft healing on tangentially excised second-degree burns, *J Burn Care Rehab* 12: 285-293, 1991.

21 Clements FR: Effect of motor neuromuscular electrical stimulation on microvascular perfusion of stimulated rat skeletal muscle, *Phys Ther* 71: 397-406, 1991.

22 Clement-Jones V: Increased B-endorphin but not met-enkephalin levels in human cerebrospinal fluid after acupuncture for recurrent pain, *Lancet* 8: 946-948, 1980.

23 Connolly JF, Hahn H, Jardon OM: The electrical enhancement of periosteal proliferation in normal and delayed fracture healing, *Clin Orthop* 124: 97-105, 1977.

24 Cosgrove KA, Alon G, Bell S, et al.: The electrical effect of two commonly used clinical stimulators on traumatic edema in rats, *Phys Ther* 72: 227-233, 1992.

25 Currier DP, Lehman J, Lightfoot P: Electrical stimulation in exercise of the quadriceps femoris muscle, *Phys Ther* 59: 1508-1512, 1979.

26 Currier DP, Mann R: Muscular strength development by electrical stimulation in healthy individuals, *Phys Ther* 63: 915-921, 1983.

27 Dallmann SL: Preference for low versus medium frequency electrical stimulation at constant: induced muscle forces, Abstract R345, *Phys Ther* 725: 5107, 1992.

28 Delitto A, Schulman A, Strube M, et al.: A study of discomfort with electrical stimulation, *Phys Ther* 72: 410-424, 1992.

29 Denegar CR: Influence of transcutaneous electrical nerve stimulation on pain, range of motion, and serum cortisol concentration in females experienceing delayed onset muscle soreness, *JOSPT* 11: 100-103, 1989.

30 Denegar C: The effects of low-volt microamperage stimulation on delayed onset muscle soreness, *J Sport Rehabil* 1: 95-102, 1993.

31 Eriksson E, Haggmark T: Comparison of isometric muscle training and electrical stimulation supplement: isometric muscle training in the recovery after major knee ligament surgery, *Am J Sports Med* 7: 169-171, 1979.

32 Fish D: Effect of anodal high voltage pulsed current on edema formation in frog hind limbs, *Phys Ther* 71: 724-733, 1991.

33 Flicker MT: *An analysis of cold intermittent compression with simultaneous treatment of electrical stimulation in the reduction of post acute ankle lymphadema,* Unpublished Masters' Thesis, Chapel Hill, NC, 1993, University of North Carolina.

34 Franklin ME: Effect of varying the ration of electrically induced muscle contraction time to rest time on serum creatin kinase and perceived soreness, *JOSPT* 13: 310-315, 1991.

35 Gault WR, Gatens PF Jr: Use of low intensity direct current in management of ischemic skin ulcers, *Phys Ther* 56: 265-269, 1976.

36 Gentzkow G: Electrical stimulation to heal dermal wounds, *J Derm Surg Oncol* 19: 753-758, 1993.

37 Gersh MR: Microcurrent electrical stimulation: putting it in perspective, *Clin Manage* 9(4): 51-54, 1989.

38 Goodgold J, Eberstein A: *Electrodiagnosis of neuromuscular diseases,* Baltimore, 1972, Williams & Wilkins.

39 Griffin JW: Reduction of chronic posttraumatic hand edema: A comparison of high voltage pulsed current intermittant pneumatic compression, and placebo treatments, *Phys Ther* 70: 279-286, 1990.

40 Griffin JW: Efficacy of high voltage pulsed current for healing of pressure ulcers in patients with spinal cord injury, *Phys Ther* 71: 433-444, 1991.

41 Guffey JS, Asmussen MD: In vitro bactericidal effects of high voltage pulsed current versus direct current against staphylococcus aureus, *J Clin Electrophysiol* 1: 5-9, 1989.

42 Guyton AC: *Textbook of medical physiology,* ed 2, Philadelphia, 1961, WB Saunders.

43 Hooker DN: *Personal communication,* January 30, 1994.

44 Howson D: *Report on neuromuscular reeducation,* Minneapolis, 1978, Medical General.

45 Howson DC: Peripheral neural excitability, *Phys Ther* 58: 1467-1473, 1978.

46 *Instruction manual for Electrostim 180-2,* Promatek, Canada, 1989.

47 Jeter JS, Valcenta DP: The effects of microcurrent electrical nerve stimulation on delayed onset muscle soreness and peak torque deficits in trained weight lifters. Abstract PO-R065-M. *Phys Ther* 735: 5-24, 1993.

48 Kahn J: *Low voltage technique,* ed 4, Syossett, NY, 1983, Joseph Kahn.

49 Karnes JL: Effects of low voltage pulsed current on edema formation in frog hind limbs following impact injury, *Phys Ther* 72: 273-278, 1992.

50 Karnes JL: Influence of high voltage pulsed current on diameters of anterioles during histamine-induced vasodilation, Abstract R341, *Phys Ther* 725: 5105, 1992.

51 Kincaid CB, Lavoie KH: Inhibition of bacterial growth in vitro following stimulation with high voltage monophasic pulsed current, *Phys Ther* 69: 651-655, 1989.

52 Kulig K: Comparison of the effects of high velocity exercise and microcurrent neuromuscular stimulation on delayed onset muscle soreness, Abstract R284, *Phys Ther* 715: 5115, 1991.

53 Lampe GN: *A clinical approach to transcutaneous electrical nerve stimulation in the treatment of chronic and acute pain,* Minneapolis, 1978, Med General.

54 Lampe GN: Introduction to the use of transcutaneous electrical nerve stimulation devices, *Phys Ther* 58: 1450-1454, 1978.

55 Laughman RK, Youdes J, Garrett T: Strength changes in the normal quadriceps femoris muscle as a result of electrical stimulation, *Phys Ther* 63: 494-499, 1983.

56 Lea JA: The effect of electrical stimulation on edematous rat hind paws, Abstract R379, *Phys Ther* 725: 5116, 1992.

56a Leffmann D, Arnall D, Holmgren P: Effect of microamperage stimulation on the rate of wound healing in rats: a histological study, *Phys Ther* 74(3): 195-200, 1994.

57 Leffmann DL: The effect of subliminal transcutaneous electrical stimulation on the rate of wound healing in rats, Abstract R166, *Phys Ther* 725: 567, 1992.

58 Malizia E: Electroaccupuncture and peripheral B-endorphin and ACTH levels, *Lancet* 8: 535-6, 1979.

59 Mannheimer J, Lampe G: *Clinical transcutaneous electrical nerve stimulation,* Philadelphia, 1984 FA Davis.

60 Marino A, Becker RO: Biologic effects of extremely low frequency electric and magnetic fields: a review, *Phys Chem Physics* 9: 131-143, 1977.

61 Maurer CL: The effectiveness of microelectrical neural stimulation on exercise-induced muscle trauma, Abstract R200, *Phys Ther* 725: 574, 1992.

62 Melzack R: *The puzzle of pain,* New York, 1973, Basic Books.

63 Melzack R: Prolonged relief of pain by brief, intense transcutaneous electrical stimulation, *Pain* 1(4): 357-373, 1975.

64 Melzack R, Stillwell DM, Fox EJ: Trigger points and acupuncture points for pain: correlations and implications, *Pain* 3(1): 3-23, 1977.

65 Mendel FC: High voltage pulsed current using surface electrodes: effect on acute edema formation after hyperflexion injury in frogs, *JOSPT* 16: 140-144, 1992.

66 Mendel FC: Influence of high voltage pulsed current on edema formation following impact injury in rats, *Phys Ther* 72: 668-673, 1992.

67 Michlovitz S: Ice and high voltage pulsed stimulation in treatment of acute lateral ankle sprains, *JOSPT* 9: 301-304, 1988.

68 Mohr T, Akers T, Landry R: Effect of high voltage stimulation on edema reduction in the rat hind limbs, *Phys Ther* 67: 1703-1707, 1987.

69 Mulder GD: Treatment of open-skin wounds with electric stimulation, *Arch Phys Med Rehabil* 72: 375-377, 1991.

70 Nelson RL, Currier DP: *Clinical electrotherapy,* Norwalk, Conn., 1987, Appleton & Lange.

71 Nessler JP, Mass PP: Direct current electrical stimulation of tendon healing in vitro, *Clin Orthop* 217: 303-312, 1987.

72 Newton RA, Karselis TC: Skin pH following high voltage pulsed galvanic stimulation, *Phys Ther* 63: 1593-1596, 1983.

73 Nikolova L: *Treatment with interferential current,* New York, 1987, Churchill Livingstone.

74 *Notes on low volt therapy.* White Plains, NY, 1966, TECA Corporation.

75 Pettine KA: External electrical stimulation and bracing for treatment of spondylolysis: case report, *Spine* 188: 436-439, 1993.

76 Picker RI: Current trends 1 and 2. low voltage pulsed microamp stimulation, *Clin Manag* 9: 11-14; 9:(3) 28-33, 1990.

77 Randall BF, Imig CJ, Hines HM: Effect of electrical stimulation upon blood flow and temperature of skeletal muscles *Arch Phys Med* 33: 73-78, 1952.

78 Rapaski D: Microcurrent electrical stimulation: comparison of two protocols in reducing delayed onset muscle soreness, Abstract R286, *Phys Ther* 715: 5116, 1991.

79 Reed B: Effect of high voltage pulsed electrical stimulation on microvascular permeability to plasma proteins: a possible mechanism in minimizing edema, *Phys Ther* 68: 491-495, 1988.

80 Rolle WC, Alon G, Nirschl RP: Comparison of subliminal and placebo stimulation in the management of elbow epicondylitis, Abstract R280, *Phys Ther* 715: 5114, 1991.

81 Salar G, Job F, Salvatore M, et al.: Effect of transcutaneous electrotherapy on CSF B-endorphin content in patients without pain problems, *Pain* 10: 169-172, 1981.

82 Selkowitz D: Improvement in isometric strength of the quadriceps femoris muscle after training with electrical stimulation, *Phys Ther* 65: 186-196, 1985.

83 Selkowitz DM: High frequency electrical stimulation in muscle strengthening, *Am J Sport Med* 17: 103-111, 1989.

84 Siff M: Applications of electrostimulation in physical conditioning: a review, *J Appl Sport Sci Res* 4: 20-26, 1990.

85 Snyder SH: Opiate receptors and internal opiates: *Sci Am* 236: 44-56, 1977.

86 Synder-Mackler L, Garrett M, Roberts M: A comparison of torque generating capabilities of three different electrical stimulating currents, *JOSPT* 10: 297,301, 1989.

87 Stanish WD, Gunnlaugson B: Electrical energy and soft tissue injury healing, *Sport Care and Fitness,* Sept/Oct: 12-14, 1988.

88 Stillwell GK: *Therapeutic electricity and ultraviolet radiation,* Baltimore, 1983, Williams & Wilkins.

89 Svacina L: Modified interferential technique, *Pain Control,* April 1978, p. 1-2, Staodynamics, Inc.

90 Szabo G, Illes T: Experimental stimulation of osteogenesis induced by bone matrix, *Orthopaedics* 14: 63-67, 1991.

91 Taylor K: Effect of electrically induced muscle contraction on post traumatic edema formation in frog hind limbs, *Phys Ther* 72: 127-132, 1992.

92 Taylor K: Effect of a single 30-minute treatment of high voltage pulsed current on edema formation in frog hind limbs, *Phys Ther* 72: 63-68, 1992.

93 Travell J, Simon D: *Myofascial pain and dysfunction: the trigger point manual,* Baltimore, 1983, Williams & Wilkins.

94 Unger PG: A randomized clinical trial of the effects of HVPC on wound healing, Abstract R294, *Phys Ther* 715: 5118, 1991.

95 Watkins AL: *A manual of electrotherapy,* ed 3, Philadelphia, 1968, Lea & Febiger.

96 Weber WD: The effect of MENS on pain and torque deficits associated with delayed onset muscle soreness, Abstract R034, *Phys Ther* 715: 535, 1991.

97 Weiss DS, Kirsner R, Eaglstein WH: Electrical stimulation and wound healing, *Arch Derm* 126: 222-225, 1990.

98 Wolcot C: A comparison of the effects of high voltage and microcurrent stimulation on delayed onset muscle soreness, Abstract R287, *Phys Ther* 715: 5116, 1991.

99 Wolf SL: Perspectives on central nervous system responsiveness to transcutaneous electrical nerve stimulation, *Phys Ther* 58: 1443-1449, 1978.

100 Wolf SL: *Electrotherapy,* New York, 1981, Churchill Livingstone.

101 Wolf SL, Gersh MR, Kutner M: Relationship of selected clinical variables to current delivered during transcutaneous electrical nerve stimulation, *Phys Ther* 58: 1478-1483, 1978.

102 Wood JM: A multicenter study on the use of pulsed low-intensity direct current for healing chronic stage II and stage III decubitus ulcers, *Arch Dermatol* 129: 999-1009, 1993.

103 Young SL: Efficacy of interferential current stimulation alone for pain reduction in patients with osteoarthritis of the knee: a randomized placebo control clinical trial, Abstract R088, *Phys Ther* 715: 552, 1991.

SUGGESTED READINGS

Alon G: High voltage stimulation: effects of electrode size on basic excitatory responses, *Phys Ther* 65: 890, 1985.

Alon G, Allin J, Inbar GE: Optimization of pulse duration and pulse charge during transcutaneous electrical stimulation, *Aust J Physiother* 29: 195, 1983.

Alon G, Bainbridge J, Croson G: High-voltage pulsed direct current effects on peripheral blood flow *Phys Ther* 61: 678, 1981.

Andersson SA: *Pain control by sensory stimulation.* In Bonica JJ, Liebeskind J, Albe-Fessard D, et al., editors: *Advances in pain research and therapy,* vol 3, New York, 1979, Raven.

Andersson SA, Hansson G, Holmgren E: Evaluation of the pain suppression effect of different frequencies of peripheral electrical stimulation in chronic pain conditions, *Acta Orthop Scand* 47: 149, 1979.

Baker LL: *Neuromuscular electrical stimulation in the restoration of purposeful limb movements.* In Wolf SL, editor: *Electrotherapy -- clinics in physical therapy,* New York, 1981, Churchill Livingstone.

Benton LA, Baker LL, Bowman BR, et al.: *Functional electrical stimulation: a practical clinical guide,* ed 2, Downey, Calif, 1981, Professional Staff Association of Rancho Los Amigos Medical Center.

Berlandt SR: Method of determining optimal stimulation sites for transcutaneous nerve stimulation *Phys Ther* 64: 924, 1984.

Brown MD, Cotter M, Hudlicka O: The effects of long-term stimulation of fast muscles on their ability to withstand fatigue *J Physiol (London)* 238: 47, 1974.

Brown MD, Cotter M, Hudlicka O: *Metabolic changes in long-term stimulated fast muscles.* In Howland H, Poortmans JR, editors: *Metabolic adaptation to prolonged physical exercise,* Basel, 1975, Birkhauser.

Burr HS, Harvey SC: Bio-electric correlates of wound healing, *Yale J Biol Med* 11: 103,1938-1939, 1939.

Burr HA, Taffel M, Harvey SC: An electrometric study of the healing wound in man, *Yale J Biol Med* 12: 483, 1940.

Campbell JA: A critical appraisal of the electrical output characteristics of ten transcutaneous nerve stimulators, *Clin Phys Physiol Meas* 3: 141, 1982.

Chan CS, Chow SP: Electroacupuncture in the treatment of post-traumatic sympathetic dystrophy (Sudek's atrophy), *Br J Anesth* 53: 899, 1981.

Chase J: Elicitation of periods of inhibition in human muscle by stimulation of cutaneous nerves, *J Bone Joint Surg (Am)* 54: 1737, 1972.

Cooperman AM: Use of transcutaneous electrical stimulation in the control of post operative pain: results of a prospective, randomized, controlled study, *Am J Surg* 133: 185, 1977.

Curico F, Berweger R: *A clinical evaluation of the pain supressor TENS,* Fairleigh Dickenson University School of Dentistry, 1983.

Currier DP, Mann R: Muscular strength development by electrical stimulation in healthy individuals, *Phys Ther* 63: 915, 1983.

Currier DP, Mann R: Pain complaint: comparison of electrical stimulation with conventional isometric exercise, *J Orthop Sports Phys Ther* 5: 318, 1984.

Currier DP, Petrilli CR, Threlkeld AJ: Effect of medium frequency electrical stimulation on local blood circulation to healthy muscle, *Phys Ther* 66: 937, 1986.

DeGirardi CQ, Seaborne D, Goulet FS: The analgesic effect of high voltage galvanic stimulation combined with ultrasound in the treatment of low back pain: a one-group pre-test/post-test study, *Physiother Can* 36: 327, 1984.

Eisenberg BR, Gilal A: Structural changes in single muscle fibers after stimulation at a low frequency *J Gen Physiol* 74: 1, 1979.

Eriksson E, Haggmark T, Kiessling KH: Effect of electrical stimulation on human skeletal muscle, *Int J Sports Med* 2: 18, 1981.

Ersek R: Transcutaneous electrical neurostimulation — a new modality for controlling pain, *Clin Orthop* 128: 314, 1977.

Fox FJ, Melzack R: Transcutaneous electrical stimulation and acupuncture: comparison of treatment for low back pain, *Pain* 2: 141, 1976.

Frank C, Schachar N, Dittrich D: Electromagnetic stimulation of ligament healing in rabbits, *Clin Orthop* 175: 263, 1983.

Geddes LA: A short history of the electrical stimulation of excitable tissue, *Physiologist* 27(suppl): 1, 1984.

Godfrey CM, Jayawardena H, Quance TA: Comparison of electrostimulation and isometric exercise in strengthening the quadriceps muscle, *Physiother Can* 31: 265, 1979.

Gould M, Donnermeyer D, Gammon GG: Transcutaneous muscle stimulation to retard disuse atrophy after open meniscectomy, *Clin Orthop* 178: 190, 1983.

Greathouse DG, Nitz AJ, Matullonis D: Effects of electrical stimulation on ultrastructure of rat skeletal muscles, *Phys Ther* 64: 755, 1984.

Halback JW, Straus D: Comparison of electromyostimulation to isokinetic training in increasing power of the knee extensor mechanism, *J Orthop Sports Phys Ther* 2: 20, 1980.

Ignelzi RJ, Nyquist JK: Excitability changes in peripheral nerve fibers after repetitive electrical stimulation: implications in pain modulation, *J Neurosurg* 61: 824, 1979.

Jones DA, Bigland-Ritchie B, Edwards RHT: Excitation and frequency and muscle fatigue: mechanical responses during voluntary and stimulated contractions, *Exper Neurol* 64: 401, 1979.

Kahn J: *Low-volt technique,* Syosset, NY, 1973, Joseph Kahn.

Kramer JF, Mendryk SW: Electrical stimulation as a strength improvement technique: a review *J Orthop Sports Phys Ther* 4: 91, 1982.

Lainey CG, Walmsley RP, Andrew GM: Effectiveness of exercise alone versus exercise plus electrical stimulation in strengthening the quadriceps muscle, *Physiother Can* 35: 5, 1983.

Lampe GN: Introduction to the use of transcutaneous electrical nerve stimulation devices, *Phys Ther* 58: 1450, 1978.

Lane JF: Electrical impedances of superficial limb tissue, epidermis, dermis and muscle sheath, *Ann NY Acad Sci* 238: 812, 1974.

Laughman RK, Youdas JW, Garrett TF: Strength changes in the normal quadriceps femoris muscle as a result of electrical stimulation, *Phys Ther* 63: 494, 1983.

LeDoux J, Quinones MA: An investigation of the use of percutaneous electrical stimulation in muscle reeducation, *Phys Ther* 61: 678, 1981.

Licht S: *History of electrotherapy.* In Stillwell GK, editor. *Therapeutic electricity and ultraviolet radiation,* ed 3, Baltimore, 1983, Williams & Wilkins.

Loeser JD: *Nonpharmacologic approaches to pain relief.* In Ng LKY, Bonica JJ, editors: *Pain, discomfort and humanitarian care,* New York, 1980, Elsevier.

Loeser JD, Black RG, Christman A: A relief of pain by transcutaneous stimulation, *J Neurosurg* 42: 308, 1975.

Long D: Cutaneous afferent stimulation for relief of chronic pain, *Clin Neurosurg* 21: 257, 1974.

Mannneimer C, Carlsson CA: The analgesic effect of transcutaneous electrical nerve stimulation (TENS) in patients with rheumatoid arthritis: a comparative study of different pulse patterns, *Pain* 6: 329, 1979.

Mannheimer C, Lund S, Carlsson CA: The effect of transcutaneous electrical nerve stimulation (TENS) on joint pain in patients with rheumatoid arthritis, *Scand J Rheumatol* 7: 13, 1978.

Mannheimer JS: Electrode placements for transcutaneous electrical nerve stimulation, *Phys Ther* 58: 1455, 1978.

Mao W, Ghia JN, Scott DS: High versus low intensity acupuncture analgesic for treatment of chronic pain: effects on platelet serotonin, *Pain* 8: 331, 1980.

Marvie KW: A major advance in the control of post-operative knee pain, *Orthopedics* 2: 129, 1979.

Massey BH, Nelson RC, Sharkey BC: Effects of high frequency electrical stimulation on the size and strength of skeletal muscle, *J Sports Med Phys Fit* 5: 136, 1965.

McMiken DF, Todd-Smith M, Thompson C: Strengthening of human quadriceps muscles by cutaneous electrical stimulation, *Scand J Rehab Med* 15: 25, 1983.

McNeal DR, Bowman BR: *Peripheral neuromuscular stimulation.* In Myklebust JB, Cusick J, Fances A, editors. *Neural stimulation,* Boca Raton, Fla, 1985, CRC Press.

Meyer GA, Fields HL: Causalgia treated by selective large fibre stimulation of peripheral nerve, *Brain* 95: 163, 1972.

Milner-Brown HS, Stein RB: The relation between the surface electromyogram and muscular force, *J Physiol* 246: 549, 1975.

Mohr T, Carlson B, Sulentic C: Comparison of isometric exercise and high volt galvanic stimulation on quadriceps, femoris muscle strength, *Phys Ther* 65: 606, 1985.

Munsat TL, McNeal DR, Waters RL: Preliminary observations on prolonged stimulation of peripheral nerve in man, *Arch Neurol* 33: 608, 1976.

Naess K, Storm-Mathison A: Fatigue of sustained tetanic contractions, *Acta Physiol Scand* 34: 351, 1955.

Owens J, Malone T: Treatment parameters of high frequency electrical stimulation as established on the electro stim 180, *J Orthop Sports Phys Ther* 4: 162, 1983.

Picaza JA, Cannon BW, Hunter SE: Pain suppression by peripheral stimulation. I. Observations with transcutaneous stimuli, *Surg Neurol* 4: 105, 1975.

Procacci P, Zoppi M, Maresca M: Transcutaneous electrical stimulation in low back pain: a critical evaluation, *Acupunct Electrother Res* 7: 1, 1982.

Rack PMH, Westbury DR: The effects of length and stimulus rate on tension in the isometric cat soleus muscle, *J Physiol* 204: 443, 1969.

Reddana P, Moortly CV, Govidappa S: Pattern of skeletal muscle chemical composition during in vivo electrical stimulations, *Ind J Physiol Pharmacol* 25: 33, 1981.

Roeser W, Meeks L, Venis R, et al.: The use of transcutaneous nerve stimulation for pain control in athletic medicine: a preliminary report, *Am J Sports Med* 4(5): 210, 1976.

Romero JA, Sanford TL, Schroeder RV: The effects of electrical stimulation of normal quadriceps on strength and girth, *Med Sci Sports Exerc* 14: 194, 1982.

Rosenberg M, Vutyid L, Bourbe D: Transcutaneous electrical nerve stimulation for the relief of post-operative pain, *Pain* 5: 129, 1978.

Rowley BA, McKenna JM, Chase GR: The influence of electrical current on an infecting microorganism in wounds, *Ann NY Acad Sci* 238: 543, 1974.

Selkowitz DM: Improvement in isometric strength of the quadricep femoris muscle after training with electrical stimulation, *Phys Ther* 65: 186, 1985.

Shealey CN, Maurer D: Transcutaneous nerve stimulation for control of pain, *Surg Neurol* 2: 45, 1974.

Sjolund BH, Eriksson MBE: The influence of naloxone on analgesia produced by peripheral conditioning stimulation, *Brain Res* 173: 295, 1979.

Sjolund BH, Terenius L, Eriksson MBE: Increased cerebrospinal fluid levels of endorphin after electroacupuncture, *Acta Physiol Scand* 100: 382, 1977.

Standish WD, Valiant GA, Bonen A: The effects of immobilization and of electrical stimulation on muscle glycogen and myofibrillar ATPase, *Can J Appl Sports Sci* 7: 267, 1982.

Szehi E, David E: The stereodynamic interferential current -- a new electrotherapeutic technique, *Electromedica* 48: 13, 1980.

Taylor P, Hallet M, Flaherty L: Treatment of osteoarthritis of the knee with transcutaneous electrical nerve stimulation, *Pain* 11: 233, 1981.

Taylor MK, Newton RA, Personius WJ: The effects of interferential current stimulation for the treatment of subjects with recurrent jaw pain, *Abstract Phys Ther* 66: 774, 1986.

Terezhalmy GT, Ross GR, Holmes-Johnson E: Transcutaneous electrical nerve stimulation treatment of TMJMPDS patients *Ear Nose Throat J* 61: 664, 1982.

Thorsteinsson G, Stonnington HH, Stillwell K, et al.: The placebo effect of transcutaneous electrical stimulation, *Pain* 5: 31, 1978.

Wheeler P, Wolcott L, Morris J: *Neural considerations in the healing of ulcerated tissue by clinical electrotherapeutic application of weak direct current: findings and theory.* In Reynolds, DV, Sjoberg AE, editors: *Neuroelectric research,* Springfield, Ill, 1971, Charles C. Thomas.

Wolf SL, Gersh MR, Rao VR: Examination of electrode placements and stimulating parameters in treating chronic pain with conventional transcutaneous nerve stimulation (TENS), *Pain* 11: 37, 1981.

Wong RA, Jette DV: Changes in sympathetic tone associated with different forms of transcutaneous electrical nerve stimulation in healthy subjects, *Phys Ther* 64: 478, 1984.

Zecca L, Ferrario P, Furia G: Effects of pulsed electromagnetic field on acute and chronic inflammation, *Trans Biol Repair Growth Soc* 3: 72, 1983.

Iontophoresis

6

William E. Prentice

OBJECTIVES

After completion of this chapter, the student will be able to do the following:

- Differentiate between iontophoresis and phonophoresis.

- Discuss the basic mechanisms of ion transfer.

- Discuss specific iontophoresis application procedures and techniques.

- Identify the different ions most commonly used in iontophoresis.

- Describe the various clinical applications for using an iontophoresis technique in a sports-medicine setting.

- Identify precautions and concerns when using iontophoresis treatment.

Iontophoresis is a therapeutic technique that involves the introduction of ions into the body tissues by means of a direct electrical current. Originally referred to as **ion transfer,** it was first described by LeDuc in 1903 as a technique of transporting chemicals across a membrane using an electrical current as a driving force.[32] Since that time there have been increases and decreases in the popularity and use of iontophoresis as a therapeutic technique. Recently in sports medicine, new emphasis has been placed on iontophoresis and it has become a commonly used technique in that setting. Iontophoresis has several advantages as a treatment technique in that it is a painless, sterile, non-invasive way to introduce specific ions into the tissue that have been demonstrated to have a positive effect on the healing process.

It is critical to point out the difference between iontophoresis and phonophoresis since the two techniques are often confused and occasionally the two terms are erroneously interchanged. Both techniques are used to deliver chemicals to various biologic tissues. Phonophoresis, which is discussed in detail in Chapter 12, involves the use of acoustic energy in the form of ultrasound to drive whole molecules across the skin into the tissues, while iontophoresis uses an electrical current to transport ions into the tissues.

BASIC MECHANISMS OF ION TRANSFER

As defined in Chapter 4, **ions** are positively or negatively charged particles. Through the process of **ionization,** soluble compounds, such as acids, alkaloids, or salts, dissociate or dissolve into ions that are suspended in some type of solution.[7] The resulting solutions in which ionic movement occurs are called **electrolytes.** Ions will move or migrate within this solution according to the electrically charged currents acting on them. The term **electrophoresis** refers to the movement of ions in solution.

At any given instant, the electrode that has the greatest concentration of electrons is negatively charged and is referred to as the negative electrode, or cathode. Conversely, the electrode with a lower concentration of electrons is called the positive electrode, or anode. Negatively charged ions will be repelled from the negative electrode, thus moving toward the positive electrode, creating an acidic reaction. Positively charged ions will tend to move toward the negative electrode and away from the positive electrode, resulting in an alkaline reaction.

The manner in which ions move in solution forms the basis for iontophoresis. Positively charged ions are driven into the tissues from the positive pole, and negatively charged ions are introduced by the negative pole. Thus knowing the correct ion polarity and matching it with the appropriate electrode polarity is of critical importance in using iontophoresis.

The force that acts to move ions through the tissues is determined by both the strength of the electrical field and the electrical impedence of tissues to current flow. The strength of the electrical field is determined by the current density. The difference in current density between the active and inactive or dispersive electrodes establishes a gradient of potential difference that produces ion migration within the electrical field. In Chapter 5 the active electrode was defined as the smaller of the two electrodes that has the greatest current density. When using iontophoresis the **active electrode** is defined as the one that is used to drive the ion into the tissues. Current density may be altered either by increasing or decreasing current intensity or by changing the size of the electrode. Increasing the size of the electrode will decrease current density under that electrode. It has been recommended that the current density be reduced at the cathode. The accumulation of positively charged ions in a small area creates an alkaline reaction that is more likely to produce tissue damage than an accumulation of negatively charged ion that produces an acidic reaction. Thus the negative electrode should be larger, perhaps twice the size of the positive electrode, to reduce current density.[7,23] This size relationship should remain the same even when the negative electrode is the active electrode.

Skin and fat are poor conductors of electrical current, offering greater resistance to current flow. Higher current intensities are necessary to create ion movement in areas where the skin and fat layers are thick, further increasing the likelihood of burns particularly around the cathode. However the presence of sweat glands decreases impedance, thus facilitating the flow of direct current and ions. The sweat ducts are the primary paths by which ions move through the skin.[22] As the skin becomes more saturated with electrolyte and blood flow increases to the area during treatment, overall skin impedance will decrease under the electrodes.[7]

The quantity of ions transferred into the tissues through iontophoresis is determined by the intensity of the current or current density at the active electrode, the duration of the current flow, and the concentration of ions in solution.[7] The number of ions absorbed is directly proportional to the current density. In addition, the longer the current flows the greater the number of ions transferred to the tissues. Therefore ion transfer may be increased by increasing the intensity and duration of the treatment. Unfortunately, as treatment duration increases the skin impedance decreases, thus increasing the likelihood of burns. Even though ion concentration affects ion transfer, concentrations greater than 1% to 2% are not more effective than medications at lower concentrations.[37,38]

Once the ions have passed through the skin, they recombine with existing ions and free radicals floating in the bloodstream, thus forming the necessary new compounds for favorable therapeutic interactions.[23]

IONTOPHORESIS TECHNIQUES
Type Of Current Required

Continuous direct current must be used for iontophoresis. Direct current ensures the unidirectional flow of ions, which cannot be accomplished using a bidirectional or alternating current. Neither high-voltage direct currents nor interferential currents may be used for iontophoresis, since the current is interrupted and the current duration is too short to produce significant ion movement.

Iontophoresis Generators

There are a variety of current generators available on the market that produce continuous direct current and are specifically used for iontophoresis (Figure 6-1). It should be emphasized that any generator that has the capability of producing continuous direct current may be used for iontophoresis. Some generators are driven by batteries and others by alternating current. Many generators produce current at a constant voltage that gradually reduces skin impedance, consequently increasing current density and thus increasing the risk of burns. The generator should deliver a constant voltage output to the athlete by adjusting the output amperage to normal variations that occur in tissue impedance, thereby reducing the likelihood of burns. For safety purposes the generator should automatically shut down if the skin impedance decreases to some preset limit.

The generator should have some type of current intensity control that can be adjusted between 1 and 5 mA. There should also be an adjustable timer that can be set for up to 25 minutes. Polarity of the terminals should be clearly marked, and a polarity reversal switch is desirable. The lead wires connecting the electrodes to the terminals should be well insulated and should be checked regularly for damage or breakdown.

Current Intensity and Treatment Duration

Low amperage currents appear to be more effective as a driving force than currents with higher intensities.[20,23,35] Higher intensity currents tend to reduce effective penetration into the tissues. Recommended current amplitudes used for iontophoresis range between 3 and 5 mA.[2,8,16,23] When initiating the treatment, the current intensity should

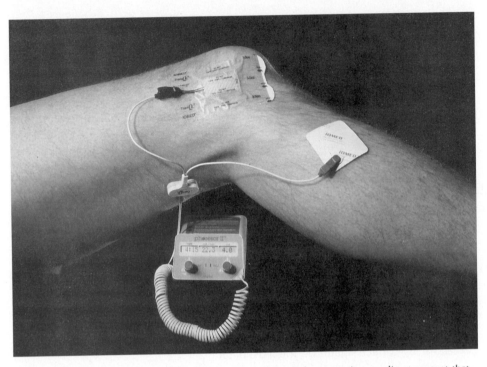

Fig. 6-1. The Phoresor® is an example of a generator that produces continuous direct current that is specifically used for iontophoresis.

always be increased very slowly until the athlete reports feeling a tingling or prickly sensation. If pain or a burning sensation is elicited, the intensity is too great and should be decreased. Likewise when terminating the treatment, current intensity should be slowly decreased to zero before the electrodes are disconnected.

It has been recommended that the maximum current intensity be determined by the size of the active electrode[36] (Figure 6-2). Current amplitude is usually set so that the current density falls between 0.1 and 0.5 mA/cm² of the active electrode surface.[7]

Recommended treatment durations range between 10 and 20 minutes, with 15 minutes as an average. During this 15-minute treatment, the athlete should be comfortable, with no reported or visible signs of pain or burning. The sports therapist should check the athlete's skin every 3 to 5 minutes during treatment, looking for signs of skin irritation. Since skin impedance usually decreases during the treatment, it may be necessary to decrease current intensity to avoid pain or burning.

Electrodes

The continuous direct electrical current must be delivered to the athlete through some type of electrode. Many different electrodes are available to the sports therapist ranging from those "borrowed" from other electrical stimulators to commercially manufactured ready-to-use disposable electrodes made specifically for iontophoresis.[2,17]

The more traditional electrodes are made of tin, copper, lead, aluminum, or

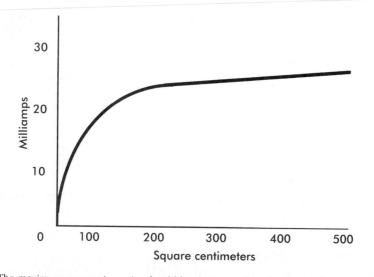

Fig. 6-2. The maximum current intensity should be determined by the size of the active electrode. Current amplitude is usually set so that the current density falls between 0.1-0.5 mA/cm² of the active electrode surface.

platinum backed by rubber and completely covered by a sponge, towel, or gauze that is in contact with the skin. The absorbent material is soaked with the ionized solution to be driven into the tissues. If the ions are contained in an ointment, it should be rubbed into the skin over the target zone and covered by some absorbent material soaked in water or saline before the electrode is applied.

The commercially produced electrodes are sold with most iontophoresis systems. These electrodes have a small chamber into which the ionized solution may be injected that is covered by some type of semipermeable membrane. The electrode self-adheres to the skin (Figure 6-3). This type of electrode has eliminated the mess and hassles that have been associated with electrode preparation for iontophoresis in the past.

Regardless of the type of electrode used, to ensure maximum contact of the electrodes the skin should be shaved and cleaned before attachment of the electrodes. Care should be taken not to excessively abrade the skin during cleaning, since damaged skin has a lower resistance to the current so that a burn may more easily occur. Also, caution should be used when treating areas that for one reason or another have reduced sensation.

Once this electrode has been prepared, it then becomes the active electrode, and the lead wire to the generator is attached such that the polarity of the wire is the same as the polarity of the ion in solution. A second electrode, the dispersive electrode, is prepared with water, gel, or some other conductive material as recommended by the manufacturer. Both electrodes must be securely attached to the skin such that uniform skin contact and pressure is maintained under both electrodes to minimize the risk of burns. Electrodes sent via the lead wires should not be connected to the generator unless both the generator and the amplitude or intensity control are turned off. At the

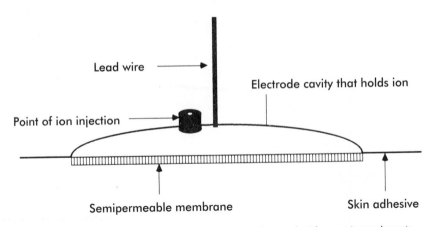

Lead wire

Electrode cavity that holds ion

Point of ion injection

Semipermeable membrane

Skin adhesive

Fig. 6-3. The commercially produced self-adhering electrodes used with most iontophoresis systems have a small chamber into which the ionized solution may be injected that is covered by some type of semipermeable membrane.

end of the treatment the intensity control should be returned to zero and the generator turned off before the electrodes are detached from the patient.

The size and shape of the electrodes can cause a variation in current density and affect the size of the area treated.[13] Smaller electrodes have a higher current density and should be used to treat a specific lesion. Larger electrodes should be used when the target treatment area is not well defined.

Recommendations for spacing between the active and dispersive electrodes vary. They should be separated by at least the diameter of the active electrode. One source has recommended spacing them at least 18 inches apart.[7] As spacing between the electrodes increases the current density in the superficial tissues will be decreased, perhaps minimizing the potential for burns.

Selecting the Appropriate Ion

It is critical that the sports therapist be knowledgeable in the selection of the most appropriate ions for treating specific conditions. For a compound to penetrate a membrane, such as the skin, it must be soluble in both fat and water. It must be water soluble if it is to remain in an ionized state in solution. However, since human skin is relatively impervious to water, ions that are soluble only in water do not diffuse in the tissues.[4] They must be fat soluble to permeate the body tissues.[17] Penetration is relatively superficial and is generally less than 1 mm.[23] The majority of the ions deposited in the tissues are found primarily at the site of the active electrode where they are stored as either a soluble or insoluble compound. They may be used locally as a concentrated source or transported by the circulating blood producing more systemic effects.[23]

The tendency of some ions to form insoluble precipitates as they pass into the tissues inhibits their ability to penetrate. This is particularly true with heavy metal ions including iron, copper, silver, and zinc.[9]

Negative ions accumulating at the anode produce an acidic reaction through the formation of hydrochloric acid. Negative ions are sclerolytic, thus they produce softening of the tissues by decreasing protein density. This is useful in treating scars or adhesions. In addition, some negative ions (salicylates) can also produce an analgesic effect.

The majority of the ions used for iontophoresis are positively charged. Positive ions that accumulate at the negative pole produce an alkaline reaction with the formation of sodium hydroxide. Positive ions are sclerotic and produce hardening of the tissues by increasing protein density.

Box 6-1 lists the ions most commonly used with iontophoresis.

CLINICAL APPLICATIONS

A relatively long list of conditions for which iontophoresis is an appropriate treatment technique has been cited in the literature. In sports medicine, iontophoresis is most often used to treat inflammatory musculoskeletal conditions. It may also be used for analgesic effects, scar modification, and wound healing and in treating edema, calcium deposits, and hyperhydrosis. Many of these published studies are case reports that attempt to establish the clinical efficacy of iontophoresis in treating various conditions.[13] Table 6-1 provides a list of studies of various conditions treated with iontophoresis.

TREATMENT PRECAUTIONS AND CONSIDERATIONS

Problems that might arise from treating an athlete using iontophoresis techniques may for the most part be avoided if the sports therapist (1) has a good understanding of the existing condition that is to be treated, (2) uses the most appropriate ions to accomplish the treatment goal, and (3) uses appropriate treatment parameters and equipment set-up. Poor treatment technique on the part of the sports therapist is most often responsible for adverse reactions to iontophoresis.

Treatment Burns

Perhaps the single most common problem associated with iontophoresis is a chemical burn that usually occurs as a result of the direct current itself and not because of the ion being used in treatment.[36] Passing a continuous direct electrical current through the tissues creates migration of ions, which alters the normal pH of the skin. The normal pH of the skin is between 3 and 4. In an **acidic reaction** the pH falls below 3, while in an **alkaline reaction** the pH is greater than 5. Although chemical burns may occur under either electrode, they most typically result from the accumulation of sodium hydroxide at the cathode. The alkaline reaction causes sclerolysis of local tissues. Initially, the burn lesion is pink and raised but within hours becomes a grayish, oozing wound.[23] Decreasing current density by increasing the size of the cathode relative to the anode can minimize the potential for chemical burn.

Heat burns may occur as a result of high resistance to current flow created by poor contact of the electrodes with the skin. Poor contact results when the electrodes are not moist enough, when there are wrinkles in the gauze or paper towels impregnated with the ionic solution, or when there is space between the skin and electrode around the perimeter of the electrode. The athlete should not be treated with body weight

BOX 6-1 RECOMMENDED IONS FOR USE BY THE SPORTS THERAPIST[30]

POSITIVE

Antibiotics Gentamycin Sulfate (+), 8 mg/ml, for suppurative ear chondritis.

Calcium (+) from calcium chloride, 2% aqueous solution, believed to stabilize the irritability threshold in either direction, as dictated by the physiologic needs of the tissues. Effective with spasmodic conditions, tics, and "snapping fingers" (joints).

Copper (+), from a 2% aqueous solution of copper sulfate crystals; fungicide, astringent, useful with intranasal conditions, e.g., allergic rhinitis ("hay fever"), sinusitis, and also dermatophytosis ("athlete's foot").

Dexamethasone (+) from Decadron, used for treating musculoskeletal inflammatory conditions.

Hyaluronidase (+), from Wydase crystals in aqueous solution as directed; for localized edema.

Lidocaine (+), from XYLOCAINE 5% ointment, anesthetic/analgesic, especially with acute inflammatory conditions, e.g., bursitis, tendinitis, tic doloreux, and TMJ pain.

Lithium (+), from lithium chloride or carbonate, 2% aqueous solution, effective as an exchange ion with gouty tophi and hyperuricemia.*

Magnesium (+), from magnesium sulfate ("Epsom Salts"), 2% aqueous solution, an excellent muscle relaxant, good vasodilator, and mild analgesic.

Mecholyl (+), familiar derivative of acetylcholine, 0.25% ointment, is a powerful vasodilator, good muscle relaxant and analgesic. Used with discogenic low back radiculopathies and sympathetic reflex dystrophy.

Priscoline (+), from benzazoline hydrochloride, 2% aqueous solution, reported effective with indolent ulcers.

Zinc (+), from zinc oxide ointment 20%, a trace element necessary for healing, especially effective with open lesions and ulcerations.

NEGATIVE

Acetate (−), from acetic acid, 2% aqueous solution; dramatically effective as a sclerolytic exchange ion with calcific deposits. +

Chlorine (−), from sodium chloride, 2% aqueous solution, good sclerolytic agent. Useful with scar tissue, keloids, and burns.

Citrate (−), from potassium citrate,2% aqueous solution, reported effective in rheumatoid arthritis.

Iodine (−), from "Iodex" ointment, 4.7%, an excellent sclerolytic agent, as well as bacteriocidal, fair vasodilator. Used successfully with adhesive capsulitis ("frozen shoulder"), scars, etc.

Salicylate (−), from "Iodex with methyl salicylate," 4.8% ointment, a general decongestant, sclerolytic, and anti-inflammatory agent. If desired without the iodine, may be obtained from MYOFLEX ointment (trolamine salicylate 10%) or a 2% aqueous solution of sodium salicylate powder. Used successfully with frozen shoulder, scar tissue, warts, and other adhesive or edematous conditions.

EITHER

Ringer's solution (+/−), with alternating polarity for open decubitus lesions.

Tap water (+/−), usually administered with alternating polarity and sometimes with glycopyrronium bromide in hyperhidrosis.

*The lithium ion replaces the weaker sodium ion in the insoluble sodium urate tophus, converting it to soluble lithium urate.
+ The acetate radical replaces the carbonate radical in the insoluble calcium carbonate calcific deposit, converting it to soluble calcium acetate.
From Kahn J: NonSteroid Iontophoresis, *Clin Manage Phys Ther* 7(1): 14-15, 1987.

TABLE 6-1 Conditions Treated with Iontophoresis

Condition	Ions Used in Treatment
INFLAMMATION	
Bertolucci 1982[2]	Hydrocortisone, salicylate dexamethasone
Chantraine et al. 1986[5]	
Delacerda 1982[8]	
Glass et al. 1980[12]	
Harris 1982[16]	
Hasson 1991[18]	
Kahn 1982[28]	
ANALGESIA	
Gangarosa 1974[10]	Lidocaine, magnesium
Garzione 1978[11]	
Russo et al. 1980[41]	
Schaeffer et al. 1971[42]	
SPASM	
Kahn 1975[24]	Calcium, magnesium
Kahn 1982[27]	
ISCHEMIA	
Kahn 1985[29]	Magnesium, mecholyl, iodine
EDEMA	
Boone 1969[3]	Magnesium, mecholyl, hyaluronidase, salicylate
Kahn 1985[29]	
Magistro 1964[34]	
Schwartz 1955[43]	
CALCIUM DEPOSITS	
Kahn 1977[25]	Acetic acid
Psaki, Carol 1955[39]	
Weider 1992[47]	
SCAR TISSUE	
Kahn 1985[29]	Chlorine, iodine, salicylate
Tannenbaum 1980[46]	
HYPERHYDROSIS	
Abell et al. 1974[1]	Tap water
Grice et al. 1972[14]	
Hill 1976[19]	
Kahn 1973[23]	
Levit 1969[33]	
Shrivastava, Sing 1977[44]	
Stolman 1987[45]	
FUNGI	
Haggard 1939[15]	Copper
Kahn 1985[29]	

Continued.

TABLE 6-1   **Conditions treated with iontophoresis—cont'd**

Condition	Ions Used in Treatment
OPEN SKIN LESIONS	
Cornwall 1981[6]	Zinc
Jenkinson et al. 1974[21]	
ALLERGIC RHINITIS	
Kahn 1985[29]	Copper
GOUT	
Kahn 1982[26]	Lithium
BURNS	
Rapperport et al. 1965[40]	Antibiotics

resting on top of the electrode, since this is likely to create some ischemia (reduced circulation) under the electrode. Instead, the electrode should be held firmly in place with adhesive tape, elastic bands, or lightweight sand bags. It is recommended that both chemical and heat burns be treated with sterile dressings and antibiotics.[23]

Sensitivity Reactions to Ions

Sensitivity reactions to ions rarely occur; however they may be very serious. The sports therapist should routinely question the athlete about known drug allergies before initiating iontophoresis treatment. During the treatment the sports therapist should closely monitor the athlete, looking for either abnormal localized reactions of the skin or systemic reactions.

Athletes who have sensitivity to aspirin may have a reaction when using salicylates. Hydrocortisone may adversely affect individuals with gastritis or an active stomach ulcer. In cases of asthma, mecholyl should be avoided. Athletes who are sensitive to metals should not be treated with copper, zinc, or magnesium. Iodine iontophoresis should not be used with individuals who have allergies to seafood or those who have had a bad reaction to intravenous pyelograms.[23]

SUMMARY

1. Iontophoresis is a therapeutic technique that involves the introduction of ions into the body tissues by means of a direct electrical current.
2. The manner in which ions move in solution forms the basis for iontophoresis. Positively charged ions are driven into the tissues from the positive pole, and negatively charged ions are introduced by the negative pole.
3. The force that acts to move ions through the tissues is determined by both the strength of the electrical field and the electrical impedance of tissues to current flow.
4. The quantity of ions transferred into the tissues through iontophoresis is determined by the intensity of the current or current density at the active electrode, the duration of the current flow, and the concentration of ions in solution.

5. Continuous direct current must be used for iontophoresis, thus ensuring the unidirectional flow of ions that cannot be accomplished using a bidirectional or alternating current.

6. Electrodes available to the sports therapist may be either borrowed from other electrical stimulators or commercially manufactured ready-to-use disposable electrodes.

7. It is critical that the sports therapist be knowledgeable in the selection of the most appropriate ions for treating specific conditions.

8. In sports medicine, iontophoresis is used to treat inflammatory musculoskeletal conditions, for analgesic effects, scar modification, wound healing, and in treating edema, calcium deposits, and hyperhydrosis.

9. Perhaps the single most common problem associated with iontophoresis is a chemical burn that usually occurs as a result of the direct current itself and not because of the ion being used in treatment.

GLOSSARY

acidic reaction The accumulation of negative ions under the positive pole, which produces hydrochloric acid.

active electrode The electrode that is used to drive ions into the tissues.

alkaline reaction The accumulation of positive ions under the negative electrode, which produces sodium hydroxide.

electrolytes Solutions in which ionic movement occurs.

electrophoresis The movement of ions in solution.

ions Positively or negatively charged particles.

ion transfer A technique of transporting chemicals across a membrane using an electrical current as a driving force.

ionization A process by which soluble compounds such as acids, alkaloids, or salts dissociate or dissolve into ions that are suspended in some type of solution.

iontophoresis A therapeutic technique that involves introducing ions into the body tissues by means of a continuous direct electrical current.

REFERENCES

1 Abell E, Morgan K: Treatment of idiopathic hyperhydrosis by glycopyrronium bromide and tap water iontophoresis, *Br J Dermatol* 91: 87, 1974.

2 Bertolucci LE: Introduction of anti-inflammatory drugs by iontophoresis: a double-blind study, *JOSPT* 4(2): 103, 1982.

3 Boone D: Hyaluronidase iontophoresis, *J Am Phys Ther Assoc* 49: 139-145, 1969.

4 Boone D: *Applications of iontophoresis.* In Wolf S, editor: *Electrotherapy*, New York, 1981, Churchill Livingstone.

5 Chantraine A, Lundy JP, Berger D: Is cortisone iontophoresis possible? *Arch Phys Med Rehabil* 67: 380, 1986.

6 Cornwall MW: Zinc oxide iontophoresis for ischemic skin ulcers, *Phys Ther* 61(3): 359, 1981.

7 Cummings J: *Iontophoresis.* In Nelson RM, Currier DP, editors: *Clinical electrotherapy*, Norwalk, Conn, 1991, Appleton & Lange.

8 Delacerda FG: A comparative study of three methods of treatment for shoulder girdle myofascial syndrome, *J Orthop Sports Phys Ther* 4(1): 51-54, 1982.

9 Gadsby PD: Visualization of the barrier layer through iontophoresis of ferric ions, *Med Instrum* 13: 281, 1979.

10 Gangarosa LP: Iontophoresis for surface local anesthesia, *J Am Dent Assoc* 88: 125, 1974.

11 Garzione JE: Salicylate iontophoresis as an alternative treatment for persistent thigh pain following hip surgery, *Phys Ther* 58(5): 570-571, 1978.

12 Glass JM, Stephen RL, Jacobsen SC: The quantity and distribution of radiolabeled dexamethasone delivered to tissues by iontophoresis, *Int J Dermatol* 19: 519, 1980.

13 Glick E, Snyder-Mackler L: *Iontophoresis.* In Snyder-Mackler L, Robinson AJ, editors: *Clinical electrophysiology and electrophysiologic testing*, Baltimore, 1989, Williams & Wilkins.

14 Grice K, Sattar H, Baker H: Treatment of idiopathic hyperhidrosis with iontophoresis of tap water and poldine methosulphate, *Br J Dermatol* 86: 72, 1972.

15 Haggard HW, Strauss MJ, Greenberg LA: Fungous infections of hand and feet treated by copper iontophoresis, *JAMA* 112: 1229, 1939.

16 Harris P: Iontophoresis: clinical research in musculoskeletal inflammatory conditions, *J Orthop Sports Phys Ther* 4(2): 109-112, 1982.

17 Harris R: *Iontophoresis.* In Licht S, (editor): *Therapeutic electricity and ultraviolet radiation*, Waverly, 1967, Baltimore.

18 Hasson SH: Exercise training and dexamethasone iontophoresis in rheumatoid arthritis: a case study, *Physiotherapy Canada* 43: 11, 1991.

19 Hill BHR: Poldine iontophoresis in the treatment of palmar and plantar hyperhidrosis, *Aust J Dermatol* 17: 92, 1976.

20 Jacobson S, Stephen R, Sears W: *Development of a new drug delivery system (iontophoresis)*, Salt Lake City, 1980, University of Utah Press.

21 Jenkinson D, McEwan J, Walton G: The potential use of iontophoresis in the treatment of skin disorders, *Vet Rec* 94: 8-12, 1974.

22 Johnson C, Shuster S: The patency of sweat ducts in normal looking skin, *Br J Dermatol* 83: 367, 1970.

23 Kahn J: *Tap-water iontophoresis for hyperhidrosis.* Reprinted in Medical Group News, August 1973.

24 Kahn J: Calcium iontophoresis in suspected myopathy, JAPTA 55(4): 276, 1975.

25 Kahn J: Acetic acid iontophoresis for calcium deposits, *JAPTA* 57(6): 658, 1977.

26 Kahn J: A case report: lithium iontophoresis for gouty arthritis, *J Orthop Sports Phys Ther* 4: 113, 1982.

27 Kahn J: Iontophoresis: practice tips, *Clin Management* 2(4): 37, 1982.

28 Kahn J: Iontophoresis with hydrocortisone for Peyronie's disease, *JAPTA* 62(7): 995, 1982.

29 Kahn J: *Clinical electrotherapy,* ed 4, Syosset, NY, 1985, Joseph Kahn.

30 Kahn J: Non-steroid iontophoresis, *Clin Manage Phys Ther* 7(1): 14-15, 1987.

31 Kahn J: *Practices and principles of electrotherapy,* New York, 1991, Churchill Livingstone.

32 LeDuc S: *Electric ions and their use in medicine,* Liverpool, 1903, Rebman.

33 Levit R: Simple device for treatment of hyperhidrosis by iontophoresis, *Arch Dermatol* 98: 505-507, 1968.

34 Magistro CM: Hyaluronidase by iontophoresis in the treatment of edema: a preliminary clinical report, *Phys Ther* 44: 169, 1964.

35 Mandleco C: *Research: iontophoresis,* Salt Lake City, 1978, Institute for Biomedical Engineering.

36 Molitor H: Pharmacologic aspects of drug administration by ion transfer, *The Merck Report* 22-9, 1943.

37 Murray W, Levine LS, Seifter E: The iontophoresis of C2 esterified glucocorticoids: preliminary report, *Phys Ther* 43: 579, 1963.

38 O'Malley E, Oester Y: Influence of some physical chemical factors on iontophoresis using radio-isotopes, *Arch Phys Med Rehabil* 36: 310, 1955.

39 Psaki C, Carol J: Acetic acid ionization: a study to determine the absorptive effects upon calcified tendinitis of the shoulder, *Phys Ther* 35: 84, 1955.

40 Rapperport AS: Iontophoresis—a method of antibiotic administration in the burn patient, *Plast Reconstr Surg* 36(5): 547-552, 1965.

41 Russo J, Lipman AG, Comstock TJ, et al.: Lidocane anesthesia: comparison of iontophoresis, injection and swabbing, *Am J Hosp Pharm* 37: 843-847, 1980.

42 Schaeffer ML, Bixler D, Yu P: The effectiveness of iontophoresis in reducing cervical hypersensitivity, *J Periodontol* 42: 695, 1971.

43 Schwartz MS: The use of hyaluronidase by iontophoresis in the treatment of lymphedema, *Arch Intern Med* 95: 662, 1955.

44 Shrivastava SN, Sing G: Tap water iontophoresis in palm and plantar hyperhidrosis, *Br J Dermatol* 96: 189, 1977.

45 Stolman LP: Treatment of excess sweating of the palms by iontophoresis, *Arch Dermatol* 123: 893, 1987.

46 Tannenbaum M: Iodine iontophoresis in reduction of scar tissue, *Phys Ther* 60(6): 792, 1980.

47 Wieder DL: Treatment of traumatic myositis ossificans with acetic acid iontophoresis, *Phys Ther* 72(2): 133-137, 1992.

SUGGESTED READINGS

Abramowitsch D, Neoussikine B: *Treatment by ion transfer,* New York, 1946, Grune & Stratton.

Abramson DI: Physiologic and clinical basis for histamine by ion transfer, *Arch Phys Med Rehabil* 48: 583-592, 1967.

Akins DL, Meisenheimer IL, Dobson RL: Efficacy of the Drionic unit in the treatment of hyperhidrosis, *J Am Acad Dermatol* 16: 828, 1987.

Brummett R, Comeau M: Local anesthesia of the tympanic membrane by iontophoresis, *Trans Am Acad Otolaryngol* 78: 453, 1974.

Comeau M, Brummett R, Vernon J, et al.: Local anesthesia of the ear by iontophoresis, *Arch Otolaryngol* 98: 114-120, 1973.

Comeau M, Brummett R: Anesthesia of the human tympanic membrane by iontophoresis of a local anesthetic, *Laryngoscope* 88: 277-285, 1978.

Falcone AE, Spadaro JA: Inhibitory effects of electrically activated silver material on cutaneous wound bacteria, *Plast Reconstr Surg* 77: 455, 1986.

Fay MF: Indications and applications for iontophoresis, *Today's OR Nurse* 11(4): 10-16, 29-31, 1989.

Gangarosa LP, Park NH, Fong BC: Conductivity of drugs used for iontophoresis, *J Pharm Sci* 67: 1439-1443, 1978.

Gordon AH: Sodium salicytate iontophoresis in the treatment of plantar warts, *Phys Ther* 49: 869-70, 1969.

Haggard HW, Strauss MJ, Greenberg LA: *Copper, electrically injected, cures fungus diseases.* Reprinted in Science Newsletter, May 6, 1939.

Henley EJ: Transcutaneous drug delivery: iontophoresis, phonophoresis, *Phys Med Rehab* 2: 139, 1991.

Jarvis CW, Voita DA: Low voltage skin burns, *Pediatrics* 48: 831, 1971.

Kahn J: Iontophoresis and ultrasound for post-surgical TMJ trismus and paresthesia, *JAPTA* 60(3): 307, 1982.

Kahn J: Iontophoresis in clinical practice, *Stimulus (APTA-SCE)* 8(3), 1983.

Kahn J: Phoresor adaptation, *Clin Manage Phys Ther* 5(4): 50-51, 1985.

Kahn J: *Iontophoresis (video tape),* AREN, Pittsburgh, 1988.

LaForest NT, Confrancisco C: Antibiotic iontophoresis in the treatment of ear chondritis, *JAPTA* 58: 32, 1978.

Langley PL: Iontophoresis to aid in releasing tendon adhesions, *Phys Ther* 64(9): 1395, 1984.

Lemming MN, Cole R, Howland WS: Low voltage direct current burns, *JAMA* 214: 1681, 1970.

Nightingale A: *Physics and electronics in physical medicine,* London, 1959, F. Bell.

Puttemans FJ, Massart DL, Gilles F, et al.: Iontophoresis: mechanism of action studied by potentiometry and x-ray fluorescence, *Arch Phys Med Rehabil* 63: 176-180, 1982.

Sawyer CJ: Cystic fibrosis of the pancreas: a study of sweat electrolyte levels in thirty-six families using pilocarpine iontophoresis, *South Med J* 59: 197-202, 1966.

Shapiro BL: Insulin iontophoresis in cystic fibrosis, *Soc Exp Biol Med* 149: 592-593, 1975.

Shriber W: A *manual of electrotherapy,* ed 4, Philadelphia, 1975, Lea & Febiger.

Sisler HA: Iontophoresis: local anesthesia for conjunctival surgery, *Ann Ophthalmol* 10: 597, 1978

Stillwell GK: *Electrotherapy.* In Kottke F, Stillwell G, Lehman J, editors: *Handbook of physical medicine and rehabilitation,* Philadelphia, 1982, WB Saunders.

Tregear RT: The permeability of mammalian skin to ions, *J Invest Dermat* 46: 16-23, 1966.

Trubatch J, Van Harrevel A: Spread of iontophoretically injected ions in a tissue, *J Theor Biol* 36: 355, 1972.

Waud DR: Iontophoretic applications of drugs, *J App Physiol* 28: 128, 1967.

Zankel HT, Cress RH, Kamin H: Iontophoresis studies with radioactive tracer, *Arch Phys Med Rehabil* 40: 193-196, 1959.

Biofeedback

7

William E. Prentice

OBJECTIVES

After completion of this chapter, the student will be able to do the following:

- Define biofeedback and identify its uses in sports medicine.

- Discuss the various types of biofeedback instruments.

- Explain physiologically how the electrical activity generated by a muscle contraction can be measured using (electromyographic activity) EMG.

- Explain how the electrical activity picked up by electrodes is amplified, processed, and converted to meaningful information by the EMG unit.

- Differentiate between visual and auditory feedback.

- Discuss the equipment set-up and clinical applications for EMG biofeedback.

Electromyographic biofeedback is a modality that seems to be gaining popularity within the sports-medicine community. It is a therapeutic procedure that uses electronic or electromechanical instruments to accurately measure, process, and feedback reinforcing information via auditory or visual signals.[5,11] In sports medicine, it is used to help the athlete develop greater voluntary control in neuromuscular relaxation or muscle reeducation after injury.

THE ROLE OF BIOFEEDBACK

The term biofeedback should be familiar because all sports therapists routinely serve as instruments of biofeedback when teaching a therapeutic exercise or coaching a movement pattern. Using feedback can help the athlete regain function of a muscle that may have been lost or forgotten after injury.[4] Feedback includes information related to the sensations associated with movement, as well as information related to the result of the action relative to some goal or objective. Feedback refers to the intrinsic information inherent to movement including kinesthetic, visual, cutaneous, vestibular, and auditory signals collectively termed as response-produced feedback. It also refers to extrinsic information or some knowledge of results that is presented verbally, mechanically, or electronically to indicate the outcome of some movement performance. Therefore feedback is ongoing, in a temporal sense, occurring before, during, and after any motor or movement task. Feedback from some measuring instrument that provides moment-to-moment information about a biologic function is referred to as biofeedback.[9]

Perhaps the biggest advantage of biofeedback is that it provides the athlete with a chance to make small corrections in performance that are immediately noted and rewarded so that eventually larger changes or improvements in performance can be accomplished. The goal is to train the athlete to perceive these changes without the use of the measuring instrument so that they can practice by themselves. Therefore athletes learn early in the rehabilitation process to do something for themselves and not to totally rely on the sports therapist. This will help them build confidence and increase their feelings of self-efficacy. Treatments using biofeedback would be useful particularly for athletes who have difficulty in perceiving the initial small correct responses or who may have a faulty perception of what they are doing. Hopefully, the rehabilitating athlete will be motivated and encouraged by seeing early signs of slight progress, thus to some extent relieving feelings of helplessness and reducing injury-related stress.[9]

To process feedback information, the athlete makes use of a complicated series of interrelated feedback loops involving very complex anatomic and neurophysiologic components.[15] An in-depth discussion of these components is well beyond the scope of this text. Thus our focus will be oriented toward how biofeedback may best be incorporated in a treatment program.

BIOFEEDBACK INSTRUMENTATION

Biofeedback instruments are designed to monitor some physiologic event, objectively quantify these monitorings, and then interpret the measurements as meaningful information.[12] There are several different types of biofeedback modalities available for use in rehabilitation. These biofeedback units cannot directly measure a physiologic event. Instead, they record some aspect that is highly correlated with the physiologic event. Thus the biofeedback reading should be taken as a convenient indication of a physiologic process but not confused with the physiologic process.[12]

The most commonly used instruments include those that record *peripheral skin temperatures* indicating the extent of vasoconstriction or vasodilation; *finger phototransmission units (photoplethysmograph)* that also measure vasoconstriction and vasodilation; units that record *skin conductance activity* indicating sweat gland activity; and units that measure *EMG* indicating amount of electrical activity during muscle contraction.

Additionally, there are other types of biofeedback units available, including electroencephalographs (EEG), pressure transducers, and electrogoniometers.

Peripheral Skin Temperature

Peripheral skin temperature is an indirect measure of the diameter of peripheral blood vessels. As vessels dilate, more warm blood is delivered to a particular area, thus increasing the temperature in that area. This effect is easily seen in the fingers and toes where the surrounding tissue warms and cools rapidly. Variations in skin temperature seem to be correlated with affective states with a decrease occurring in response to stress or fear. Temperature changes are usually measured in degrees Farenheit.[12]

Finger Phototransmission

The degree of peripheral vasoconstriction can also be measured indirectly using a photoplethysmograph. This instrument monitors the amount of light that can pass through a finger or toe, reflect off a bone, and pass back through the soft tissue to a light sensor. As the volume of blood in a given area increases, the amount of light detected by the sensor decreases, thus giving some indication of blood volume. Only changes in blood volume can be detected, since there are no standardized units of measure. These instruments are used most often to monitor pulse.[6]

Skin Conductance Activity

Sweat gland activity can be indirectly measured by determining electrodermal activity most commonly referred to as the galvanic skin response. Sweat contains salt, which increases electrical conductivity. Thus sweaty skin is more conductive than dry skin. This instrument applies a very small electrical voltage to the skin, usually on the palmar surface of the hand or the volar surface of the fingers where there are a lot of sweat glands, and measures the impedance of the electrical current in microhm units. Measuring skin conductance is a technique useful in objectively assessing psychophysiologic arousal and is most often used in "lie detector" testing.[12]

EMG BIOFEEDBACK

EMG biofeedback is certainly the most typically used of all the biofeedback modalities in a sports-medicine setting. Muscle contraction results from the more or less syncronous contraction of individual muscle fibers that compose a muscle. Individual muscle fibers are innervated by nerves that collectively comprise a motor unit. The axon of that motor unit conducts an action potential to the neuromuscular junction where a neurotransmitter substance (acetylcholine) is released. As this neurotransmitter binds to receptor sites on the sarcolemma, depolarization of that muscle fiber occurs in both directions along the muscle fiber, creating movement of ions and thus an electrochemical gradient around the muscle fiber. Changes in potential difference or voltage associated with depolarization can be detected by an electrode placed in close proximity to the muscle fiber (Figure 7-1).

Motor Unit Recruitment

The amount of tension developed in a muscle is determined by the number of active motor units. As more motor units are recruited and as the frequency of discharge increases, muscle tension increases.

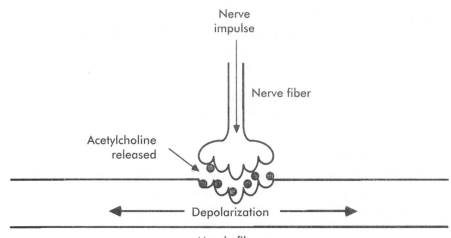

Fig. 7-1. The nerve fiber conducts an impulse to the neuromuscular junction, triggering the release of acetylcholine into the synaptic cleft. The acetylcholine binds to receptor sites on the sarcolemma causing a depolarization of the muscle fiber that creates movement of ions and thus an electrochemical gradient around the muscle fiber.

The pattern of motor unit recruitment varies depending on the inherent properties of specific motorneurons, the force required during the activity, and the speed of contraction. Smaller motor units are recruited first and are somewhat limited in their ability to generate tension. Larger motor units generate greater tension since more muscle fibers are recruited. Motor units are recruited based on the force required in an activity and not on the type of contraction performed. Thus the firing rate and recruitment of the motor units depend on the external force required. The speed of contraction also influences motor unit recruitment. Fast contractions tend to excite larger motor units and depress smaller motor units.

Measuring Electrical Activity

Although EMG is used to determine muscle activity, it does not measure muscle contraction directly. Instead, it measures electrical activity associated with muscle contraction. Movement of ions across the membrane creates a depolarization of the muscle membranes, resulting in a reversal in polarity, followed by repolarization. The various stages of membrane activity generate a triphasic electrical signal.[1] Electrical activity of the muscle is measured in volts or, more precisely, microvolts. (1 V = 1,000,000 μV)

Electrical activity is measured in standard quantitative units. Monitoring is useful in detecting changes in electrical activity, although changes cannot be quantified. The advantage of measurement over monitoring is that an objective scale is used on which comparisons can be made between different individuals, occasions, and instruments. Measurement allows *procedures* to be replicated.

Unfortunately with EMG biofeedback units there is no universally accepted standardized measurement scale. Each brand of EMG unit serves as its own reference standard. Different brands of EMG equipment may give different readings for the same

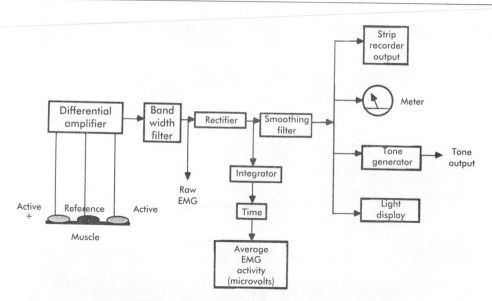

Fig. 7-2. The anatomy of a typical EMG biofeedback unit.

degree of muscle contraction. Consequently, EMG readings can be compared only when the same equipment is used for all readings.[12]

The EMG biofeedback unit receives small amounts of electrical energy generated during muscle contraction through some type of electrode. It then separates or filters this electrical energy from other extraneous electrical activity on the skin and amplifies the EMG electrical energy. The amplified EMG activity is then converted to some type of information that has meaning to the user. Figure 7-2 is a diagram of the various components of an EMG biofeedback unit.

ELECTRODES. Skin surface electrodes are most often used in EMG biofeedback. Fine-wire indwelling electrodes may also be used that permit localized highly accurate measurement of electrical activity. However these electrodes must be inserted percutaneously and thus are relatively impractical in a sports-medicine setting.

Various types of surface electrodes are available for use with EMG biofeedback units. Electrodes are most often made of stainless steel or nickel-plated brass recessed in a plastic holder. These less expensive electrodes are effective in EMG biofeedback applications. More expensive electrodes made of gold or silver/silver chloride have also been used.[14]

The size of the electrodes may range between 4 mm in diameter for recording small muscle activity and 12.5 mm for use with larger muscle groups. Increasing the size of the electrode will not cause an increase in the amplitude of the signal.[8]

Regardless of whether electrodes are disposable or nondisposable, some type of conducting gel, paste, or cream with high salt content is necessary to establish a highly conductive connection with the skin. Disposable electrodes come with the appropriate amount of gel and an adhesive ring already applied so that the electrode can be easily connected to the skin. Nondisposable electrodes need to have a double-sided adhesive ring applied. Then enough conducting gel must be added such that it is level with the surface of the adhesive ring before the electrode is applied to the skin.

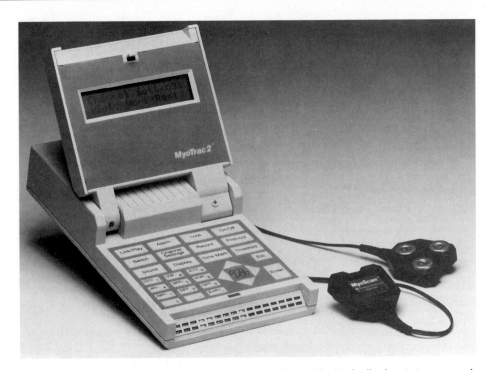

Fig. 7-3. MyoTrac 2 dual channel, portable EMG unit is shown. The biofeedback unit is connected via a series of electrodes to the skin over the contracting muscle.

Before attachment of the surface electrodes, the skin must be appropriately prepared by removing oil and dead skin along with excessive hair from the surface to reduce skin impedance. Scrubbing with an alcohol-soaked prep pad is recommended.[14] However, if the skin is cleaned until it becomes irritated it may interfere with EMG recording.

Some surface electrodes are permanently attached to cable wires, while others may snap onto the wire. Some biofeedback units include a set of three electrodes preplaced on a velcro band that may be easily attached to the skin.

Electrode placement. The electrodes should be placed as near to the muscle being monitored as possible to minimize recording extraneous electrical activity. They should be secured with the body part in the position in which it will be monitored so that movement of the skin will not alter the positioning of the electrodes over a particular muscle[4] (Figure 7-3).

The electrodes should be parallel to the direction of the muscle fibers to ensure that a better sample of muscle activity is monitored while reducing extraneous electrical activity.

Spacing of the electrodes is also a critical consideration. Electrodes generally detect measurable signals from a distance equal to that of the interelectrode spacing. Therefore as the distance between the electrodes increases, the EMG signal will include electrical activity not only from muscles directly under the electrodes but also from other nearby muscles.[1]

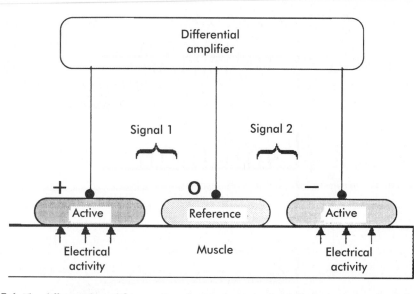

Fig. 7-4. The differential amplifier monitors the two separate signals from the active electrodes and amplifies the difference, thus eliminating extraneous noise.

SEPARATION AND AMPLIFICATION OF EMG ACTIVITY. Once electrical activity is detected by the electrodes, the extraneous electrical activity or **noise** must be eliminated before the EMG activity is amplified and subsequently objectified. This is accomplished by using two **active electrodes** and a single ground or **reference electrode** in a **bipolar arrangement** to create three separate pathways from the skin to the biofeedback unit (Figure 7-4). The active electrodes should be placed in close proximity to one another, while the reference electrode may be placed anywhere on the body. Typically in biofeedback, the reference electrode is placed between the two active electrodes.

The active electrodes pick up electrical activity from motor units firing in the muscles beneath the electrodes. The magnitude of the small voltages detected by each active electrode will differ with respect to the reference electrode, creating two separate signals. These two signals are then fed to a **differential amplifier** that basically subtracts the signal from one active electrode from the other active electrode. This in effect cancels out or rejects any components that the two signals coming from the active electrodes have in common, thus amplifying the difference between the signals. The differential amplifier uses the reference electrode to compare the signals of the two active or recording electrodes (see Figure 7-4).

There will always be some degree of extraneous electrical activity created by power lines, motors, lights, appliances, etc., that is picked up by the body and eventually is detected by the surface electrodes on the skin. Assuming that this extraneous noise is detected equally by both active electrodes, the differential amplifier will subtract the noise detected by one active electrode from the noise detected by the other active electrode, leaving only the true difference between the active electrodes. The ability of the differential amplifier to eliminate the common noise between the active electrodes is called the **common mode rejection ratio (CMRR).**

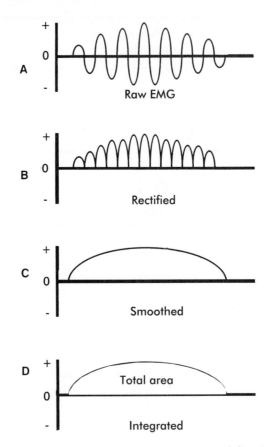

Fig. 7-5. Processing an EMG signal involves taking **A**, raw EMG and then **B**, rectifying, **C**, smoothing, and **D**, integrating it so that the information can be presented in some meaningful format.

External noise can be further reduced by using **filters** that essentially make the amplifier more sensitive to some incoming frequencies and less sensitive to others. Therefore the amplifier will pick up signals only at those frequencies produced by electrical activity in the muscle within a specific frequency range or **bandwidth.** In general, the wider the bandwidth, the higher the EMG and noise readings.

The sports therapist is interested in measuring the electrical activity within the muscle. Excessive external noise that is not eliminated by the biofeedback instrument will mask true EMG activity and will significantly decrease the reliability of the information being generated by that device.

Converting EMG Activity to Meaningful Information

After amplification and filtering, the EMG signal is indicative of the true electrical activity within the muscles being monitored. This is referred to as raw EMG activity. **Raw EMG** is an alternating voltage, which means that the direction or polarity is constantly reversing (Figure 7-5, *A*). The amplitude of the oscillations increases to a maximum and then diminishes. Biofeedback measures the overall increase and decrease in electrical activity. To obtain this measurement the deflection toward the negative pole must be flipped upward toward the positive pole, otherwise the sum total of the deflections would be zero, since they would cancel out one another (Figure 7-5, *B*). This process, referred to as **rectification,** essentially creates a pulsed direct current.

PROCESSING THE EMG SIGNAL. The rectified EMG signal can be smoothed and integrated. **Smoothing** the EMG signal means eliminating the peaks and valleys or eliminating the high frequency fluctuations that are produced with a changing electrical signal (Figure 7-5, *C*). Once the EMG has been smoothed, the signal may be **integrated** by measuring the area under the curve for a specified period of time. Integration forms the basis for quantification of EMG activity (Figure 7-5, *D*).

At this point it is necessary to take this rectified, smoothed, and integrated EMG signal and display this information in a form that has some meaning. Biofeedback units generally provide either visual or auditory feedback relative to the quantity of electrical activity. Some biofeedback units can provide both visual and auditory feedback depending on the output mode selected.

VISUAL FEEDBACK. Raw EMG activity is usually displayed visually on an oscilloscope. On most biofeedback units, integrated EMG activity is visually presented as a line travelling across a monitor, as a light or series of lights that go on and off, or as a bar graph that changes dimension, all of which change in response to the incoming integrated signal. Some of the newer EMG units have incorporated video games as part of their visual feedback systems. If a biofeedback unit uses some type of meter, it may either be calibrated in objective units such as microvolts or given some relative scale of measure.[14]

Meters may also be either analogue or digital. Analogue meters have a continuous scale and a needle that indicates the level of electrical activity within a particular range. Digital meters display only a number. They are very simple and easy to read. However, the disadvantage of a digital meter is that it is more difficult to tell where in a given range the signal falls.

AUDIO FEEDBACK. On some biofeedback units, raw EMG activity is presented in an audio format. The majority of biofeedback units have audio feedback, which produces some tone, buzzing, beeping, or clicking. An increase in the pitch of a tone, buzz, or beep or an increase in the frequency of clicking indicates an increase in the level of EMG activity. This would be most useful for individuals who need to strengthen muscle contractions. Conversely, decreases in pitch or frequency indicating a decrease in EMG activity would be most useful in teaching athletes to relax.

SETTING SENSITIVITY. Signal sensitivity or **signal gain** may be set by the sports therapist on many biofeedback units. If a high gain is chosen the biofeedback unit will have a high sensitivity for the muscle activity signal. Sensitivity may be set at 1 μV, 10 μV, or 100 μV. A 1 μV setting is sensitive enough to detect the smallest amounts of electrical activity and thus has the highest signal gain. High sensitivity levels should be used during relaxation training. Comparatively lower sensitivity levels would be more useful in muscle-reeducation during which the athlete may produce several hundred μV of EMG activity. Generally, when adjusting the sensitivity range it should be set at the lowest level that does not elicit feedback at rest.

EQUIPMENT SET-UP AND APPLICATION

It is imperative that the sports therapist have some understanding of how biofeedback units monitor and record the electrical activity being produced in a muscle before attempting to set-up and use the biofeedback unit in treatment of an athlete. Specific treatment protocols involve skin preparation, application of electrodes, selection of feedback or output modes, and selection of sensitivity settings. Once these are complete, the sports therapist should choose to have the athlete sitting, lying, or occasionally standing in a comfortable position depending on the treatment objectives. Generally the sports therapist should begin with easier tasks and progressively make the activities more difficult. Teaching the athlete how to appropriately use the biofeedback unit and briefly explaining what is being measured are essential. In most cases, it is recommended that the sports therapist attach the biofeedback unit to themselves and then demonstrate to the athlete exactly what is to be done during the treatment.[8]

There are essentially three treatment objectives for using biofeedback: muscle reeducation, which involves regaining neuromuscular control or increasing strength of a muscle; relaxation of muscle spasm or muscle guarding; and pain reduction.

Muscle Reeducation

The goal in muscle reeducation is to provide feedback that will reestablish or promote the ability of that muscle to contract. EMG biofeedback is used to indicate the electrical activity associated with that muscle contraction.

When biofeedback is being used to elicit a muscle contraction, the sensitivity setting should be chosen by having the athlete perform a maximum isometric contraction of the target muscle. The gain should then be adjusted such that the athlete will be able to achieve the maximum on about two thirds of the muscle contractions. If the athlete cannot produce a muscle contraction, the sports therapist should attempt to facilitate a contraction by stroking or tapping the target muscle. It is also helpful to have the athlete look at the muscle when trying to contract. It may be necessary to move the active electrodes to the contralateral limb and have the athlete practice the muscle contraction you hope to achieve on the opposite side.

The athlete should maximally contract the target muscle isometrically for 6 to 10 seconds. During this contraction, the visual or auditory feedback should be at a maximum and should be closely monitored by both the sports therapist and the athlete. Between each contraction the athlete should be instructed to completely relax the muscle such that the feedback mode returns to baseline or zero before initiating another contraction. A period of 5 to 10 minutes working with a single muscle or muscle group is most desirable, since longer periods tend to produce fatigue and boredom, neither of which is conducive to optimal learning.[7]

As increases in EMG activity occur, the athlete should develop the ability to rapidly activate motor units. This can be accomplished by setting the sensitivity level to 60% to 80% of maximum isometric activity and instructing the athlete to reach that level as many times as possible during a given time period (i.e., 10 or 30 seconds). Again, total relaxation must occur between contractions.

For the athlete, it is essential that the treatment be functionally relevant. Attention to mobility and muscle power cannot be neglected in favor of biofeedback therapy.[7]

The sports therapist should have the athlete perform functional movements while simultaneously observing body mechanics and the related EMG activity. Then recommendations can be made as to how movements can be altered to elicit normal EMG responses.[8] It must be stressed that for the athletic patient population, biofeedback is most useful in patients who perform poorly on manual muscle tests. If the athlete can only elicit a fair, trace, or zero grade, then biofeedback should be incorporated. Stronger muscles should generally be given resistive exercises rather than biofeedback,[7] although biofeedback has been recommended for increasing the strength of healthy muscle.[3]

Relaxation of Muscle Guarding

The majority of athletes demonstrate a protective response in muscle that occurs because of pain or fear of movement that is most accurately described as **muscle guarding.**

Muscle guarding must be differentiated from those neuromuscular problems arising from central nervous system deficits that result in a clinical condition known as muscle spasticity. The sports therapist must usually treat athletes exhibiting muscle guarding. Thus the goal is to induce relaxation of the muscle by reducing EMG activity through the use of biofeedback.[7]

Since muscle guarding most often involves fear of pain that may result when the muscle moves, perhaps the most important goal in treatment is to modulate pain. This is best accomplished through the use of other modalities such as ice or electrical stimulation.

Biofeedback treatments should be designed so that the athlete experiences success from the first treatment. The athlete is now attempting to reduce the visual or auditory feedback to zero. Initially, positioning of the athlete in a comfortable relaxed position is critical to reducing muscle guarding. A high sensitivity setting should be selected so that any electrical activity in the muscle will be easily detected.

During relaxation training the athlete should be given verbal cues that will enhance relaxation of either individual muscles, muscle groups, or body segments. For example, with individual muscles or small muscle groups, the athlete may be instructed to contract then relax a specific muscle or to imagine a feeling of warmth within the muscle. For larger muscle groups, using mental imagery or deep-breathing exercises may be useful.

As relaxation progresses, the spacing between the electrodes should be increased. Also, the sensitivity setting should move from low to high. Both of these changes will require the athlete to relax more muscles, thus achieving greater relaxation. The athlete must then apply this newly learned relaxation technique in different positions that are potentially more uncomfortable. Again, the goal is to eliminate muscle guarding during functional activities.[7]

Pain Reduction

A number of therapeutic modalities discussed in this text are used to reduce or modulate pain. As mentioned in the section on muscle guarding, biofeedback can be used to relax muscles that are tense because of fear of pain on movement. If the muscle can be relaxed, then chances are that pain will also be reduced by breaking the "pain-guarding-pain" cycle. It has been experimentally demonstrated to reduce pain in headaches,[2] and low back pain.[10] Pain modulation is often associated with techniques of imagery and progressive relaxation.

SUMMARY

1. Biofeedback is a therapeutic procedure that uses electronic or electromechanical instruments to accurately measure, process, and feedback reinforcing information via auditory or visual signals.
2. Perhaps the biggest advantage of biofeedback is that it provides the athlete with a chance to make small corrections in performance that are immediately noted and rewarded so that eventually larger changes or improvements in performance can be accomplished.
3. Several different types of biofeedback modalities are available for use in rehabilitation, with EMG biofeedback being the most widely used in sports medicine.
4. An EMG biofeedback unit measures the electrical activity produced by depolarization of a muscle fiber as an indicator of the quality of a muscle contraction.
5. The EMG biofeedback unit receives small amounts of electrical energy generated during muscle contraction through active electrodes, then separates or filters extraneous electrical energy via a differential amplifier before it is processed and subsequently converted to some type of information that has meaning to the user.
6. Biofeedback information is displayed either through visual, using lights or meters, or auditory, using tones, beeps, buzzes, or clicks, means.
7. High sensitivity levels should be used during relaxation training while comparatively low sensitivity levels would be more useful in muscle reeducation.
8. In sports medicine, biofeedback is most typically used for muscle reeducation, to decrease muscle guarding, or for pain reduction.

GLOSSARY

active electrode An electrode attached directly to the skin over a muscle that picks up the electrical activity produced by a muscle contraction.

bandwidth A specific frequency range in which the amplifier will pick up signals produced by electrical activity in the muscle.

bipolar arrangement Two active recording electrodes placed in close proximity to one another.

common mode rejection ratio (CMRR) The ability of the differential amplifier to eliminate the common noise between the active electrodes.

differential amplifier Monitors the two separate signals from the active electrodes and amplifies the difference, thus eliminating extraneous noise.

electromyographic biofeedback A therapeutic procedure that uses electronic or electromechanical instruments to accurately measure, process, and feedback reinforcing information via auditory or visual signals.

filters Devices that help to reduce external noise that essentially makes the amplifier more sensitive to some incoming frequencies and less sensitive to others.

integration An EMG signal processing technique that measures the area under the curve for a specified period of time, thus forming the basis for quantification of EMG activity.

muscle guarding A protective response in muscle that occurs because of pain or fear of movement.

noise Extraneous electrical activity that may be produced by any source other than the contracting muscle.

raw EMG A form in which the electrical activity produced by muscle contraction may be displayed or recorded before the signal is processed.

rectification A signal processing technique that changes the deflection of the waveform from the negative pole to the positive pole, essentially creating a pulsed direct current.

reference electrode Also referred to as the ground electrode, serves as a point of reference to compare the electrical activity recorded by the active electrodes.

signal gain Determines the signal sensitivity. If a high gain is chosen the biofeedback unit will have a high sensitivity for the muscle activity signal.

smoothing An EMG signal processing technique that eliminates the high frequency fluctuations that are produced with a changing electrical signal.

REFERENCES

1 Basmajian JV: *Description and analysis of EMG signal.* In Basmajian JV, Deluca C, editors: *Muscles alive: their functions revealed by electromyography,* Baltimore, 1985, Williams & Wilkins.

2 Budzynski C: *Biofeedback strategies in headache treatment.* In Basmajian JV, editor: *Biofeedback: principles and practice for clinicians,* Baltimore, 1989, Williams & Wilkins.

3 Croce RV: The effects of EMG biofeedback on strength acquisition, *Biofeedback Self Regul* 9: 395, 1986.

4 Draper V: Electromyographic feedback and recovery in quadriceps femoris muscle function following anterior cruciate ligament reconstruction, *Phys Ther* 70: 25, 1990.

5 Fogel ER: *Biofeedback-assisted musculoskeletal therapy and neuromuscular reeducation.* In Schwartz MS, editor: *Biofeedback: a practitioners guide,* New York, 1987, The Guilford Press.

6 Jennings JR, Tahmoush AJ, Redmond DD: *Non-invasive measurement of peripheral vascular activity.* In Martin I, Venables PH, editors: *Techniques in psychophysiology,* New York, 1980, Wiley.

7 Krebs DE: *Neuromuscular re-education and gait training.* In Schwartz MS, editor: *Biofeedback: a practitioners guide.* New York, 1987, The Guilford Press.

8 LeCraw DE, Wolf SL: *Electromyographic biofeedback (EMGBF) for neuromuscular relaxation and re-education.* In Gersh MR, editor: *Electrotherapy in rehabilitation,* Philadelphia, 1992, FA Davis.

9 Miller NE: *Biomedical foundations for biofeedback as a part of behavioral medicine.* In Basmajian JV, editor: *Biofeedback principles and practice for clinicians,* Baltimore, 1989, Williams & Wilkins.

10 Nouwen A, Bush C: The relationship between paraspinal EMG and chronic low back pain, *Pain* 20: 109-123, 1984.

11 Olson RP: *Definitions of biofeedback.* In Schwartz MS, editor: *Biofeedback: a practitioners guide,* New York, 1987, The Guilford Press.

12 Peek CJ: *A primer of biofeedback instrumentation.* In Schwartz MS, editor: *Biofeedback: a practitioners guide,* New York, 1987, The Guilford Press.

13 Wolf SL: *Treatment of neuromuscular problems, Treatment of musculoskeletal problems.* In Sandweiss J, editor: *Biofeedback review seminars,* Los Angles, 1982, University of California.

14 Wolf SL, Binder-Macleod SA: *Electromyographic feedback in the physical therapy clinic.* In Basmajian JV, editor: *Biofeedback: principles and practice for clinicians,* Baltimore, 1989, Williams & Wilkins.

15 Wolf SL, Binder-Macleod SA: *Neurophysiological factors in electromyographic feedback for neuromotor disturbances.* In Basmajian JV, editor: *Biofeedback: principles and practice for clinicians,* Baltimore, 1989, Williams & Wilkins.

SUGGESTED READINGS

Amato A, Hermomeyer CA, Kleinman KM: Use of electromyographic feedback to increase control of spastic muscles, *Phys Ther* 53: 1063, 1973.

Andrews JM: Neuromuscular reeducation of the hemiplegic with the aid of the electromyograph, *Arch Phys Med Rehabil* 45: 530, 1964.

Asato H, Twiggs DG, Ellison S: EMG biofeedback training for a mentally retarded individual with cerebral palsy, *Phys Ther* 61: 1447-1451, 1981.

Baker MP, Hudson JE, Wolf SL: ''Feedback'' cane to improve the hemiplegic patient's gait: suggestion from the field, *Phys Ther* 59: 170, 1979.

Baker MP, Regenos E, Wolf SL, et al.: Developing strategies for biofeedback: applications in neurologically handicapped patients, *Phys Ther* 57: 402-408, 1977.

Balliet R, Levy B, Blood KMT: Upper extremity sensory feedback therapy in chronic cerebrovascular accident patients with impaired expressive aphasia and auditory comprehension, *Arch Phys Med Rehabil* 67: 304, 1986.

Basmajian JV: *Learned control of single motor units.* In Schwartz GE, Beatty J, editors: *Biofeedback: theory and research,* New York, 1977, Academic Press.

Basmajian JV: Biofeedback in rehabilitation: a review of principles and practices, *Arch Phys Med Rehabil* 62: 469, 1981.

Basmajian JV: *Biofeedback: principles and practice for clinicians,* Baltimore, 1989, Williams & Wilkins.

Basmajian JV, Blumenthal R: *Electroplacement in electromyographic biofeedback.* In Basmajian JV, editor: *Biofeedback: principles and practice for clinicians,* ed 3, Baltimore, 1989, Williams & Wilkins.

Basmajian JV, Kukulka CG, Narayan MG, et al.: Biofeedback treatment of foot drop after stroke compared with standard rehabilitation technique: effects on voluntary control and strength, *Arch Phys Med Rehabil* 56: 231-236, 1975.

Basmajian JV, Regenos EM, Baker MP: Rehabilitating stroke patients with biofeedback, *Geriatrics* 32: 85, 1977.

Basmajian JV, Samson J: Special review: standardization of methods in single motor unit training, *Am J Phys Med* 52: 250-256, 1973.

Beal MS, Diefenbach G, Allen A: Electromyographic biofeedback in the treatment of voluntary posterior instability of the shoulder, *Am J Sports Med* 15: 175, 1987.

Biedermann HJ: Comments on the reliability of muscle activity comparisons in EMG biofeedback research with back pain patients, *Biofeedback Self Regul* 9: 451-458, 1984.

Biedermann HJ, McGhie A, Monga TN, et al.: Perceived and actual control in EMG treatment of back pain, *Behav Res Ther* 25: 137-147, 1987.

Bowman BR, Baker LL, Waters RL: Positional feedback and electrical stimulation: an automated treatment for the hemiplegic wrist, *Arch Phys Med Rehabil* 60: 497, 1979.

Brudny J, Grynbaum BL, Korein J: Spasmodic torticollis: treatment by feedback display of EMG, *Arch Phys Med Rehabil* 55: 403-408, 1974.

Burke RE: *Motor unit recruitment: what are the critical factors?* In Desmedt JE, editor: *Progress in clinical neurophysiology,* vol 9, Basel, Switzerland, 1981, Karger.

Burnside IG, Tobias HS, Bursill D: Electromyographic feedback in the rehabilitation of stroke patients: a controlled trial, *Arch Phys Med Rehabil* 63: 217, 1982.

Burnside IG, Tobias HS, Bursill D: Electromyographic feedback in the remobilization of stroke patients: a controlled trial, *Arch Phys Med Rehabil* 63: 1393, 1983.

Bush C, Ditto B, Feuerstein M: A controlled evaluation of paraspinal EMG biofeedback in the treatment of chronic low back pain, *Health Psychol* 4: 307-321, 1985.

Carlsson SG: Treatment of temporo-mandibular joint syndrome with biofeedback training, *J Am Dent Assoc* 91: 602-605, 1975.

Chapman SL: A review and clinical perspective on the use of EMG and thermal biofeedback for chronic headaches, *Pain* 27: 1, 1986.

Christie DJ, Dewitt RA, Kaltenbach P, et al.: Using EMG biofeedback to signal hyperactive children when to relax, *Except Child* 50: 547-548, 1984.

Cox RJ, Matyas TA: Myoelectric and force feedback in the facilitation of isometric strength training: a controlled comparison, *Psychophysiology* 20: 35-44, 1983.

Cummings MS, Wilson VE, Bird EI: Flexibility development in sprinters using EMG biofeedback and relaxation training, *Biofeedback Self Regul* 9: 395-405, 1984.

Debacher GA: *Feedback goniometers for rehabilitation.* In Basmajian JV, editor: *Biofeedback: principles and practice for clinicians,* Baltimore, 1983, Williams & Wilkins.

Deluca C: *Apparatus, detection, and recording techniques.* In Basmajian JV, Deluca C, editors: *Muscles alive: their functions revealed by electromyography,* Baltimore, 1985, Williams & Wilkins.

English AW, Wolf SL: The motor unit: anatomy and physiology, *Phys Ther* 62: 1763, 1982.

Fields RW: Electromyographically triggered electric muscle stimulation for chronic hemiplegia, *Arch Phys Med Rehabil* 68: 407-414, 1987.

Flom RP, Quast JE, Boller JD, et al.: Biofeedback training to overcome post stroke footdrop, *Geriatrics* 31: 47-51, 1976.

Flor H, Haag G, Turk DC, et al.: Efficacy of EMG biofeedback, pseudotherapy, and conventional medical treatment for chronic rheumatic back pain, *Pain* 17: 21-31, 1983.

Flor H, Haag G, Turk DC: Long-term efficacy of EMG biofeedback for chronic rheumatic back pain, *Pain* 27: 195-202, 1986.

Gaarder KR, Montgomery PS: *Clinical biofeedback: a procedural manual,* Baltimore, 1977, Williams & Wilkins.

Goodgold JE, Eberstein A: *Electrodiagnosis of neuromuscular diseases,* Baltimore, 1972, Williams & Wilkins.

Green EE, Walters ED, Green AM, et al.: Feedback technology for deep relaxation, *Psychophysiology* 6: 371-377, 1969.

Hijzen TH, Slangen JL, van Houweligen HC: Subjective, clinical and EMG effects of biofeedback and splint treatment, *J Oral Rehabil* 13: 529-539, 1986.

Hirasawa Y, Uchiza Y, Kusswetter W: EMG biofeedback therapy for rupture of the extensor pollicis longus tendon, *Arch Orthop Trauma Surg* 104: 342, 1986.

Honer L, Mohr T, Roth R: Electromyographic biofeedback to dissociate an upper extremity synergy pattern: a case report, *Phys Ther* 62: 299-303, 1982.

Ince LP, Leon MS: Biofeedback treatment of upper extremity dysfunction in Guillain-Barré syndrome, *Arch Phys Med Rehabil* 67: 30-33, 1986.

Ince LP, Leon MS, Christidis D: Experimental foundations of EMG biofeedback with the upper extremity: a review of the literature, *Biofeedback Self Regul* 9: 371-383, 1984.

Ince LP, Leon MS, Christidis D: EMG biofeedback with upper extremity musculature for relaxation training: a critical review of the literature, *J Behav Ther Exp Psychiatry* 16: 133-137, 1985.

Inglis J, Donald MW, Monga TN, et al.: Electromyographic biofeedback and physical therapy of the hemiplegic upper limb, *Arch Phys Med Rehabil* 65: 755-759, 1984.

Johnson HE, Garton WH: Muscle reeducation in hemiplegia by use of electromyographic device, *Arch Phys Med Rehabil* 54: 322-323, 1973.

Johnson HE, Hockersmith V: *Therapeutic electromyography in chronic back pain.* In Basmajian JV, editor: *Biofeedback: principles and practice for clinicians,* ed 2, Baltimore, 1983, Williams & Wilkins.

Johnson R, Lee K: Myofeedback: a new method of teaching breathing exercise to emphysematous patients, *J Am Phys Ther Assoc* 56: 826-829, 1976.

Kelly JL, Baker MP, Wolf SL: Procedures for EMG biofeedback training in involved upper extremities of hemiplegic patients, *Phys Ther* 59: 1500, 1979.

King AC, Ahles TA, Martin JE, et al.: EMG biofeedback-controlled exercise in chronic arthritic knee pain, *Arch Phys Med Rehabil* 65: 341-343, 1984.

Kleppe D, Groendijk HE, Huijing PA, et al.: Single motor unit control in the human mm. abductor pollicis brevis and mylohyoideus in relation to the number of muscle spindles, *Electromyogr Clin Neurophysiol* 22: 21-25, 1982.

Krebs DE: *Biofeedback in neuromuscular reeducation and gait training.* In Schwartz MS, editor: *Biofeedback: a practitioner's guide,* New York, 1987, The Guilford Press.

Large RG: Prediction of treatment response in pain patients: the illness self-concept repertory grid and EMG feedback, *Pain* 21: 279-287, 1985.

Large RG, Lamb AM: Electromyographic (EMG) feedback in chronic musculoskeletal pain: a controlled trial, *Pain* 17: 167-177, 1983.

Lucca JA, Recchiuti SI: Effect of electromyographic biofeedback on an isometric strengthening program, *Phys Ther* 63: 200-203, 1983.

Marinacci AA, Horande M: Electromyogram in neuromuscular reeducation, *Bull LA Neurol Soc* 25, 57-67, 1960.

Mims HW: Electromyography in clinical practice, *South Med J* 49: 804, 1956.

Morasky RL, Reynolds C, Clarke G: Using biofeedback to reduce left arm extensor EMG of string players during musical performance, *Biofeedback Self Regul* 6: 565-572, 1981.

Mulder T, Hulstijn W: Delayed sensory feedback in the learning of a novel motor task, *Psychol Res* 47: 203-209, 1985.

Mulder T, Hulstijn W, van der Meer J: EMG feedback and the restoration of motor control: a controlled group study of 12 hemiparetic patients, *Am J Phys Med* 65: 173-188, 1986.

Nafpliotis H: EMG feedback to improve ankle dorsiflexion, wrist extension and hand grasp, *Phys Ther* 56: 821-825, 1976.

Nouwen A: EMG biofeedback used to reduce standing levels of paraspinal muscle tension in chronic low back pain, *Pain* 17: 353-360, 1983.

Nouwen A, Bush C: The relationship between paraspinal EMG and chronic low back pain, *Pain* 20: 109-123, 1984.

Poppen R, Maurer JP: Electromyographic analysis of relaxed postures, *Biofeedback Self Regul* 7: 491-498, 1982.

Regenos EM, Wolf SL: Involuntary single motor unit discharges in spastic muscles during EMG biofeedback training, *Arch Phys Med Rehabil* 60: 72-73, 1979.

Russell G, Woolbridge CP: Correction of a habitual head tilt using biofeedback techniques—a case study, *Physiotherapy Canada* 27: 181-184, 1975.

Studkey SJ, Jacobs A, Goldfarb J: EMG biofeedback training, relaxation training, and placebo for the relief of chronic back pain, *Percept Mot Skills* 63: 1023, 1986.

Swaan D, van Wiergen PCW, Fokkema SD: Auditory electromyographic feedback therapy to inhibit undesired motor activity, *Arch Phys Med Rehabil* 55: 251, 1974.

Winchester P: Effects of feedback stimulation training and cyclical electrical stimulation on knee extension in hemiparetic patients, *Phys Ther* 63: 1097, 1983.

Wolf SL: Essential considerations in the use of EMG biofeedback, *Phys Ther* 58: 25, 1978.

Wolf SL: EMG biofeedback application in physical rehabilitation: an overview, *Physiotherapy Canada* 31: 65, 1979.

Wolf SL: Electromyographic biofeedback in exercise programs, *Phys Sports Med* 8: 61-69, 1980.

Wolf SL: *Fallacies of clinical EMG measures from patients with musculoskeletal and neuromuscular disorders.* Paper presented at the 14th annual meeting of the Biofeedback Society of America, Denver, 1983.

Wolf SL: *Biofeedback.* In Currier DP, Nelson RM, editors: *Clinical electrotherapy,* ed 2, Norwalk, Conn, 1991, Appleton & Lange.

Wolf SL, Baker MP, Kelly JL: EMG biofeedback in stroke: effect of patient characteristics, *Arch Phys Med Rehabil* 60: 96-102, 1979.

Wolf SL, Baker MP, Kelly JL: EMG biofeedback in stroke: a 1-year follow-up on the effect of patient characteristics, *Arch Phys Med Rehabil* 61: 351-355, 1980.

Wolf SL, Binder-Macleod SA: Electromyographic biofeedback applications to the hemiplegic patient: changes in lower extremity neuromuscular and functional status, *Phys Ther* 63: 1404-1413, 1983.

Wolf SL, Binder-Macleod SA: Electromyographic biofeedback applications to the hemiplegic patient: changes in upper extremity neuromuscular and functional status, *Phys Ther* 63: 1393, 1983.

Wolf SL, Edwards DI, Shutter LA: Concurrent assessment of muscle activity (CAMA): a procedural approach to assess treatment goals, *Phys Ther* 66: 218, 1986.

Wolf SL, Hudson JE: Feedback signal based upon force and time delay: modification of the Krusen limb load monitor: suggestion from the field, *Phys Ther* 60: 1289, 1980.

Wolf SL, LeCraw DE, Barton, LA: A comparison of motor copy and targeted feedback training techniques for restitution of upper extremity function among neurologic patients, *Phys Ther* 69: 719, 1989.

Wolf SL, Nacht M, Kelly JL: EMG feedback training during dynamic movement for low back pain patients, *Behav Ther* 13: 395, 1982.

Wolf SL, Regenos E, Basmajian JV: Developing strategies for biofeedback applications in neurologically handicapped patients, *Phys Ther* 57: 402-408, 1977.

Shortwave and Microwave Diathermy

8

William E. Prentice and Phillip B. Donley

OBJECTIVES

After completion of this chapter, the student will be able to do the following:

- Discuss how the diathermies may best be used in a sports-medicine setting.

- Explain the physiologic effects of diathermy.

- Explain the difference between capacitance and induction shortwave diathermy techniques, and identify the associated electrodes.

- Describe treatment techniques for continuous shortwave and pulsed shortwave diathermy.

- Explain the equipment set-up and treatment technique for microwave diathermy.

- Discuss the various clinical applications and indications for using continuous shortwave, pulsed shortwave, and microwave diathermy.

- Identify the treatment precautions and contraindications for using the diathermies.

Diathermy is the application of high-frequency electromagnetic energy that is primarily used to generate heat in body tissues. Heat is produced by resistance of the tissue to the passage of the energy. Diathermy may also be used to produce nonthermal effects.

Diathermy as a therapeutic agent may be classified as two distinct modalities: shortwave diathermy and microwave diathermy. Shortwave diathermy may be either continuous or pulsed. Continuous shortwave diathermy has been used in the treatment of a variety of conditions for some time. Pulsed shortwave diathermy has recently received renewed interest, although research documenting its clinical efficacy has been extremely limited.[9]

The effectiveness of a shortwave or microwave diathermy treatment depends on the sports therapist's ability to tailor the treatment to the athlete's needs. This requires that the sports therapist have an accurate evaluation or diagnosis of the athlete's condition and knowledge of the heating patterns produced by various electrodes or applicators. Many sports therapists feel that neither shortwave nor microwave diathermy produces heating at the depths desired for the treatment of athletic injuries, although the depth of penetration is greater than with any of the infrared modalities. Sports therapists who are knowledgable in the physics and biophysics of diathermy, as well as its applications to a variety of cases, tend to achieve good results. Sports therapists who work with shortwave and microwave diathermy units must spend considerable time experimenting with equipment set-up and the application of different types of electrodes on a variety of uninjured parts of the body if they are to develop the skills necessary to use diathermy effectively on injured tissue.

PHYSIOLOGIC RESPONSES TO DIATHERMY

The diathermies are not capable of producing depolarization and contraction of skeletal muscle since the wavelengths are much too short in duration.[2] Thus the physiologic effects of continuous shortwave and microwave diathermy are primarily thermal, resulting from high-frequency vibration of molecules.

The primary benefits of diathermy are those of heat in general, such as tissue temperature rise, increased blood flow, dilation of the blood vessels, increased filtration and diffusion through the different membranes, increased tissue metabolic rate, changes in some enzyme reactions, alterations in the physical properties of fibrous tissues (such as those found in tendons, joints, and scars), a certain degree of muscle relaxation, and a heightened pain threshold.[14,15] The tissue temperature must be elevated to between 40° and 45° C (104° and 113° F) if the diathermy is to be effective.[15] Diathermy treatment doses are not precisely controlled, and the amount of heating the patient receives cannot be accurately prescribed or directly measured. Heating occurs in proportion to the square of the current density and in direct proportion to the resistance of the tissue.

$$Heating = Current^2 \times Resistance$$

Why certain pathologic conditions respond better to diathermy than other forms of deep heat is not well understood or documented. It probably is more directly related to the skill of the operator applying the modality or to some placebo effects associated with tissue temperature increase than it is to the specific effects of diathermy itself.

Pulsed shortwave diathermy has been used for its nonthermal effects in the treatment of soft-tissue injuries and wounds.[9]

The mechanism of its effectiveness has been theorized to occur at the cellular level, relating specifically to cell-membrane potential.[10] Damaged cells undergo depolarization resulting in cell dysfunction, which might include loss of cell division and proliferation and loss of regenerative capabilities. Pulsed shortwave diathermy has repolarized damaged cells, thus correcting cell dysfunction.[17]

It has also been suggested that sodium tends to accumulate in the cell due to a decrease in activity of the sodium pump during the inflammatory process, creating a negatively charged environment. When a magnetic field is induced, the sodium pump is reactivated, thus allowing the cell to regain normal ionic balance.[20]

SHORTWAVE DIATHERMY

A shortwave diathermy unit is basically a radio transmitter. The **Federal Communications Commission (FCC)** assigned three frequencies to shortwave diathermy units: 27.12 MHz with a wavelength of 11 meters; 13.56 MHz with a wavelength of 22 meters; and 40.68 MHz with a wavelength of 7.5 meters (see Figure 1-2). The third frequency is rarely used.

Equipment

The shortwave diathermy unit consists of a power supply that provides power to a radio frequency oscillator (Figure 8-1). This radio frequency oscillator provides stable, drift-free oscillations at the required frequency. The power amplifier generates the power required to drive the different types of electrodes. The output resonant tank tunes in the patient as part of the circuit and allows maximum power to be transferred to the patient.

Figure 8-2, *A* and *B* diagrammatically shows the control panel of a shortwave diathermy unit. The output intensity knob controls the percentage of maximum power transferred to the patient circuit. This is similar to the volume control on a radio. The tuning control adjusts the output circuit for maximum energy transfer from the radio frequency oscillator, which is similar to tuning in a station on a radio. The power output meter monitors only the current that is drawn from the power supply and not the energy being delivered to the patient. Thus it is only an indirect measure of the energy reaching the patient.

The power output of a shortwave diathermy unit should produce sufficient energy to raise the tissue temperature into a therapeutic range, 40° to 45° C. The specific absorption rate (SAR) represents the rate of energy absorbed per unit area of tissue mass. Most shortwave units have a power output of between 80 and 120 watts. Some units are not capable of this output, making them safe but ineffective. It is important to remember that the tissue temperature rise with diathermy units can be

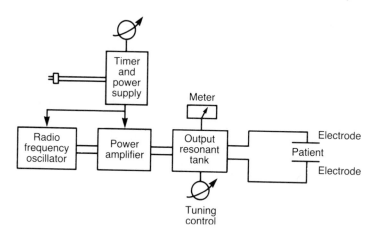

Fig. 8-1. The component parts of a shortwave diathermy unit.

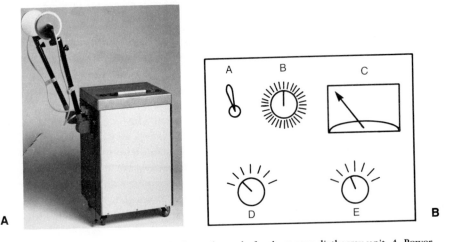

Fig. 8-2 A, Shortwave diathermy unit. **B,** Control panel of a shortwave diathermy unit. *A,* Power switch; *B,* timer; *C,* output power meter (monitors current drawn from power supply only and not in patient circuit); *D,* output intensity (controls the percentage of maximum power transferred to the patient); *E,* tuning control (tunes the output circuit for maximum energy transfer from radio frequency oscillator).

offset dramatically by an increase in blood flow, which has a cooling effect in the tissue being energized. Therefore units should be able to generate enough power to provide for an excess of the SAR.

Patient sensation provides the basis for recommendations of continuous shortwave diathermy dosage and thus varies considerably with different patients.[12,21] The following dosage guidelines have been recommended:

Dose I (Lowest) — No sensation of heat
Dose II (Low) — Mild heating sensation
Dose III (Medium) — Moderate (pleasant) heating sensation
Dose IV (Heavy) — Vigorous heating that is tolerable below the pain threshold

Some shortwave diathermy units have manual tuning, others have an automatic tuning device. If the machine is not an automatically tuning type, it is necessary to tune the patient's circuit to resonance with the oscillating circuit of the unit. This is accomplished by placing the electrodes over the area to be treated and then setting the output intensity at 30% to 40%. Then, the variable capacitor in the generator's circuitry can be adjusted by using the meter on the generator to determine the peak tuning readings. These readings should not be confused as an indication of the power received by the patient. The tuning control should be adjusted until the output power meter moves to the maximum, and then it should be adjusted down to patient tolerance, which is usually about 50% of maximum output. If more than 50% of the available power on the meter is used, then the patient's set-up is out of tune or out of resonance. Shortwave diathermy units with automatic tuning turn off the power when the patient circuit is out of tune.

A shortwave diathermy unit that generates a high frequency electrical current will produce both an **electrical field** and a **magnetic field** in the tissues.[6] The ratio of the

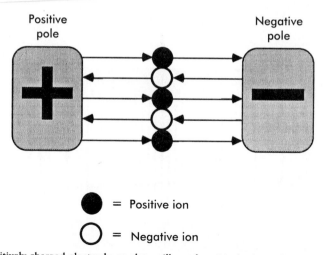

Positive pole

Negative pole

⬤ = Positive ion

◯ = Negative ion

Fig. 8-3. A positively charged electrode or plate will repel positively charged ions and attract negatively charged ions. Conversely, the negative electrode will repel negative ions and attract positive ions.

electrical field to the magnetic field depends on the characteristics of the different units as well as on the characteristics of electrodes or applicators. Shortwave units with a frequency of 13.56 MHz tend to produce a stronger magnetic field than those with a frequency of 27.12 MHz, which produces a stronger electric field. The latter is the more commonly found frequency on shortwave diathermy units.

Shortwave Diathermy Electrodes

Shortwave diathermy may be delivered to the patient via either capacitance or induction techniques. Each of these techniques can affect different biologic tissues, and selection of the appropriate electrodes is essential for effective treatment. The shortwave diathermy uses several types of applicators or electrodes including air space plates, pad electrodes, cable electrodes, or drum electrodes.

CAPACITOR ELECTRODES. The capacitance technique, using **capacitor electrodes,** creates a stronger electrical field than a magnetic field. As discussed in Chapter 6, within the body there are many free ions that are positively or negatively charged. A positively charged electrode or plate will repel positively charged ions and attract negatively charged ions. Conversely, the negative electrode will repel negative ions and attract positive ions (Figure 8-3).

An electrical field is essentially the lines of force exerted on these charged ions by the electrodes that cause charged particles to move from one pole to the other (Figure 8-4). The intensity of the electrical field is determined by the spacing of the electrodes and is greatest when they are close together. The center of this electrical field has a higher current density than regions at the periphery. When using capacitance electrodes the patient is placed between two electrodes or plates and becomes part of the circuit. Thus the tissue between the two electrodes is in a series circuit arrangement (see Chapter 4).

As the electrical field is created in the biologic tissues, the tissue that offers the

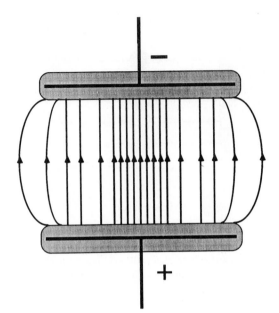

Fig. 8-4. An electrical field is essentially the lines of force exerted on these charged ions by the electrodes that cause charged particles to move from one pole to the other.
From Michlovitz S: *Thermal agents in rehabilitation,* Philadelphia, 1990, FA Davis.)

greatest resistance to current flow tends to develop the most heat. Tissues that have a high fat content tend to insulate and resist the passage of an electrical field. These tissues, particularly subcutaneous fat, tend to overheat when an electrical field is used, which is characteristic of a capacitance type of electrode application.

Air space plates. Air space plates are an example of a capacitance technique or a capacitor electrode. This type of electrode consists of two metal plates with a diameter of 7.5 to 17.5 cm surrounded by a glass or plastic plate guard. The metal plates may be adjusted approximately 3 cm within the plate guard, thus changing the distance from the skin[10] (Figure 8-5). Air space plates produce high-frequency oscillating current that is passed through each plate millions of times per second. When one plate is overloaded, it discharges to the other plate of the lower potential, and this is reversed millions of times per second.[5]

When air space plates are used, the area to be treated is placed between the electrode and becomes part of the external circuit (Figure 8-6). The sensation of heat tends to be in direct proportion to the distance of the plate from the skin. The closer the plate is to the skin, the better the energy transmission because there will be less reflection of the energy. However, it should be remembered that the closer plate will also generate more surface heat in the skin and the subcutaneous fat in that area (Figure 8-7). The greatest surface heat will be under the electrodes. Parts of the body that are low in subcutaneous fat content (e.g., hands, feet, wrists, and ankles) are best treated by this method. Athletes who have a very low subcutaneous fat content can be effectively treated in other body areas.[4] This technique is also very effective for treating the spine and the ribs.

Pad electrodes. Pad electrodes are seldom used in sports medicine; however,

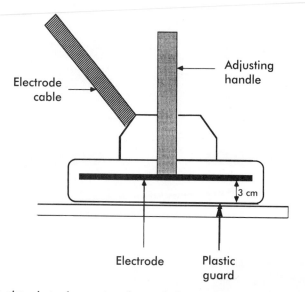

Fig. 8-5. Air space plate electrodes consists of a metal plate enclosed in a glass or plastic plate guard. The metal plate may be adjusted approximately 3 cm within the plate guard, thus changing the distance from the skin.

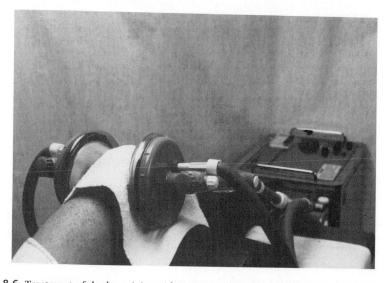

Fig. 8-6. Treatment of the knee joint with air space plates. The patient is in a series set-up.

they may be available for some units. They are true capacitor electrodes, and they must have uniform contact pressure on the body part if they are to be effective in producing deep heat, as well as to avoid skin burns (Figure 8-8). The patient is part of the external circuit. Several layers of toweling are necessary to make sure that there is sufficient spacing between the skin and the pads. The pads should be separated such that they are at least as far apart as the cross-sectional diameter of the pads. In other words, if the pads are 15 cm across, then there should be at least 15 cm between the pads. The

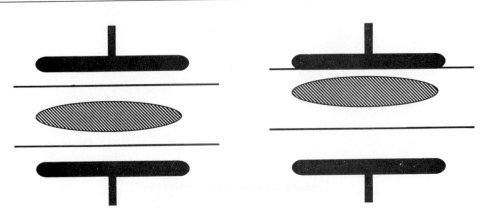

Fig. 8-7. As the plate moves closer to the surface of the skin the electrical field shifts, generating more surface heat in the skin and the subcutaneous fat.

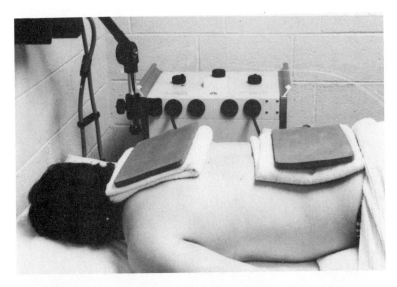

Fig. 8-8. Pad electrodes showing correct placement and spacing.

closer the spacing of the pads, the higher the current density in the superficial tissues. Increasing the spacing between the pads will increase the depth of penetration in the tissues (Figure 8-9, *A* and *B*). The part of the body to be treated should be centered between the pads.[5,6,8,14]

INDUCTION ELECTRODES. The inductance technique, using **induction electrodes,** creates a stronger magnetic field than an electrical field. When the induction technique is used in shortwave diathermy, a cable or coil is either wrapped circumferentially around an extremity or it is coiled within an electrode. In either case, when current is passed through a coiled cable, a magnetic field is generated that can affect surrounding tissues by inducing localized secondary currents, called **eddy currents,** within the tissues[10] (Figure 8-10). Eddy currents are small circular electrical fields, and the **intramolecular oscillation (vibration)** of tissue contents causes heat generation.

In the induction technique, the patient is in a magnetic field and is not part of

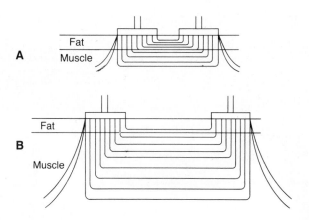

Fig. 8-9. Pad electrodes should be separated by at least the diameter of the electrodes. **A,** Electrodes placed close together produce more superficial heating. **B,** As spacing increases the current density increases in the deeper tissues.

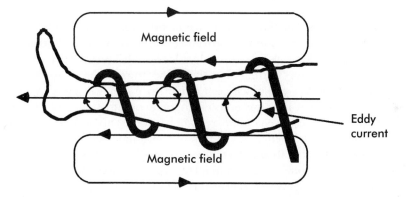

Fig. 8-10. When current is passed through a coiled cable a magnetic field is generated that can affect surrounding tissues by inducing eddy currents within the tissues.
(Modified from Michlovitz S: *Thermal agents in rehabilitation,* Philadelphia, 1990, FA Davis.)

the circuit. The tissues are in a parallel circuit (see Chapter 4), thus the greatest current flow is through the tissues with least resistance. When a magnetic field is used with an induction type set-up, the fat does not provide nearly as much resistance to the flow of the energy.

Therefore tissues that are high in electrolytic content (i.e., muscle and blood) respond best to the magnetic field by producing heat. If the energy is due primarily to generation of a magnetic field, heating may not be as obvious to the patient because the magnetic field will not provide nearly as much sensation of warmth in the skin as an electrical field.

Cable electrodes. The **cable electrode** is an induction electrode that produces a magnetic field (Figure 8-11). There are two basic types of arrangements: the pancake coil and the wraparound coil. If a pancake coil is used, the size of the smaller circle should be greater than 6 inches in diameter. In either arrangement, there should be at least 1 cm of toweling between the cable and the skin. Stiff spacers should be used

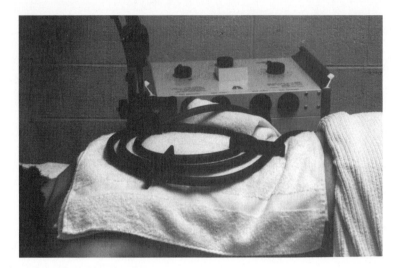

Fig. 8-11. Pancake cable electrode.

to keep the coils or the turns of the pancake or the wraparound coil between 5 and 10 cm between turns of the cable, thus providing spacing consistency. Both the pancake coils and the wraparound coils often provide more even heating because they are more able to follow the contours of the skin than are the drum or the air space plates. It is important that the cables not touch each other, since they will short out and cause excessive heat build-up. Diathermy units that operate on a frequency of 13.56 MHz are probably best suited to cable electrode type applications. This is primarily because the lower frequency provides better production of a magnetic field.[4]

Drum electrodes. The **drum electrode** also produces a magnetic field. The drum electrode is made up of one or more monoplanar coils that are rigidly fixed inside some kind of housing (Figure 8-12). If a small area is to be treated, particularly a small flat area, then a one-drum set-up is fine. However, if the area is contoured, then two or more drums, which may be on a hinged apparatus or hinged arm, may be more suitable.

Penetration into the tissues tends to be on the order of 2 to 3 cm if the skin is no more than 1 to 2 cm away from the drum.[1] The magnetic field may be significant up to 5 cm away from the drum. A light towel must be kept in contact with the skin and between the drum and the skin. The towel is used to absorb moisture because an accumulation of water droplets would tend to overheat and cause hot spots on the surface. If there is more than 2 cm of fat, there probably will be no great tissue temperature rise under the fat with a drum set-up. The maximum penetration of shortwave diathermy with a drum electrode is 3 cm, provided there is no more than 2 cm of fat beneath the skin. For best absorption of energy, the housing of the drum should be in contact with the towel that is covering the skin.[4]

Pulsed Shortwave Diathermy

Pulsed shortwave diathermy also referred to in the literature as pulsed electromagnetic energy (PEME), pulsed electromagnetic field (PEMF), or pulsed electromagnetic energy treatment (PEMET) is a relatively new form of diathermy.[9] Pulsed diathermy is created by simply interrupting the output of continuous shortwave diathermy at

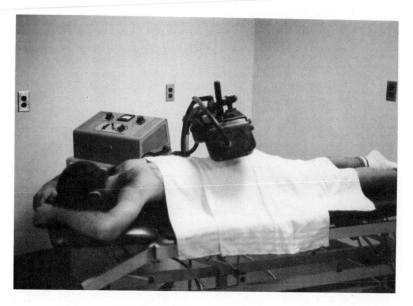

Fig. 8-12. Drum electrodes.

consistent intervals (Figure 8-13). Energy is delivered to the patient in a series of high frequency bursts or pulse trains. Pulse duration is short, ranging from 20 to 400 μsec with an intensity of up to 1000 watts per pulse. The interpulse interval or off-time depends on the pulse repetition rate, which ranges between 1 and 7000 Hz. The pulse repetition rate may be selected using the pulse-frequency control on the generator control panel.[10] Generally the off-time is considerably longer than the on-time. Therefore even though the power output during the on-time is sufficient to produce tissue heating, the long off-time interval allows the heat to dissipate. This reduces the likelihood of any significant tissue temperature increase and reduces the patient's perception of heat.

With pulsed shortwave diathermy, mean power provides a measure of heat production. Mean power may be calculated by dividing peak pulse power by the pulse repetition frequency to determine the pulse period (on-time plus off-time).

$$\text{Pulse period} = \frac{\text{Peak pulse power (watts)}}{\text{Pulse repetition frequency (Hz)}}$$

The percentage on-time is calculated by dividing the pulse duration by pulse period.

$$\text{Percentage on-time} = \frac{\text{Pulse duration (msec)}}{\text{Pulse period (msec)}}$$

The mean power is then determined by dividing the peak pulse power by the percentage on-time.

$$\text{Percentage on-time} = \frac{\text{Peak pulse power (watts)}}{\text{Percentage on-time}}$$

With pulsed shortwave diathermy the highest mean power output is usually lower than the power delivered with continuous shortwave diathermy.

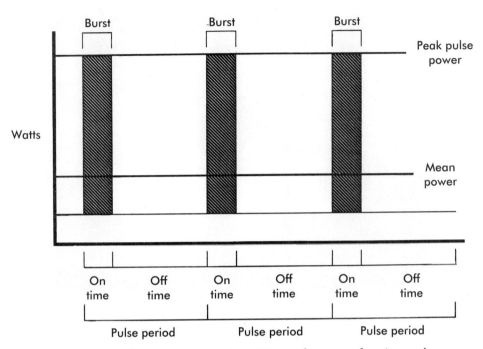

Fig. 8-13. Pulsed diathermy is created by simply interrupting the output of continuous shortwave diathermy at consistent intervals.

Generators that deliver pulsed shortwave diathermy typically use a drum type of electrode (Figure 8-14). As with continuous shortwave diathermy the drum electrode is made of a coil wrapped in a flat circular spiral pattern and housed within a plastic case. The energy is induced in the treatment area via the production of a magnetic field.

Pulsed diathermy is claimed to have therapeutic value and to produce nonthermal effects with minimal thermal physiologic effects, depending on the intensity of the application. When pulsed diathermy is used in intensities that create an increase in tissue temperature, its effects are no different from those of continuous shortwave diathermy. Studies that use pulsed shortwave diathermy do not normally compare it with continuous shortwave diathermy but rather with a control group that has received no heat treatment.[14]

Treatment Time

A 20-to-30-minute treatment for one body area is probably all that is necessary to reach maximum physiologic effects.[4] The physiologic effects seem to last for about 30 minutes. This is particularly true of the circulatory effects. Treatments in excess of 30 minutes or those that are in excess of 45 to 60 minutes may create a circulatory rebound phenomenon in which the digital temperature may drop after the treatment because of reflex vasoconstriction.[15] If a sports therapist finds that a diathermy unit has been left on in excess of 30 minutes, it would be wise to check the temperature of the toes or the fingers, depending on which extremity has been treated.

It is important to remember that as skin temperature rises, impedance falls.

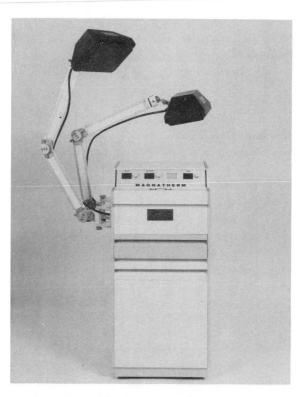

Fig. 8-14. The Magnatherm is an example of a generator capable of producing pulsed shortwave diathermy. Energy is delivered to the patient through a drum electrode. (Courtesy International Medical Electronics)

Therefore the unit should be returned to baseline level after 5 to 10 minutes of treatment.

MICROWAVE DIATHERMY

Microwave diathermy has two FCC-assigned frequencies in this country, 2456 MHz and 915 MHz. Microwave has a much higher frequency and a shorter wavelength than shortwave diathermy. Microwave diathermy units generate a strong electrical field and relatively little magnetic field.

With appropriate set-up of the microwave diathermy unit, less than 10% of the energy is lost from the machine as it is applied to the athlete. The microwave applicator beams energy toward the patient, creating the potential for much of the energy to be reflected. Heating is caused by the intramolecular vibration of molecules that are high in polarity. If the subcutaneous fat is greater than 1 cm, the fat temperature will rise to a level that is too uncomfortable before there is a tissue temperature rise in the deeper tissues.[5] This is less of a problem if the microwave diathermy is of the frequency of 915 MHz. However, there are very few commercial units operating on that frequency. Almost all of the older units have the higher frequency of 2456 MHz. If the

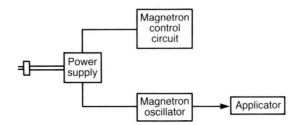

Fig. 8-15. Component parts of a microwave diathermy unit.

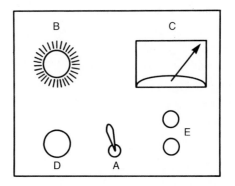

Fig. 8-16. Control panel of a microwave diathermy unit *A,* power switch; *B,* timer; *C,* output meter (indicates relative output in watts of transmitted energy); *D,* power output level; *E,* indicator lamps (amber-standby, magnetron accelerating, red- microwaves available for output).

subcutaneous fat is 0.5 cm or less, microwave diathermy can penetrate and cause a tissue temperature rise up to 5 cm deep in the tissue. Bone tends to absorb more shortwave and microwave energy than any type of soft tissue.

Equipment

The microwave diathermy unit consists of a power supply that energizes the magnetron and timing circuitry. The magnetron control regulates output power by varying the magnetron operating voltage. The magnetron oscillator uses a magnetic field to produce high-frequency currents (Figure 8-15).

Figure 8-16 represents the control panel of a microwave unit. The power output can be adjusted to patient tolerance. The output meter indicates the relative output in watts or the amount of transmitted and unabsorbed energy. There are two indicator lamps: the amber lamp indicates that the machine is still warming up, and the red lamp indicates that the machine is ready to output energy.

Microwave Diathermy Applicators

Electrodes for microwave diathermy are called **applicators.** The microwave energy can only be beamed to one surface at a time. The contour of that surface must be very flat, otherwise there will be considerable reflection of the energy.

Those microwave diathermy units operating on the frequency 2456 MHz will have a specified air space required between the applicator and the skin. The manufacturer-suggested distances and power output should be followed closely. A directional

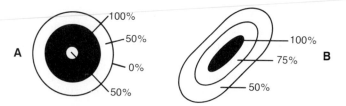

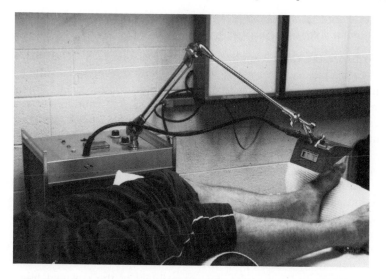

Fig. 8-17. **A,** Circular shaped microwave electrode. **B,** Rectangular shaped microwave electrode.

Fig. 8-18. Typical microwave diathermy unit with rectangular applicator.

antenna is attached to the applicator perpendicular to the face of the applicator to ensure that spacing is correct and that the energy generated from the microwave unit is striking the target treatment area at the correct angle. Units that operate on the higher frequency may have one or more applicators of various shapes and configurations.

There are two types of applicators that may be used with microwave diathermy: circular shaped and rectangular shaped. The circular-shaped applicators are either 4 or 6 inches in diameter. With circular-shaped electrodes, the maximum temperature is produced at the periphery of each radiation field (Figure 8-17, *A*).

Rectangular-shaped applicators are either 4 ½ × 5 inches or 5 × 21 inches and produce the maximum temperature at the center of the radiation field (Figure 8-17, *B*).

In units that have a frequency of 915 MHz, the applicators are placed at a distance of 1 cm from the skin, and the air space between the antenna and the skin is built into the applicator, thus minimizing energy reflection.[14]

Microwave Treatment Technique

Microwave diathermy units require a period of time to warm up. This is normally built into the circuitry so that the unit power cannot be turned on until the unit is sufficiently warmed. This warm-up time is a good time for the sports therapist to position the director and the athlete (Figure 8-18). The director should be located so that the maximum amount of energy will be penetrating at a right angle or perpendicular to the skin. Any angle greater or less than perpendicular will create reflection of the energy and significant loss of absorption (cosine law). Microwave diathermy is best used to treat conditions that exist in those areas of the body that are covered with low subcutaneous fat content. The tendons of the foot, hand, and wrist are well treated, as are the acromioclavicular and sternoclavicular joints, the patellar tendon, the distal tendons of the hamstrings, the Achilles tendon, and the costochondral joints and sacroiliac joints in lean individuals.

CLINICAL APPLICATIONS FOR DIATHERMY

For the most part, the clinical applications for the diathermies are similar to those of other physical agents that are capable of producing thermal effects resulting in a tissue temperature increase. In addition to the diathermies, the infrared modalities discussed in Chapter 9 and ultrasound discussed in Chapter 12 are commonly used as heating modalities. As with pulsed shortwave diathermy, there have been nonthermal effects documented with microwave diathermy; however, there does not appear to be any evidence that these nonthermal effects have any significant role in the medical application of microwave diathermy.[7]

The diathermies have been used to treat a variety of musculoskeletal conditions including muscle strains, contusions, ligament sprains, tendinitis, tenosynovitis, bursitis, joint contractures, and myofascial trigger points.

Continuous shortwave and microwave diathermy are most often used for a variety of thermal effects including inducing local relaxation by decreasing muscle guarding and pain, [14] selectively heating joint structures to improve joint range of motion by decreasing stiffness and increasing the extensibility of the collagen fibers and the resiliance of contracted soft tissues,[10] increasing circulation and improving blood flow to an injured area to facilitate resolution of hemorrhage and edema as well as removal of the byproducts of the inflammatory process;[14] and in reducing both subacute and chronic pain.[18]

The majority of recent clinical studies relative to diathermy have focused primarily on the efficacy of pulsed shortwave diathermy in facilitating tissue healing. To date, results have been at best inconclusive. Various claims have been made as to the specific mechanisms that facilitate healing including an increase in the number and activity of the cells in the area, reduced swelling and inflammation, resorption of hematoma, increased rate of collagen deposition and organization, and increased nerve growth and repair. These claims are based on a limited number of clinical studies and even fewer experimental studies.[9]

There are a number of conditions that may potentially occur in sports medicine that would make diathermy the treatment of choice.

1. If for any reason the skin or some underlying soft tissue is very tender and will not tolerate the loading of a moist heat pack or pressure from an ultrasound transducer, then diathermy should be used.
2. Both continuous shortwave and microwave diathermy are more capable of increasing temperatures to a greater tissue depth than any of the infrared modalities.

3. When the treatment goal is to increase tissue temperatures in a large area (i.e., throughout the entire shoulder girdle, in the low back region), the diathermies should be used.

4. In areas where subcutaneous fat is thick and deep heating is required, the induction technique using either cable or drum electrodes should be used to minimize heating of the subcutaneous fat layer. Both the capacitance technique with shortwave diathermy and microwave diathermy are more likely to selectively heat more superficial subcutaneous fat.

5. The sports therapist should never underestimate the placebo effects that a treatment with any large machine may be capable of producing.

Sports therapists should take the opportunity to examine several different types of diathermy units, as well as the different applicators available with each unit. They should not only practice using the different applicators on healthy tissue, but they should also experience the sensation themselves. In particular, they should recognize or experience the difference between the energy flow with an induction type application as opposed to the capacitor type application.

DIATHERMY TREATMENT PRECAUTIONS AND CONTRAINDICATIONS

There are probably more treatment precautions and contraindications for the use of either shortwave or microwave diathermy than for any of the other physical agents used in a sports-medicine setting.

Diathermy produces a tissue temperature rise and may be contraindicated in any condition where this increased temperature may produce negative or undesired effects including traumatic musculoskeletal injuries with acute bleeding,[3] acute inflammatory conditions,[16] areas with reduced blood supply (ischemia),[3] and areas with reduced sensitivity to temperature or pain.[10] It is important to keep in mind that the power meter on the diathermy units does not indicate the energy entering the tissues. Therefore the sports therapist must rely on the sensation of pain for a warning that the athlete's tolerance levels have been exceeded.[13]

Because diathermy selectively heats tissues that are high in water content, caution must be exercised when using diathermy over fluid-filled areas or organs. Joint effusion may be exacerbated by heating with diathermy. The increase in temperature may cause an increase in synovitis.[16] Because of the high fluid content, it should not be used around the eyes for any prolonged periods of time or for repeated treatments,[11] nor should it be used with contact lenses.[22]

Toweling should be used to absorb perspiration.[5] A single layer of toweling should be used with both the drum and air space plates. However, with other types of applicators, such as pads and cables, the toweling should be more dense and thick, up to about 1 cm or more.[3] Toweling is not necessary with microwave diathermy. There should be no overlapping of skin surfaces. If the buttocks area is to be treated, then a towel should be placed in the cleavage between the buttocks. If the shoulder area is to be treated, a towel should be placed between the skinfolds in the axilla.

It is also important that no clothing be permitted in the exposed area. Many of the synthetic fabrics worn today allow for no evaporation of moisture. These fabrics serve as a vapor barrier and allow moisture to accumulate. Similarly, moisture can accumulate in athletes taped with adhesive tape or wearing compressive wraps or supportive braces. This moisture can create extremely hot spots with diathermy treatments.[19] Diathermy should not be used over moist wound dressings again due to potential for rapid heating of moisture.[14]

Diathermy should not be applied to the pelvic area of the female who is menstruating. The application of diathermy during menstruation has increased blood flow.[14]

Exposure of the gonads to diathermy should be avoided.[25] The testes are more superficial and thus are more susceptible to injury from microwave treatment than the ovaries. Minimal evidence exists that diathermy may potentially cause damage to the human fetus, however it is recommended that caution be used in treating the pregnant female.[23]

Caution should be used when using diathermy over bony prominences to avoid burning of the overlying soft tissue.[12] There should be no vigorous heating of the epiphysis in children.[14]

The patient should not come in contact with any of the cables connecting the generator with the air space plates, pad, cable, or drum electrodes. There should be no crossover of the lead cables with any electrode set-up. At no time should the antenna within the microwave applicator ever come in contact with the skin. This would cause a build-up of energy sufficient to cause a severe burn.

It is very important to use diathermy units at a safe distance from other types of medical electrical devices or equipment that is transistorized. Transcutaneous electrical nerve stimulation (TENS) units and other low-frequency current units often have transistor type circuits, and these can be damaged by the reflected or stray radiation that is produced by shortwave and microwave diathermy units.[14] Unshielded cardiac pacemakers may also be damaged by diathermy.[24]

There should be no metal chairs or metal tables used to support the athlete during treatment. The area being treated should also be free of metal implants. Women wearing intrauterine devices should not be treated in the low back or lower abdomen. There should be no watches or jewelry in the area because the electromagnetic energy will tend to magnetize the watch and the electromagnetic energy may heat up the jewelry.[14]

The athlete must remain in a reasonably comfortable position for the duration of the treatment so that the field does not change because of movement during treatment.

The skin should be inspected before and after a diathermy treatment. It is recommended that the part being treated either be horizontal or elevated during the treatment.

SUMMARY

1. Diathermy is the application of high-frequency electromagnetic energy that is primarily used to generate heat in body tissues. Diathermy as a therapeutic agent may be classified as two distinct modalities, shortwave diathermy and microwave diathermy. Shortwave diathermy may be continuous or pulsed.

2. The physiologic effects of continuous shortwave and microwave diathermy are primarily thermal resulting from high-frequency vibration of molecules.

Pulsed shortwave diathermy has been used for its nonthermal effects in the treatment of soft-tissue injuries and wounds.

3. A shortwave diathermy unit that generates a high frequency electrical current will produce both an electrical field and a magnetic field in the tissues. The ratio of the electrical field to the magnetic field depends on the characteristics of the different units as well as on the characteristics of electrodes or applicators.

4. The capacitance technique, using capacitor electrodes (air space plates and pad electrodes), creates a strong electrical field, which is essentially the lines of force exerted on charged ions by the electrodes that cause charged particles to move from one pole to the other.

5. The inductance technique, using induction electrodes (cable and drum electrodes), creates a strong magnetic field when current is passed through a coiled cable. It may affect surrounding tissues by inducing localized secondary currents, called eddy currents, within the tissues.

6. Pulsed diathermy is created by simply interrupting the output of continuous shortwave diathermy at consistant intervals. Generators that deliver pulsed shortwave diathermy typically use a drum type of electrode to induce energy in the treatment area via the production of a magnetic field.

7. Microwave diathermy units generate a strong electrical field and relatively little magnetic field through either circular shaped and rectangular shaped applicators that beam energy to the treatment area.

8. The diathermies have been used to treat a variety of musculoskeletal conditions including muscle strains, contusions, ligament sprains, tendinitis, tenosynovitis, bursitis, joint contractures, and myofascial trigger points.

9. There are probably more treatment precautions and contraindications for the use of either shortwave or microwave diathermy than for any of the other physical agents used in a sports-medicine setting.

10. Effective treatments using the diathermies require practice in application and adjustment of techniques to the individual patient.

GLOSSARY

air space plate A capacitor type electrode in which the plates are separated from the skin by the space in a glass case. Used with shortwave diathermy.

applicator The electrode used to transfer energy in microwave diathermy.

cable electrodes An inductance type electrode in which the electrodes are coiled around a body part, creating an electromagnetic field.

capacitor electrodes Air space plates or pad electrodes that create a stronger electrical field than a magnetic field.

diathermy The application of high-frequency electrical energy that is used to generate heat in body tissues resulting from tissue resistance to the passage of energy. It may also be used to produce nonthermal effects.

drum electrodes Induction electrodes that produce a strong magnetic field. Primarily used with pulsed shortwave diathermy.

eddy currents Small circular electrical fields induced when a magnetic field is created that result in intramolecular oscillation (vibration) of tissue contents, causing heat generation.

electrical field The lines of force exerted on charged ions in the tissues by the electrodes that cause charged particles to move from one pole to the other.

Federal Communications Commission (FCC) Federal agency charged with assigning frequencies for all radio transmitters including diathermies.

induction electrodes Cable or drum electrodes that create a stronger magnetic field than electrical field.

intermolecular oscillation (vibration) Movement between molecules that produces friction and thus heat.

magnetic field Field created when current is passed through a coiled cable that affects surrounding tissues by inducing localized eddy currents within the tissues.

pad electrodes Capacitor type electrode used with shortwave diathermy to create an electrical field.

pulsed shortwave diathermy Created by simply interrupting the output of continuous shortwave diathermy at consistant intervals, it is used primarily for nonthermal effects.

REFERENCES

1 DeLateur BJ, Lehmann JF, Stonebridge JB, et al.: Muscle heating in human subjects with 915 MHz microwave contact applicator, *Arch Phys Med Rehabil* 51: 147-151, 1970.

2 Delpizzo V, Joyner KH: On the safe use of microwave and shortwave diathermy units, *Aust J Physiother* 33(3): 152-162, 1987.

3 Fischer C, Solomon S: *Physiologic responses to heat and cold.* In Licht S, editor: *Therapeutic heat and cold,* New Haven, 1965, Elizabeth Licht.

4 Griffin JE: *Update on selected physical modalities,* Paper presented in Chicago, December 1981.

5 Griffin JE, Karselis TC: *The diathermies.* In: *Physical agents for physical therapists,* ed 2, Springfield, Ill, 1982, Charles C. Thomas.

6 Griffin JE, Santiesleban AJ, Kloth L: *Electrotherapy for instructors,* Paper presented in Lacrosse, Wis, August 1982.

7 Guy AW, Lehmann JF: On the determination of an optimum microwave diathermy frequency for a direct contact applicator, *Biomedical Engineering* 13: 76-87, 1966.

8 *Health devices shortwave diathermy units.* Proceedings of the Emergency Care Research Institute, Meeting in Plymouth, Penn, June 1979.

9 Kitchen S, Partridge C: Review of shortwave diathermy continuous and pulsed patterns, *Physiotherapy,* 78(4): 243-252, 1992.

10 Kloth L, Ziskin M: *Diathermy and pulsed electromagnetic fields.* In Michlovitz SL, editor: *Thermal agents in rehabilitation,* ed 2., Philadelphia, 1990, FA Davis.

11 Konarska I, Michneiwicz L: Shortwave diathermy of diseases of the anterior portion of the eye, *Klin Oczna* 25: 185, 1955.

12 Lehmann JF: Comparison of relative heating patterns produced in tissues by exposure to microwave energy with exposures at 2450 and 900 megacycles, *Arch Phys Med Rehabil* 46: 307, 1965.

13 Lehmann JF: *Diathermy.* In Krusen FH, editor: *Handbook of physical medicine and rehabilitation,* Philadelphia, 1965, WB Saunders.

14 Lehmann JF: *Therapeutic heat and cold,* ed 4, Baltimore, 1990, Williams & Wilkins.

15 Lehmann JF, DeLateur BJ: *Diathermy and superficial heat and cold.* In Krusen FH, editor: *Handbook of physical medicine and rehabilitation,* ed 3, Philadelphia, 1982, WB Saunders.

16 Lehmann JF, Warren CG, Scham SM: Therapeutic heat and cold, *Clin Orthop* 99: 207, 1974.

17 Low JL: The nature and effects of pulsed electromagnetic radiations, *NZ Physiotherapy* 6: 18, 1978.

18 Low J, Reed A: *Electrotherapy explained: principles and practice,* London, 1990, Butterworth-Heinemann.

19 *Progress report,* American Physical Therapy Association, June 1980.

20 Sanseverino EG: *Membrane phenomena and cellular processes under the action of pulsating magnetic fields,* Presented at the Second International Congress for Magneto Medicine, Rome, 1980.

21 Schliephake E: *Carrying out treatment.* In Thom H, editor: *Introduction to shortwave and microwave diathermy,* ed 3, Springfield, Ill, 1966, Charles C. Thomas.

22 Scott BO: Effect of contact lenses on shortwave field distribution, *Br J Opthalmology* 40: 696, 1956.

23 Smith DW, Clarren SK, Harvey MA: Hyperthermia as a possible teratogenic agent, *J Pediatrics* 92: 878, 1978.

24 Smyth H: The pacemaker patient and the electromagnetic environment, *JAMA* 227: 1412, 1974.

25 Van Demark NL, Free MJ: *Temperature effects.* In Johnson AD, editor: *The testis,* vol 3, New York, 1973, Academic Press.

SUGGESTED READINGS

Abramson DL: Physiologic basis for the use of physical agents in peripheral vascular disorders, *Arch Phys Med Rehabil* 46: 216, 1965.

Abramson DL, Bell Y, Rejal H, et al.: Changes in blood flow, oxygen uptake and tissue temperatures produced by therapeutic physical agents, *Am J Phys Med* 39: 87-95, 1960.

Abramson DL, Chu LSW, Tuck S, et al.: Effect of tissue temperature and blood flow on motor nerve conduction velocity, *J Am Med Assoc* 198: 1082-1088, 1966.

Adey WR: Electromagnetic field effects on tissue, *Physiological Review* 61(3): 436-514, 1981.

Adey WR: *Physiological signaling across cell membranes and co-operative influences of extremely low frequency electromagnetic fields.* In Frohlich H, editor: *Biological coherence and response to external stimuli,* Heidleberg, 1988, Springer Verlag.

Allberry J: Shortwave diathermy for herpes zoster, *Physiotherapy* 60: 386, 1974.

Aronofsky D: Reduction of dental post-surgical symptoms using non-thermal pulsed high-peak-power electromagnetic energy, *Oral Surgery* 32(5): 688-696, 1971.

Babbs CF, Dewitt DP: Physical principles of local heat therapy for cancer, *Medical Instrumentation (USA),* 15: 367-373, 1981.

Bansal PS, Sobti VK, Roy KS: Histomorphochemical effects of shortwave diathermy on healing of experimental muscle injury in dogs, *Ind J Exp Biol* 28: 766-770, 1990.

Barclay V, Collier RJ, Jones A: Treatment of various hand injuries by pulsed electromagnetic energy, *Physiotherapy* 69(6): 186-188, 1983.

Barker AT, Barlow PS, Porter J, et al.: A double-blind clinical trial of low-power pulsed shortwave therapy in the treatment of a soft tissue injury, *Physiotherapy* 71(12): 500-504, 1985.

Barnett M: SWD for herpes zoster, *Physiotherapy* 61: 217, 1975.

Benson TB, Copp EP: The effect of therapeutic forms of heat and ice on the pain threshold of the normal shoulder, *Rheumatology Rehabilitation* 13: 101-104, 1974.

Bentall RH, Eckstein HB: A trial involving the use of pulsed electromagnetic therapy on children undergoing orchidopexy, *Kinderchirurgie* 17(4): 380-389, 1975.

Brown M, Baker RD: Effect of pulsed shortwave diathermy on skeletal muscle injury in rabbits, *Phys Ther* 67(2): 208-214, 1987.

Brown-Woodnan PDC, Hadley JA, Richardson L, et al.: Evaluation of reproductive function of female rats exposed to radio frequency fields (27.12 MHz) near a shortwave diathermy device, *Health Physics* 56(4): 521-525, 1989.

Burr B: *Heat as a therapeutic modality against cancer,* Report 16, US National Cancer Institute, Bethesda, Maryland, 1974.

Cameron BM: Experimental acceleration of wound healing, *Am J Orthop* 3: 336-343, 1961.

Chamberlain MA, Care G, Gharfield B: Physiotherapy in osteoarthrosis of the knee, *Ann Rheum Dis* 23: 389-391, 1982.

Constable JD, Scapicchio AP, Opitz B: Studies of the effects of Diapulse treatment on various aspects of wound healing in experimental animals, *J Surg Res* 11: 254-257, 1971.

Currier DP, Nelson RM: Changes in motor conduction velocity induced by exercise and diathermy, *Phys Ther* 49(2): 146-152, 1969.

Daels J: Microwave heating of the uterine wall during parturition, *J Microwave Power* 11: 166, 1976.

Department of Health: Evaluation report: shortwave therapy units, *J Med Eng Technol* 11(6): 285-298, 1987.

Department of Health and Welfare (Canada): *Canada wide survey of non-ionising radiation-emitting medical devices,* 80-EHD-52, 1980.

Department of Health and Welfare (Canada): *Safety code 25 — Shortwave diathermy guidelines for limited radio frequency exposure,* 80-EHD-98, 1983.

Doyle JR, Smart BW: Stimulation of bone growth by shortwave diathermy, *J Bone Joint Surg* 45[A]: 15, 1963.

Engel JP: The effects of microwaves on bone and bone marrow and adjacent tissues, *Arch Phys Med Rehabil* 31: 453, 1950.

Erdman WJ: Peripheral blood flow measurements during application of pulsed high frequency currents, *Am J Orthop* 2: 196-197, 1960.

Feibel H, Fast H: Deep heating of joints: a reconsideration, *Arch Phys Med Rehabil* 57: 513, 1976.

Fenn JE: Effect of pulsed electromagnetic energy (Diapulse) on experimental haematomas, *Can Med Assoc J* 100: 251-253, 1969.

Foley-Nolan D Barry C, Coughlan RJ, et al.: Pulsed high frequency (27 MHz) electromagnetic therapy for persistent neck pain, *Orthopaedics* 13(4): 445-451, 1990.

Gibson T, Grahame R, Harkness J, et al.: Controlled comparison of shortwave diathermy treatment with osteopathic treatment in non-specific low back pain, *Lancet* 1: 1258-1261, 1985.

Ginsberg AJ: Pulsed shortwave in the treatment of bursitis with calcification, *Int Rec Med* 174(2): 71-75, 1961.

Goldin JH, Broadbent NRG, Nancarrow JD, et al.: The effect of Diapulse on healing of wounds: a double blind randomized controlled trial in man, *Br J Plast Surg* 34: 267-270, 1981.

Grant A, Sleep J, McIntosh J, et al.: Ultrasound and pulsed electromagnetic energy treatment for peroneal trauma: a randomised placebo-controlled trial, *Br J Obstet Gynaecol* 96: 434-439, 1981.

Guy AW: Analyses of electromagnetic fields induced in biological tissues by thermographic studies on equivalent phantom models, *IEEE Trans Microwave Theory Tech* Vol MTT 19: 205, 1971.

Guy AW: Biophysics of high frequency currents and electromagnetic radiation. In Lehmann JF, editor: *Therapeutic heat and cold,* 4 ed, Baltimore, 1990, Williams & Wilkins.

Guy AW, Lehmann JF, Stonebridge JB: Therapeutic applications of electromagnetic power, *Proc IEEE* 62: 55-75, 1974.

Guy AW, Lehmann JF, Stonebridge JB, et al.: Development of a 915 MHz direct contact applicator for therapeutic heating of tissues, *IEEE Trans Microwave Theory Techniques* 26: 550-556, 1978.

Hall EL: Diathermy generators, *Arch Phys Med Rehabil* 33: 28, 1952.

Hansen TI, Kristensen JH: Effect of massage, shortwave diathermy and ultrasound upon 133Xe disappearance rate from muscle and subcutaneous tissue in the human calf, *Scand J Rehabil Med* 5: 179-182, 1973.

Harris R: Effect of shortwave diathermy on radio-sodium clearance from the knee joint in the normal and in rheumatoid arthritis, *Arch Phys Med Rehabil* 42: 241, 1961.

Hayne R: Pulsed high frequency energy: its place in physiotherapy, *Physiotherapy* 70(12): 459-466, 1984.

Herrick JF, Jelatis DG, Lee GM: Dielectric properties of tissues important in microwave diathermy, *Fed Proc* 9: 60, 1950.

Herrick JF, Krusen FH: Certain physiologic and pathologic effects of microwaves, *Electrical Engineers* 72: 239, 1953.

Hollander JL: Joint temperature measurement in evaluation of antiarthritic agents, *J Clin Invest* 30: 701, 1951.

Hutchinson WJ, Burdeaux BD: The effects of shortwave diathermy on bone repair, *J Bone Joint Surg* 33[A]: 155, 1951.

Johnson CC, Guy AW: Nonionizing electromagnetic wave effects in biological materials and systems, *Proc IEEE* 66: 692, 1972.

Jones SL: Electromagnetic field interference and cardiac pacemakers, *Phys Ther* 56: 1013, 1976.

Kantor G: Evaluation and survey of microwave and radio frequency applicators, *J Microwave Power* 16(2): 135, 1981.

Kantor G, Witters DM: *The performance of a new 915 MHz direct contact applicator with reduced leakage — a detailed analysis,* HHS Publication (FDA) S3-8199, April, 1983.

Kaplan EG, Weinstock RE: Clinical evaluation of Diapulse as adjunctive therapy following foot surgery, *J Am Ped Assoc* 58: 218-221, 1968.

Kloth LC, Morrison M, Ferguson B: *Therapeutic microwave and shortwave diathermy: a review of thermal effectiveness, safe use, and state-of-the-art-1984,* Center for Devices and Radiological Health, DHHS, FDA 85-8237, December 1984.

Krag C, Taudorf U, Siim E, et al.: The effect of pulsed electromagnetic energy (Diapulse) on the survival of experimental skin flaps, *Scand J Plasti Reconstr Hand Surg,* 13: 377-380, 1979.

Lehmann JF: *Review of evidence for indications, techniques of application, contraindications, hazards and clinical effectiveness for shortwave diathermy,* DHEW/FDA HFA510, Rockville, MD 20852, 1974.

Lehmann JF: Microwave therapy: stray radiation, safety and effectiveness, *Arch Phys Med Rehabil* 60: 578, 1979.

Lehmann JF, DeLateur BJ, Stonebridge JB: Selective muscle heating by shortwave diathermy with a helical coil, *Arch Phys Med Rehabil* 50: 117, 1969.

Lehmann JF, Guy AW, DeLateur BJ, et al.: Heating patterns produced by shortwave diathermy using helical induction coil applicators, *Arch Phys Med Rehabil* 49: 193-198, 1968.

Lehmann JF, McDougall JA, Guy AW, et al.: Heating patterns produced by shortwave diathermy applicators in tissue substitute models, *Arch Phys Med Rehabil* 64: 575-577, 1983.

Licht S, editor: *Therapeutic heat and cold,* ed 2, New Haven, Conn, 1972, Elizabeth Licht.

McDowell AD, Lunt MJ: Electromagnetic field strength measurements on Megapulse units, *Physiotherapy* 77(12): 805-809, 1991.

McGill SN: The effect of pulsed shortwave therapy on lateral ligament sprain of the ankle, *NZ J Physiother* 10: 21-24, 1988.

McNiven DR, Wyper DJ: Microwave therapy and muscle blood flow in man *J Microwave Power* 11: 168-170, 1976.

Michaelson SM: Effects of high frequency currents and electromagnetic radiation. In Lehmann JF, editor: *Therapeutic heat and cold,* ed 4, Baltimore, 1990, Williams & Wilkins.

Millard JB: Effect of high frequency currents and infrared rays on the circulation of the lower limb in man, *Ann Phys Med* 6(2): 45-65, 1961.

Morrissey LJ: Effects of pulsed shortwave diathermy upon volume blood flow through the calf of the leg: plethysmography studies, *J Am Phys Ther Assoc* 46: 946-952, 1966.

Mosely H, Davison M: Exposure of physiotherapists to microwave radiation during microwave diathermy treatment, *Clin Phys Physiol Meas* 3:(2): 217, 1981.

Nadasdi M: Inhibition of experimental arthritis by athermic pulsing shortwave in rats, *Am J Orthop* 2: 105-107, 1960.

Nelson AJM, Holt JAG: Combined microwave therapy, *Med J Aust* 2: 88-90, 1978.

Nicolle FV, Bentall RM: The use of radiofrequency pulsed energy in the control of post-operative reaction to blepharoplasty, *Anaesth Plast Surg* 6: 169-171, 1982.

Nielson NC, Hansen R, Larsen T: Heat induction in copper bearing IUDs during shortwave diathermy, *Acta Obstet Gynaecol Scand* 58: 495, 1972.

Nwuga GB: *A study of the value of shortwave diathermy and isometric exercise in back pain management,* Proceedings of the IXth International Congress of the WCPT, Legitimerader Sjukgymnasters Riksforbund, Stockholm, Sweden, 1982.

Osborne SL, Coulter JS: Thermal effects of shortwave diathermy on bone and muscle, *Arch Phys Ther* 38: 281-284, 1938.

Paliwal BR: Heating patterns produced by 434 MHz erbotherm UHF69, *Radiology* 135: 511, 1980.

Pasila M, Visuri T, Sundholm A: Pulsating shortwave diathermy: value in treatment of recent ankle and foot sprains, *Arch Phys Med Rehabil* 59: 383-386, 1978.

Patzold J: Physical laws regarding distribution of energy for various high frequency methods applied in heat therapy, *Ultrasonics Bio Med* 2: 58, 1956.

Quirk AS, Newman RJ, Newman KJ: An evaluation of interferential therapy, shortwave diathermy and exercise in the treatment of osteo-arthrosis of the knee, *Physiotherapy* 71(2): 55-57, 1985.

Rae JW, Herrick JF, Wakim KG, et al.: A comparative study of the temperature produced by MWD and SWD, *Arch Phys Med Rehabil* 30: 199, 1949.

Raji AM: An experimental study of the effects of pulsed electromagnetic field (Diapulse) on nerve repair, *J Hand Surg* 9[B](2): 105-112, 1984.

Reed MW, Bickerstaff DR, Hayne CR, et al.: Pain relief after inguinal herniorrhaphy: ineffectiveness of pulsed electromagnetic energy, *Br J Clin Pract* 41(6): 782-784, 1987.

Richardson AW: The relationship between deep tissue temperature and blood flow during electromagnetic irradiation, *Arch Phys Med Rehabil* 31: 19, 1950.

Rubin A, Erdman W: Microwave exposure of the human female pelvis during early pregnancy and prior to conception, *Am J Phys Med* 38: 219, 1959.

Ruggera PS: *Measurement of emission levels during microwave and shortwave diathermy treatments,* Bureau of Radiological Health Report, HHS Publication (FDA), 80-8119, 1980.

Schwan HP: *Interaction of microwave and radio frequency radiation with biological systems.* In Cleary SF, editor: *Biological effects and health implications of microwave radiation,* Washington, D.C., 1970, US Department of Health, Education and Welfare.

Schwan HP, Piersol GM: The absorption of electromagnetic energy in body tissues. I. *Am J Phys Med* 33: 371, 1954.

Schwan HP, Piersol GM: The absorption of electromagnetic energy in body tissues. II. *Am J Phys Med* 34: 425, 1955.

Silverman DR, Pendleton LA: A comparison of the effects of continuous and pulsed shortwave diathermy on peripheral circulation, *Arch Phys Med Rehabil* 49: 429-436, 1968.

Stuchly MA, Repacholi MH, Lecuyer DW, et al.: Exposure to the operator and patient during shortwave diathermy treatments, *Health Physics* 42(3): 341-366, 1982.

Svarcova J, Trnavsky K, Zvarova J: The influence of ultrasound, galvanic currents and shortwave diathermy on pain intensity in patients with osteo-arthritis, *Scand J Rheumatol* supplement 67: 83-85, 1988.

Taskinen H, Kyyronen P, Hemminki K: The effects of ultrasound, shortwaves and physical exertion on pregnancy outcome in physiotherapists, *J Epidemiol Community Health* 44: 96-201, 1990.

Thom H: *Introduction to shortwave and microwave therapy,* ed 3, Springfield, Ill 1966, Charles C. Thomas.

Van Ummersen CA: *The effect of 2450 mc radiation on the development of the chick embryo.* In Peyton MF, editor: *Biological effects of microwave radiation,* vol 1, New York, 1961, Plenum Press.

Vanharanta H: *Effect of shortwave diathermy on mobility and radiological stage of the knee in the* development of experimental osteo-arthritis *Am J Phys Med* 61(2): 59-65, 1982.

Verrier M, Falconer K, Crawford JS: A comparison of tissue temperature following two shortwave diathermy techniques, *Physiotherapy Canada* 29(1): 21-25, 1977.

Wagstaff P, Wagstaff S, Downie M: A pilot study to compare the efficacy of continuous and pulsed magnetic energy (shortwave diathermy) on the relief of low back pain, *Physiotherapy* 72(11): 563-566, 1986.

Ward AR: *Electricity fields and waves in therapy,* Science Press, Australia, 1980, NSW.

Wilson DH: Treatment of soft tissue injuries by pulsed electrical energy, *Br Med J* 2: 269-270, 1972.

Wilson DH: Comparison of shortwave diathermy and pulsed electromagnetic energy in treatment of soft tissue injuries, *Physiotherapy* 60(10): 309-310, 1974.

Wilson DH: The effects of pulsed electromagnetic energy on peripheral nerve regeneration, *Ann NY Acad Sci* 238: 575, 1975.

Wise CS: The effect of diathermy on blood flow, *Arch Phys Med Rehabil* 29: 17, 1948.

Witters DM, Kantor G: An evaluation of microwave diathermy applicators using free space electric field mapping, *Phys Med Biol* 26: 1099, 1981.

Worden RE: The heating effects of microwaves with and without ischemia, *Arch Phys Med Rehabil* 29: 751, 1948.

Wyper DJ, McNiven DR: Effects of some physiotherapeutic agents on skeletal muscle blood flow, *Physiotherapy* 63(3): 83-85, 1976.

Infrared Modalities

9

Gerald W. Bell and William E. Prentice

OBJECTIVES

After completion of this chapter, the student will be able to do the following:

- Understand how the infrared modalities are classified in the electromagnetic spectrum.

- Differentiate between the physiologic effects of therapeutic heat and cold.

- Describe the contemporary modalities of the infrared spectrum in thermotherapy and cryotherapy.

- Describe the indications and contraindications for each infrared modality discussed.

- Given a clinical diagnosis, select the most effective infrared modalities.

- Explain how the sports therapist can use the infrared modalities to reduce pain.

Of the therapeutic modalities discussed in this text, perhaps none are more commonly used than **infrared** modalities. As indicated in Chapter 1, the infrared region of the electromagnetic spectrum falls between the microwave diathermy and the visible light portions of the spectrum in terms of wavelength and frequency. There is a great deal of misunderstanding among sports therapists regarding which of the modalities used in a sports-medicine setting are actually classified as infrared modalities. Traditionally, the term infrared heating conjures up visions of infrared lamps and bakers. However, it must be reemphasized that most of the heat and cold modalities, such as hydrocollator packs, paraffin baths, hot and cold whirlpools, and ice packs, as well as infrared lamps, produce forms of radiant energy that have wavelengths and frequencies that fall into the infrared region. (see Figure 1-2). This chapter will include a discussion of all the modalities that fall into the infrared portion of the electromagnetic spectrum.

MECHANISMS OF HEAT TRANSFER

Easy application and convenience of use of hot and cold modalities provide the sports therapist with the necessary tools for primary care of sports injuries. Heat is defined as the internal vibration of the molecules within a body. The transmission of heat occurs by three mechanisms: **conduction, convection,** and **radiation.** A fourth mechanism of heat transfer, **conversion,** is discussed in Chapter 12.

Conduction occurs when the body is in direct contact with the heat or cold source. Convection occurs when particles (air or water) move across the body, thus creating a temperature variation. Radiation is the transfer of heat from a warmer source to a cooler source through a conducting medium, such as air (e.g., infrared lamps). The body may either gain or lose heat through any of these three processes of heat transfer. The infrared modalities discussed in this chapter use these three methods of heat transfer to effect a tissue temperature increase or decrease.

APPROPRIATE USE OF THE INFRARED MODALITIES

Infrared modalities are often abused by sports therapists who use a modality randomly without reviewing its benefits. Placing the athlete in the whirlpool or a slush bucket of ice simply because these two modalities are available is not an acceptable treatment technique.

Heating techniques used for therapeutic purposes are referred to as **thermotherapy.** Thermotherapy is used when a rise in tissue temperature is the goal of treatment. The use of cold, or **cryotherapy,** is most effective in the acute stages of the healing process immediately following injury, when a loss of tissue temperature is the goal of therapy. Cold applications can be continued into the reconditioning stage of athletic injury management. Thermotherapy and cryotherapy are included in this section on the basis of their classification in the electromagnetic spectrum. The term **hydrotherapy** can be applied to any cryotherapy or thermotherapy technique that uses water as the medium for tissue temperature exchange.

The electromagnetic spectrum has a relatively large region of radiations designated as infrared. The infrared wavelength provides the radiant energy that is used therapeutically (see Figure 3-2). Penetration of the energy is dependent on the source but is generally considered to be a superficial form of treatment.

While this chapter is concerned primarily with application of the infrared modalities and their physiologic effects, several of the other modalities discussed in this text (e.g., the diathermies and ultrasound) cause similar physiologic responses. Specifically, the effects of heat and cold therapy discussed in this chapter may be applied to any modality that alters tissue temperature.

Heating and cooling agents can be used successfully to treat athletic injuries and trauma.[14] The sports therapist must know the injury mechanism and specific pathology, as well as the physiologic effects of the heating and cooling agents, to establish a consistent treatment schedule.

PHYSIOLOGIC EFFECTS OF TISSUE HEATING

Local superficial heating (infrared heat) is recommended in subacute conditions for reducing pain and inflammation through analgesic effects. Superficial heating produces lower tissue temperatures at the site of the pathology (injury) relative to the higher temperatures in the superficial tissues, resulting in **analgesia.** During the later stages of injury healing, a deeper heating effect is usually desirable; it can be achieved by using the diathermies or ultrasound.

Heat dilates blood vessels, causing the resting capilaries (patent small blood vessels) to open up and increase circulation. The skin is supplied with sympathetic vasoconstrictor fibers that secrete norepinephrine at their endings (especially evident in feet, hands, lips, nose, and ears). At normal body temperature the sympathetic vasoconstrictor nerves keep vascular anastomoses (blood vessel junctions) almost totally closed, but when the superficial tissue is heated, the number of sympathetic impulses is greatly reduced so that the anastomoses dilate and allow large quantities of blood to flow into the venous plexuses (a group of veins). This increases blood flow about twofold which can promote heat loss from the body.[19]

The **hyperemia** (increased blood flow) created by heat has a beneficial effect on athletic injury. This is based on increases of blood flow and pooling of blood during the metabolic processes. Recent hematomas (blood clots) should never be treated with heat until resolution of bleeding is completed. Some sports therapists have advocated never using heat during any therapeutic modality application.[22,24,26,28]

The rate of metabolism of tissues depends partly on temperature. The metabolic rate has increased approximately 13% for each 1° C (1.8° F) increase in temperature.[22] A similar decrease in metabolism has been demonstrated when temperatures are lowered.

A primary effect of local heating is an increase in the local metabolic rate with a resulting increase in the production of **metabolites** and additional heat. These two factors lead to an increased intravascular hydrostatic pressure, causing arteriolar **vasodilation** and increased capilary blood flow.[48] However, with increased hydrostatic pressure, there is a tendency toward formation of edema, which may increase the time required for rehabilitation of a particular injury. Increased capilary blood flow is important with many types of injury in which there is mild or moderate inflammation, since it causes an increase in the supply of oxygen, antibodies, leukocytes, and other necessary **nutrients** and enzymes, along with an increased clearing of metabolites. With higher heat intensities, vasodilation and increased blood flow will spread to remote areas, causing increased metabolism in the unheated area. This is known as **consensual heat vasodilation** and may be useful in many conditions where local heating is contraindicated.[16]

The application of heat can produce an analgesic effect, resulting in a reduction in the intensity of pain. The analgesic effect is the most frequent **indication** for the use of heat.[48] Although the mechanisms underlying this phenomenon are not well understood, current thinking is that it is in some way related to the gate control theory of pain modulation.

Heat is applied in musculoskeletal and neuromuscular disorders, such as sprains, strains, articular (joint-related) problems, and muscle spasms, which all describe various types of muscle pain.[16] Heat generally is considered to produce a relaxation effect and a reduction in guarding in skeletal muscle. It also increases the elasticity and decreases the viscosity of connective tissue, which is an important consideration in postacute joint injuries or after long periods of immobilization.

Many sports therapists empirically (through observation and experience) believe that in these types of disorders heat has little effect on the disease itself but serves

---

PHYSIOLOGIC EFFECTS OF HEAT AND COLD

EFFECTS OF HEAT

Increased local temperature superficially
Increased local metabolism
Vasodilation of arterioles and capillaries
Increased blood flow to part heated
Increased leukocytes and phagocytosis
Increased capillary permeability
Increased lymphatic and venous drainage
Increased metabolic wastes
Increased axon reflex activity
Increased elasticity of muscles, ligaments, and capsule fibers
Analgesia
Increased formation of edema
Decreased muscle tone
Decreased muscle spasm

EFFECTS OF COLD

Decreased local temperature, in some cases to a considerable depth
Decreased metabolism
Vasoconstriction of arterioles and capillaries (at first)
Decreased blood flow (at first)
Decreased nerve conduction velocity
Decreased delivery of leukocytes and phagocytes
Decreased lymphatic and venous drainage
Decreased muscle excitability
Decreased muscle spindle depolarization
Decreased formation and accumulation of edema
Extreme anesthetic effects

---

merely to facilitate further treatment by producing relaxation.[16] This is accomplished by relieving pain, lessening hypertonicity (excessive tension) of muscles, producing sedation (which decreases spasticity, tenderness, and spasm), and decreasing tightness in muscles and related structures. The physiologic effects of heat are summarized in Box 9-1.

PHYSIOLOGIC EFFECTS OF TISSUE COOLING

The physiologic effects of cold are for the most part opposite those of heat, the primary effect being a local decrease in temperature. Cold has its greatest benefit in acute athletic injury.[5,18,23,26,40] There is general agreement that the use of cold is the initial treatment for most conditions in the musculoskeletal system. The primary reason for using cold in acute injury is to lower the temperature in the injured area, thus reducing the metabolic rate with a corresponding decrease in production of metabolites and metabolic heat. This helps the injured tissue survive the hypoxia and limits further tissue injury that may occur.[24,26] It is also used immediately after injury to decrease pain and promote local **vasoconstriction,** thus controlling hemorrhage and **edema** (swelling).[39,45] It is also used in the acute phase of inflammatory conditions, such as bursitis, tenosynovitis, and tendinitis, in which heat may cause additional pain and swelling.[35] Cold is also used to reduce pain and the reflex muscle spasm and spastic conditions that accompany it.[40] Its analgesic effect is probably one of its greatest benefits.[13,36,46] One explanation of the analgesic effect is that cold decreases the velocity of nerve conduction, although it does not entirely eliminate it.[11,36,37] It is also possible that cold bombards central pain receptor areas with so many cold impulses that pain impulses are lost through the gate control theory of pain modulation. With ice treatments, the patient usually reports an uncomfortable sensation of cold followed by stinging or burning, then an aching sensation, and finally complete numbness.[27]

Cold also has been demonstrated to be effective in the treatment of **myofascial pain**.[50] This type of pain is referred from active myofascial trigger points with various symptoms, including pain on active movement and decreased range of motion. Trigger points may result from muscle strain or tension, which sensitizes nerves in a localized area. A trigger point may be palpated as a small nodule or as a strip of tense muscle tissue.[51]

Cold depresses the excitability of free nerve endings and peripheral nerve fibers, and this increases the pain threshold.[31] This is of great value in short-term treatment. Cold applications can also enhance voluntary control in spastic conditions, and in acute traumatic conditions they may decrease painful spasms that result from local muscle irritability.[3]

Reduction in muscle spasm relative to acute athletic trauma has been observed by all active sports therapists. Literature reviewed indicates various reasons behind reduced muscle spasms with the common thought of decreased muscle spindle activity.[30]

The initial reaction to cold is local vasoconstriction of all smooth muscle by the central nervous system to conserve heat.[45] Localized vasoconstriction is responsible for the decrease in the tendency toward formation and accumulation of edema,[48] probably as a result of a decrease in local hydrostatic pressure. There is also a decrease in the amount of nutrients and phagocytes (cells that eliminate debris) delivered to the area, thus reducing phagocytic activity.[48]

It has been hypothesized that when local temperature is lowered considerably for a period of about 30 minutes, intermittent periods of vasodilation occur, lasting 4 to 6 minutes. Then vasoconstriction recurs for a 15- to 30-minute cycle, followed again by vasodilation. This phenomenon is known as the **hunting response** and is necessary to prevent local tissue injury caused by cold.[9,10,34] The hunting response has been accepted for a number of years as fact; in reality, however, these investigations have talked about measured temperature changes rather than circulatory changes. Thus the hunting response is more likely a measurement artifact than an actual change in blood flow in response to cold.[2,27]

If a large area is cooled, the hypothalamus (the temperature-regulating center in the brain) will reflexly induce shivering, which raises the core temperature as a result of increased production of heat. Cooling of a large area might also cause arterial vasoconstriction in other remote parts of the body, resulting in an increased blood pressure.[48]

Because of the low thermal conductivity of underlying subcutaneous fat tissue, applications of cold for short periods of time will probably be ineffective in cooling deeper tissues. It has also been shown that using cold for too long may be detrimental to the healing process.[18]

The length of treatment time needed to cool tissue effectively depends on differences in subcutaneous tissue thickness. Patients with thick subcutaneous tissue should be treated with cold applications for longer than 5 minutes to produce a significant drop in intramuscular temperature. Grant[17] treated acute and chronic conditions of the musculoskeletal system and found that thin people require shorter icing periods and that response was more successful. McMaster[39] supported these findings. Recommended treatment times range from direct contact of 5 to 45 minutes to obtain adequate cooling.

It is generally believed that cold treatments are more effective in reaching deep tissue than most forms of heat. Cold applied to the skin is capable of significantly lowering the temperature of tissue at a considerable depth. The extent of this lowered tissue temperature is dependent on the type of cold applied to the skin, the duration of its application, the thickness of the subcutaneous fat, and the region of the body on which it is applied.[5]

The application of cold decreases cell permeability, decreases cellular metabolism, and decreases accumulation of edema and should be continued in 5- to 45-minute applications for up to 72 hours after initial trauma.[24] Care should be taken to avoid aggressive cold treatment to prevent disruption of the healing sequence.

If edema continues into the subacute phase, **contrast baths** (hot and cold immersion technique) may be incorporated to facilitate a capillary response for edema reduction. This consists of alternating hot and cold immersions and will be discussed in greater detail in the clinical section.

The physiologic effects of cold are summarized in Box 9-1 on p. 178.

EFFECTS OF TISSUE TEMPERATURE CHANGE ON CIRCULATION

Local application of heat or cold is indicated for **thermal** physiologic effects. The main physiologic effect is on superficial circulation because of the response of the temperature receptors in the skin and the sympathetic nervous system.

Circulation through the skin serves two major functions: (1) nutrition of the skin tissues and (2) conduction of heat from internal structures of the body to the skin so that heat can be removed from the body.[19] The circulatory apparatus is composed of *two major vessel types:* (1) arteries, capillaries, and veins and (2) vascular structures for heating the skin. Two types of vascular structures are the subcutaneous venous plexus, which holds large quantities of blood that heat the surface of the skin, and the arteriovenous anastomosis, which provides vascular communication between arteries and venous plexuses.[32] The walls of the plexuses have strong muscular coats innervated by sympathetic vasoconstrictor nerve fibers that secrete norepinephrine. When constricted, blood flow is reduced in the venous plexus to almost nothing. When maximally dilated, there is an extremely rapid flow of blood into the plexuses. The arteriovenous anastomoses are found principally in the volar or palmar surfaces of the hands and feet, the lips, the nose, and the ears.

When cold is applied directly to the skin, the skin vessels progressively constrict to a temperature of about 15° C (59° F), at which point they reach their maximum constriction.[19] This constriction results primarily from increased sensitivity of the vessels to nerve stimulation, but it probably also results at least partly from a reflex that passes to the spinal cord and then back to the vessels. At temperatures below 15° C (59° F), the vessels begin to dilate. This dilation is caused by a direct local effect of the cold on the vessels themselves, producing paralysis of the contractile mechanism of the vessel wall or blockage of the nerve impulses coming to the vessels. At temperatures approaching 0° C (32° F), the skin vessels frequently reach maximum vasodilation.

Skin plexuses are supplied with sympathetic vasoconstrictor innervation. In times of circulatory stress, such as exercise, hemorrhage, or anxiety, sympathetic stimulation of these skin plexuses forces large quantities of blood into internal vessels. Thus the subcutaneous veins of the skin act as an important blood reservoir, often providing blood to serve other circulatory functions when needed.[19]

Three types of sensory receptors are found in the subepithelial tissue: cold, warm, and pain. The pain receptors are free nerve endings. Temperature and pain are transmitted to the brain via the lateral spinothalamic tract (see Chapter 1). The nerve fibers respond differently at different temperatures. Both cold and warm receptors discharge minimally at 33° C (91.4° F). Cold receptors discharge between 10° and 41° C (50° and 105.8° F) with a maximum discharge in the 37.5° to 40° C (99.5° to 104° F) range. Above 45° C (113° F), cold receptors begin to discharge again and pain receptors are stimulated. Nerve fibers transmitting sensations of pain respond to the temperature extremes. Both warm and cold receptors adapt rapidly to temperature change; the more rapid the temperature change, the more rapid the receptor adaptation. The number of warm and cold receptors in any given small surface area is thought to be few. Therefore small temperature changes are difficult to perceive in localized areas. Larger surface areas stimulate summation of thermal signals. These larger patterns of excitation activate the vasomotor centers and the hypothalamic center.[33,35] Stimulation of the anterior hypothalamus causes cutaneous vasodilation, while stimulation of the posterior hypothalamus causes cutaneous vasoconstriction.[19,47]

The cutaneous blood flow depends on the discharge of the sympathetic nervous system. These sympathetic impulses are transmitted simultaneously to the blood vessels for cutaneous vasoconstriction and to the adrenal medulla. Both norepinephrine and epinephrine are secreted into the blood vessels and induce vessel constriction.[19] Most of the sympathetic constriction influences are mediated chemically through these neural transmitters. General exposure to cold elicits cutaneous vasoconstriction, shivering, piloerection, and an increase in epinephrine secretion, so vascular contraction occurs. Simultaneously, metabolism and heat production are increased to maintain the body temperature.[19]

Increased blood flow supplies additional oxygen to the area, thus explaining the analgesic and relaxation effects on muscle spasm. An increased proprioceptive reflex mechanism may explain these effects. Receptor end organs located in the muscle spindle are inhibited by heat temporarily, while sudden cooling tends to excite the receptor end organ.[33,35]

EFFECTS OF TISSUE TEMPERATURE CHANGE ON MUSCLE SPASM

Numerous studies deal with the effects of heat and cold in the treatment of many musculoskeletal conditions. While it is true that the use of heat as a therapeutic modality has long been accepted and documented in the literature, it is apparent that most recent research has been directed toward the use of cold. There seems to be general agreement that the physiologic mechanisms underlying the effectiveness of heat and cold treatments in reducing muscle spasm lie at the level of the muscle spindle (receptors sensitive to changes in the length of a muscle), Golgi tendon organs (receptors sensitive to changes in the tension of a muscle), and the gamma system.

Heat is believed to have a relaxing effect on skeletal muscle tone.[16] Local application of heat relaxes muscles throughout the skeletal system by simultaneously lessening the stimulus threshold of muscle spindles and by decreasing the gamma efferent firing rate. This suggests that the muscle spindles are more easily excited. Consequently, the muscles may be electromyographically silent while at rest during the application of heat, but the slightest amount of voluntary or passive movement may cause the Ia efferents to fire, thus increasing muscular resistance to stretch. If this is indeed the case, then it seems logical that decreasing the afferent impulses by raising the threshold of the muscle spindles might be effective in facilitating muscle relaxation as long as there is no movement.

The rate of firing of both primary and secondary endings is directly proportional to temperature. Local applications of cold decrease local neural activity. Annulospiral, flower-spray (small fibers located in the muscle spindle that detect changes in muscle position), and Golgi tendon organ endings all fire more slowly when cooled. Cooling actually decreases the rate of afferent activity even more, with an increase in the amount of tension on the muscle. Thus cold appears to raise the threshold stimulus of muscle spindles, and heat tends to lower it.[15] While firing of the primary spindle afferents increases abruptly with the application of cold, a subsequent decrease in spindle afferent activity occurs and persists as the temperature is lowered.[36]

Simultaneous use of heat and cold in the treatment of muscle spasm has also been studied.[12] Local cooling with ice, while maintaining body temperature to prevent shivering, results in a significant reduction of muscle spasm, greater than that which occurs with the use of heat or cold independently. This effect was attributed to maintenance of body temperature, which decreases efferent activity while local cooling decreases afferent activity. If the core temperature of the body were not maintained, the reflex shivering would result in increased muscle tone, thus inhibiting relaxation.

There is a substantial reduction in the frequency of action potential (stimulus intensity necessary for firing muscle fibers) firing of the motor unit when the muscle temperature is reduced. Muscle spindle activity is most significantly reduced when the muscle is cooled while normal body temperature is maintained.

Miglietta[41] presented a slightly different perspective on the effect of cold in reducing muscle spasm. He performed an electromyographic analysis of the effects of cold on the reduction of clonus (increased muscle tone) or spasticity in a group of 15 patients. After immersion of the spastic extremity in a cold whirlpool for 15 minutes, it was observed that electromyographic activity dropped significantly and in some cases disappeared altogether. The cold was thought to induce an afferent bombardment of cold impulses, which modify the cortical excitatory state and block the stream of painful impulses from the muscle. Thus relaxation of skeletal muscle is assumed to occur with the disappearance of pain.[49] It is not certain whether it is the excitability of the motor neurons or the hyperactivity of the gamma system, which is changed either at the muscle-spindle level or at the spinal cord level, that is responsible for the reduction of spasticity. However, it is certain that cold is effective in reducing spasticity by reducing or modifying the highly sensitive stretch-reflex mechanism in muscle.

Another factor that may be important to the reduction of spasticity is reduction in the nerve conduction velocity as a result of the application of cold.[11] These changes may result from a slowing of motor and sensory nerve conduction velocity and a decrease of the afferent discharges from cutaneous receptors.

Several studies investigated the use of cold followed by some type of exercise in the treatment of various injuries to the musculotendinous unit.[17,29] Each of these studies indicated that the use of cold and exercise was extremely effective in the treatment of acute pathologies of the musculoskeletal system that produced restrictions of muscle action.

CLINICAL USE OF THE INFRARED MODALITIES

The physiologic effects of heat and cold discussed previously are rarely the result of direct absorption of infrared energy. There is general agreement that no form of infrared energy can have a depth of penetration greater than 1 cm.[1] Thus the effects of the infrared modalities are primarily superficial and directly affect the cutaneous blood vessels and the cutaneous nerve receptors.[38]

Absorption of infrared energy cutaneously increases and decreases circulation subcutaneously in both the muscle and fat layers. If the energy is absorbed cutaneously over a long enough period of time to raise the temperature of the circulating blood, the hypothalamus will reflexively increase blood flow to the underlying tissue. Likewise, absorption of cold cutaneously can decrease blood flow via a similar mechanism in the area of treatment.[1]

Thus if the primary treatment goal is a tissue temperature increase with a corresponding increase in blood flow to the deeper tissues, it is perhaps wiser to choose a modality, such as diathermy or ultrasound, that produces energy that can penetrate the cutaneous tissues and be directly absorbed by the deep tissues.

If the primary treatment goal is to reduce tissue temperature and decrease blood flow to an injured area, the superficial application of ice or cold is the only modality capable of producing such a response.

Perhaps the most effective use of the infrared modalities should be to provide analgesia or reduce the sensation of pain associated with injury. The infrared modalities stimulate primarily the cutaneous nerve receptors. Through one of the mechanisms of pain modulation discussed in Chapter 3, most likely the gate control theory, hyperstimulation of these nerve receptors by heating or cooling reduces pain. Within the philosophy of an aggressive program of rehabilitation, as is standard in most sports-medicine settings, the reduction of pain as a means of facilitating therapeutic exercise is a common practice. As emphasized in the preface to this text, therapeutic modalities are perhaps best used as an adjunct to therapeutic exercise. Certainly, this should be a prime consideration when selecting an infrared modality for use in any treatment program.

Continued investigation and research into the use of heat and cold is warranted to provide useful data for the sports therapist. Heat and cold applications, when used properly and efficiently, will provide the sports therapist with the tools to enhance recovery and provide the athlete with optimal health-care management. Thermotherapy and cryotherapy are only two of the tools available to assist in the well-being and reconditioning of the injured athlete.

CRYOTHERAPY TECHNIQUES

Cryotherapy is the use of cold in the treatment of acute trauma and subacute injury and for the decrease of discomfort after athletic reconditioning and rehabilitation.[25] Tools of cryotherapy include ice packs, cold whirlpool, ice whirlpool, ice massage, commercial chemical cold spray, and contrast baths. Application of cryotherapy produces a three- to four-stage sensation. First there is an uncomfortable sensation of cold followed by a stinging, then a burning or aching feeling, and finally numbness. Each stage is related to the nerve endings as they temporarily cease to function as a result of decreased blood flow. The time required for this sequence varies, but several authors indicate that it occurs within 5 to 15 minutes.* After 12 to 15 minutes the hunting response is sometimes demonstrated with intense cold (10° C [50° F]).[9,28,42,45] Thus a minimum of 15 minutes is necessary to achieve extreme analgesic effects.

Application of ice is safe, simple, and inexpensive. Cryotherapy is contraindicated in patients with cold allergies (hives, joint pain, nausea), Raynaud's phenomenon (arterial spasm), and some rheumatoid conditions.[2,14,17,19,22]

Depth of penetration depends on the amount of cold and the length of the treatment time because the body is well-equipped to maintain skin and subcutaneous tissue viability through the capillary bed by reflex vasodilation of up to 4 times normal blood flow. The body has the ability to decrease blood flow to the body segment that is supposedly losing too much body heat by shunting the blood flow. Depth of penetration is also related to intensity and duration of cold application and the circulatory response to the body segment exposed. If the person has normal circulatory responses, frostbite should not be a concern. Even so, caution should be exercised when applying intense cold directly to the skin. If deeper penetration is desired, ice therapy is most effective using ice towels, ice packs, ice massage, and ice whirlpools. Patients should be advised of the four stages of cryotherapy and the discomfort they will experience. The sports therapist should explain this sequence and advise the athlete of the expected outcome, which may include a rapid decrease in pain.[2,11,17,21]

Ice Massage

Ice massage can be applied by the sports therapist or the athlete if the athlete can reach the area of application to administer self-treatment. It is best for the first three treatments to be administered by the sports therapist to give the athlete the full benefit of the treatment. When positioning the athlete's body segment to be treated, it should be relaxed and the athlete should be made comfortable. Appropriate seating and positioning should be taken into consideration with the application of ice. Administration must be thorough to get maximal treatment. Ice massage is perhaps best indicated in conditions in which some type of stretching activity is to be used.

---

*References 2, 4, 17, 20, 27, 42-45.

EQUIPMENT NEEDED (FIGURES 9-1 AND 9-2)

A. Styrofoam cups. A regular 6- to 8-ounce styrofoam cup should be filled with water and placed in the freezer. After it is frozen, all the styrofoam on the sides should be removed down to 1 inch from the bottom. This device is preferred because it has a handle with which to hold the block of ice.

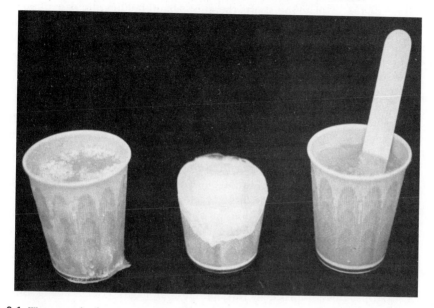

Fig. 9-1. Water may be frozen in a paper cup, styrofoam cup, or on a popsicle stick for the purpose of ice massage.

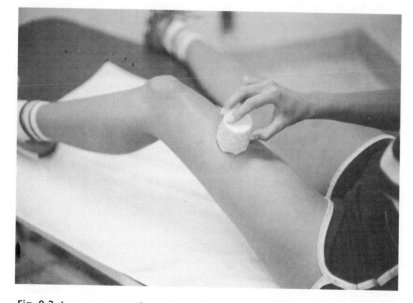

Fig. 9-2. Ice massage may be applied using either circular or longitudinal strokes.

B. Popsicle ice cups. Cups are filled with water, and a wooden popsicle stick (tongue blade) is placed in each cup. The cups are then placed in the freezer. After it is frozen the paper cup is torn off. A block of ice on a stick is now ready to be used for massage purposes.

C. Paper cups. Same technique as the styrofoam cups, except toweling may be needed to insulate the sports therapist's hand holding the paper cup.

D. Towels. These are used for positioning and absorbing the melting water in the area of the ice massage application.

TREATMENT

A. Athlete position. Sidelying, prone, supine, hooklying, or sitting, depending on the area to be treated.

B. Self-treatment. Used when athletes can comfortably reach the area to be treated by themselves.

C. Circular motion. Application of ice massage in a circular pattern with each succeeding stroke covering half the previous stroke.

D. Longitudinal strokes. Application of ice massage in a longitudinal motion with each stroke overlapping half the previous stroke.

E. Peripheral coverage. Ice should be applied for 15 to 20 minutes; consistent patterning of circular and longitudinal strokes includes the sequence described in the clinical uses section.

PHYSIOLOGIC RESPONSES

A. Cold progression proceeds through the four stages: cold, stinging, burning, and numbness.

B. Reddening of the skin (erythema) occurs as a result of blanching or lack of blood in the capillary bed. A common example occurs when one works outside in the cold without gloves or appropriate footwear and returns inside to find the toes beet-red. The body is attempting to pool blood in the area to prevent further temperature loss.

C. Ice applications of 5 to 15 minutes and greater than 10° C (50° F) will not stimulate the hunting response and do not stimulate the reflex vasodilation that creates the body's own physically induced heat or increased blood flow.

CONSIDERATIONS

A. The time necessary for the surface area to be numbed will depend on the body area to be massaged. Approximate time will depend on how fast the ice melts and what thermopane develops between the skin and ice massage.

B. Athlete comfort should be considered at all times.

C. If adequate circulation is present, frostbite should not be a concern. However, if the athlete has diabetes, the extremities, especially the toes, may require reduced temperature and adjustment of the intensity and duration of the cold.

APPLICATION. After the type of cold applicator for ice massage is selected, the athlete should be positioned comfortably and clothing should be removed from the area to be treated. The area should be set up before positioning the athlete. Remove the top two thirds of paper from the ice-filled paper or styrofoam cup, leaving 1 inch on the bottom of the cup as a handle for the therapist or athlete to use as a handgrip. The therapist should smooth the rough edges of the ice cup by gently rubbing along the edges. Ice should be applied to the athlete's exposed skin in circular or longitudinal strokes, with each stroke overlapping the previous stroke. The application should be continued until the athlete goes through the cold progression sequence of cold, stinging, burning or aching, and numbness. Once the skin is numb to fine touch, ice application can be terminated. The cold progression is the response of the sensory nerve fibers in the skin. The difference between cold and burning is primarily between the dropping out (sensory deficit) of the cold and warm nerve endings. *Standard* treatments allow the athlete to place cold applications every other 20 minutes, thus facilitating the hunting response. Some thermobarrier is developed during the ice massage in the layer of water directly on the skin, but this allows the ice cup to move smoothly over the skin. The time from application to numbing of the body segment depends on the size of the segment, but progression to numbing should be around 7 to 10 minutes.

Commercial (Cold) Hydrocollator Packs

Cold **hydrocollator packs** (Figure 9-3) are indicated in any acute injury to a musculoskeletal structure.

EQUIPMENT NEEDED
A. Hydrocollator cold pack. This must be cooled to 8° F (− 15° C); a 120 V cycle is commercially available. It needs plastic liners or protective toweling for placement on a body segment. Petroleum distillate gel is the substance contained in the plastic pouch design.
B. Moist cold towels. Towels may be immersed in ice water and molded to the

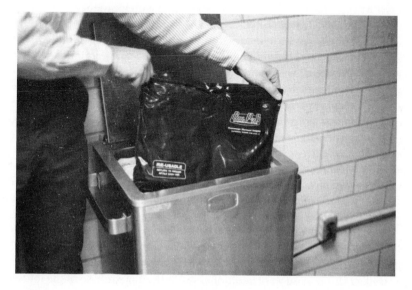

Fig. 9-3. Commercial cold pack.

skin surface, or they can be packed in ice and allowed to remain in place. The commercial cold pack should be placed on top of a moist towel.

C. Plastic bag. The hydrocollator should be placed in the bag. Air should be removed from the bag. The plastic bag may then be molded around the body segment.

D. Dry towel. To prevent the cold hydrocollator from losing heat rapidly, the towel is used as a covering to insulate the cold pack.

TREATMENT

A. Athlete position. Sidelying, prone, supine, hooklying, or sitting, depending on the area to be treated.

B. The patient must remain still during the treatment to maintain appropriate positioning of the cold pack.

C. Cold pack must be molded onto the skin.

D. The pack should be covered with a towel to limit loss of cold.

E. A timer should be set, or time should otherwise be noted.

F. Treatment time should be 20 minutes.

PHYSIOLOGIC RESPONSES

A. Cold progression proceeds through the four stages.

B. Erythema occurs.

CONSIDERATIONS

A. Body area should be covered to prevent unnecessary exposure.

B. The physiologic response to cold treatment is immediate.

C. Athlete comfort should be considered at all times.

D. Frostbite should not be a concern unless circulation is inadequate.

APPLICATION. The athlete should be positioned with treatment area exposed and towel draped to protect clothing. The commercial cold pack should be placed against wet toweling to enhance transfer of cold to the body segment. If the injury is acute or subacute, the body segment should be elevated to reduce gravity-dependent swelling. Pack the cold pack around the joint in a manner designed to remove all air and ensure placement directly against wet toweling. Cold progression will be the same as with ice massage but not as quick because of the toweling between the skin and cold pack. General treatment time required for numbing is about 20 minutes. The importance of a comfortable, properly positioned athlete is evident. Checking the sensory area after application is important. Again, frostbite should not be a concern if circulation is intact. If swelling is a concern, a wet compression (elastic) wrap could be applied under the cold pack. A sequence of 20 minutes on and 20 minutes off should be repeated for 2 hours; the same sequence can be used in home treatment. Elevation is a key adjunct therapy during the sleeping hours.

Ice Packs

Like cold hydrocollator packs, ice packs (Figure 9-4) are indicated in acute stages of injury, as well as for prevention of additional swelling after exercise of the injured part.

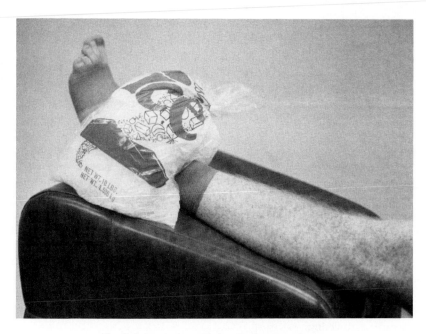

Fig. 9-4. Ice pack molded to fit the injured part.

EQUIPMENT NEEDED

A. Small plastic bags. Vegetable or bread bags may be used.
B. Ice flaker machine. Flaked or crushed ice is easier to mold than cubed ice.
C. Moist towels. These are used to facilitate cold transmission and should be placed directly on the skin.
D. Elastic bandaging. Bandaging holds the plastic ice pack in place and applies compression. The body segment may be elevated.
E. Salt solution. This is used to increase melting temperature. Melting ice has more thermal energy than stable ice and is therefore colder.

TREATMENT

A. Athlete position. Position depends on the part to be treated.
B. The patient must remain still during treatment.
C. Pack must be placed on skin.
D. Pack should be secured in place with toweling or elastic bandage.
E. Pack should be covered with towel to limit cold loss.
F. A timer should be set, or time should otherwise be noted.
G. Treatment time should be 20 minutes.

PHYSIOLOGIC RESPONSES

A. Cold progression proceeds through the four stages.
B. Erythema occurs.

CONSIDERATIONS

A. Body area should be covered to prevent unnecessary exposure.

B. The physiologic response to cold is immediate.

C. Athlete comfort should be considered at all times.

D. Frostbite should not be a concern unless circulation is inadequate.

APPLICATION. Application of ice packs is similar to the use of commercial cold hydrocollator packs; the equipment to be set up in the treatment area consists of flaked or cubed ice in a plastic bag large enough for the area to be treated. The plastic bag can be applied directly to the skin and held in place by a moist or dry elastic wrap. Patient comfort is of the utmost importance during this application to facilitate patient relaxation. The sports therapist may want to add salt to the ice to facilitate melting of the ice to create a colder slush mixture. Melting ice gives off more energy because of its less stable state, and it is therefore colder. A towel should be placed over the ice pack to decrease the warming effect of the environmental air, thus facilitating the cold application. The normal physiologic response will be cold-stinging-burning-numbness, at which time the set-up can be terminated. Because of the pliability of the flaked ice pack, it can be molded to the body segment treated. If cubed ice is used instead of flaked ice, it can still be molded, but it will not readily hold its position and will need to be secured via elastic wrap or toweling.

Cold Whirlpool

The cold whirlpool (Figure 9-5) is indicated in acute and subacute conditions in which exercise of the injured part during a cold treatment is desired.

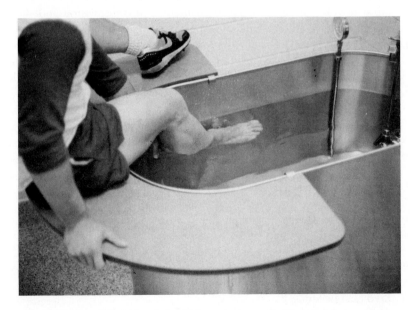

Fig. 9-5. The cold whirlpool should have the ice melted before it is turned on.

EQUIPMENT NEEDED

A. Whirlpool. The appropriate size whirlpool must be filled with cold water or ice to lower the temperature to 50° to 60° F. The therapist should use flaked ice and make sure the ice melts completely, since pieces of ice could become projectiles if a body segment is in the pool.

B. Ice machine. Flaked ice acts faster than cubed to lower the water temperature.

C. Toweling. Sufficient toweling is needed for padding the body segment on the whirlpool and for drying off after treatment.

D. Appropriate set-up in area. A chair, whirlpool, and a bench in the whirlpool must be arranged before treatment.

TREATMENT

A. Temperature should be set at 50° to 60° F.

B. Body segment must be immersed.

C. For total body immersion the water temperature should be set at 65° to 80° F.

D. Treatment time should be 5 to 15 minutes.

PHYSIOLOGIC RESPONSES

A. Cold progression proceeds through the four stages.

B. Erythema occurs.

CONSIDERATIONS

A. Caution: Gravity-dependent positions should be avoided with acute and subacute injuries. Cold wet compression or elastic wrap should be put in place before treatment.

B. The body area treated should be completely immersed.

C. A cold whirlpool allows exercises to be done during treatment.

D. Athlete comfort should be considered at all times.

E. Frostbite should not be a concern unless circulation is inadequate.

F. A toe cap made of neoprene can be used to make the athlete more comfortable in the cold whirlpool.

APPLICATION. The unit should be turned on after it has been established that the ground fault interrupter (GFI) is functioning. The athlete should be positioned in the whirlpool area, and appropriate padding should be provided for the athlete's comfort. The timer should be set for the amount of time desired, depending on the size of the body part to be treated. Treatment should continue until the body segment becomes numb (approximately 15 minutes). Numbness is the cutaneous (skin or superficial) response. Frostbite should not be a concern unless the individual has a history of circulatory deficiencies or has diabetes. Treatment time will be between 7 and 15 minutes to allow the complete circulatory response. Caution is indicated in the gravity-dependent position because of the likelihood of additional swelling if the body segment is already swollen.[10] This is the most intense application of cold of the cryotherapy techniques listed. Therefore the first two or three treatments should be administered with the sports therapist remaining in the area. One of several reasons for the intensity of cold is that the body cannot develop a **thermopane** (insulating layer of water) on the skin because of the convection effect of the whirlpool. Additional benefits include the massaging and vibrating effect of the water flow. Removal of the part being treated from the whirlpool will necessitate a review of the skin surface and an assessment of edema in the extremities. If total body immersion is used, care should be taken for the intensity and duration of the whirlpool and for protection of the genitals from direct water flow. Applications can be repeated following rewarming of the body segment after sensation has returned. If the cold application is administered before practice, it should be done before the application of preventive strapping. Enough time should also be allowed for sensation to return before taping. Studies have indicated that the reflex vasodilation lasts up to 2 hours. An athlete could practice, then return to the training room and receive additional treatment without additional edema created by **congestion** as a result of vascular and capillary insufficiency occurring during the healing process. Increased heart rate and blood pressure are associated with cold application. Conditioned athletes should not have a problem with dizziness after cold applications, but care should be taken when transferring the athlete from the whirlpool area. To keep bacterial growth under control, whirlpool cultures of the tank and jet should be taken monthly.

Cold Spray

Cold sprays, such as Fluori-Methane or ethyl chloride, do not provide adequate deep penetration, but they do provide adjunctive therapy for acupressure techniques to reduce muscle spasm. Physiologically this is accomplished by stimulating the A fibers involved in the gate control theory. The primary action of a cold spray is reduction of the pain spasm sequence secondary to direct trauma. It will, however, not reduce hemorrhage because it works on the superficial nerve endings to reduce the spasm via the stimulation of A fibers to reduce the so-called painful arc. Cold spray is an extremely effective technique in the treatment of myofascial trigger points. Precautions concerning the use of cold spray include protecting the the patient's face from the fumes and spraying the skin at an acute angle rather than at a perpendicular angle.[50] Cold spray is indicated when stretching of an injured part is desired along with cold treatment.

EQUIPMENT NEEDED
A. Fluori-Methane.
B. Toweling.
C. Padding.

TREATMENT
A. The area to be treated should be sprayed and then stretched.
B. Spasm should be reduced.
C. Treatment should be distal to proximal.
D. A quick jetstream spray or stroking motion should be used.
E. Cooling should be superficial; no frosting should occur.
F. Cold sprays may be used in conjunction with acupressure.
G. Treatment time should be set according to body segment.

PHYSIOLOGIC RESPONSES
A. Muscle spasm is reduced.
B. Golgi tendon organ response is facilitated.

C. Muscle spindle response is inhibited.

D. Ligament and other musculoskeletal structures may be stimulated.

CONSIDERATIONS

A. Both the acute and the subacute response should be positive.

B. The room should be well ventilated to avoid the accumulation of fumes.

C. Athlete comfort should be considered at all times.

APPLICATION. The application of Fluori-Methane (Figure 9-6) is typical of the application of other cold sprays. The following application procedures apply specifically to Fluori-Methane, but they provide an outline of the procedures, indications, and precautions applicable to all cold sprays. The sports therapist should follow the manufacturer's instructions in the use of any cold spray.

Fluori-Methane is a topical vapocoolant that produces a "touch cold sensation," acting as a counterirritant to block pain impulses of muscles in spasm. When used in conjunction with the spray-and-stretch technique. Fluori-Methane can break the pain cycle, allowing the muscle to be stretched to its normal length (pain-free state). The application of spray-and-stretch technique is a therapeutic modality that involves three stages: evaluation, spraying, and stretching. The therapeutic value of spray and stretch becomes most effective when the practitioner has mastered all stages and applies them in the proper sequence.

1. Evaluation: During the evaluation phase the cause of pain is determined as local spasm of an irritated trigger point. The method of applying spray and stretch to a muscle spasm differs slightly from application to a trigger point. The trigger point is a deep hypersensitive localized spot in a muscle that causes a referred pain pattern. With trigger points the source of pain is seldom the site of the pain. A trigger point may be detected by a snapping palpation over

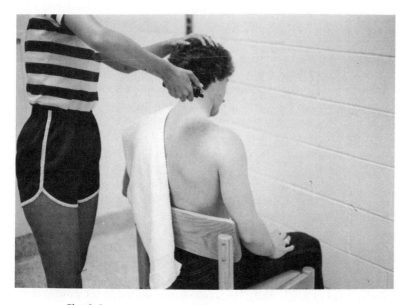

Fig. 9-6. Spray and stretch technique using Fluori-Methane.

the muscle, causing the muscle in which the irritated trigger point is situated to "jump." In the case of muscle spasm, the source and site of pain are identical.

2. Spraying: To apply Fluori-Methane: (a) Patients should assume a comfortable position. (b) Take precautions to cover the patient's eyes, nose, and mouth if spraying near face. (c) Hold bottle in an upside-down position 12 to 18 inches away from the treatment surface, allowing the jetstream of vapocoolant to meet the skin at an acute angle to lessen the shock of impact. (d) Apply the spray in one direction only—not back and forth—at a rate of 4 inches (10 cm) per second. Three or four sweeps of the spray in one direction only are sufficient to extinguish the trigger point or to overcome painful muscle spasms. The skin must not be frosted because the intense cold ($-15°$ C) of the Fluori-Methane can freeze the skin, cause a first degree burn similar to frostbite, and result in superficial tissue necrosis. In the case of trigger point, spray should be applied from the trigger point to the area of referred pain. If there is no trigger point, the spray should be applied from the affected muscle to its insertion. The spray should be applied in an even sweep. About two to four parallel, but not overlapping, sweeps of spray should be enough to cover this skin representation of the affected muscle.

3. Stretching: The stretch should begin as you start spraying from the origin to the insertion (simple muscle spasm pain) or from the trigger point to the referred pain when the trigger point is present. Spray and stretch until the muscle reaches its maximal or normal resting length. You will usually feel a gradual increase in range of motion. The spraying and stretching may require two to four spray applications to achieve the therapeutic results in any treatment session. An athlete may have multiple treatment sessions in any one day.

The spray-and-stretch technique outlined above must be considered a therapeutic system. The practitioner should spend some time each day practicing until the technique is mastered.

4. Composition: Fluori-Methane is a combination of two chlorofluorocarbons— 15% dichlorodifluoromethane and 85% trichloromonofluoromethane. The combination is not flammable and at room temperature is only volatile enough to expel the contents from the inverted container. Fluori-Methane is supplied in amber Dispenseal bottles that emit a jetstream from a calibrated nozzle.

5. Indications: Fluori-Methane is a vapocoolant intended for topical application in the management of myofascial pain, restricted motion, and muscle spasm. Clinical conditions that may respond to spray and stretch include low back pain (caused by muscle spasm), acute stiff neck, torticollis, acute bursitis of shoulder, muscle spasm associated with osteoarthritis, ankle sprain, tight hamstring, masseter muscle spasm, certain types of headache, and referred pain from trigger points.

6. Precautions: Federal law prohibits dispensing without a prescription. Although Fluori-Methane is safe for topical application to the skin, care should be taken to minimize inhalation of vapors, especially when it is being applied to the head or neck. Fluori-Methane is not intended for production of local

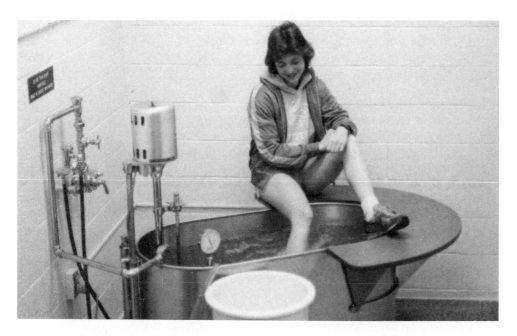

Fig. 9-7. Contrast bath using a warm whirlpool and ice immersion cylinder.

anesthesia and should not be applied to the point of frost formation. Freezing can occasionally alter pigmentation.*

Contrast Bath

Contrast baths are used to treat subacute swelling, gravity-dependent swelling, and vasodilation-vasoconstriction response.

EQUIPMENT NEEDED (FIGURE 9-7)
A. Two containers. One container is used to hold cold water (50° to 60° F), and the other is used to hold warm water (104° to 106° F). Whirlpools may be used for one or both containers.
B. Ice machine.
C. Towels.
D. Chair.

TREATMENT
A. Hot and cold immersions are alternated.
B. Treatment time should be at least 20 minutes. Treatments should consist of five 1-minute cold immersions and five 3-minute warm immersions, although the exact ratio of cold to hot treatment is highly variable.

*Modified with permission of the Gebauer Chemical Company, Cleveland, Ohio, 44104, (800) 321-9348; Ohio, (216) 271-5252.

PHYSIOLOGIC RESPONSES
A. Vasoconstriction and vasodilation occur.
B. There is a reduction of necrotic cells at the cellular level.
C. Edema is decreased.

CONSIDERATIONS
A. The temperatures of the baths must be maintained.
B. A large area is required for treatment.
C. Athlete comfort must be considered at all times.

APPLICATION. After the area is set up, a whirlpool can be used for either hot or cold application, with the opposite method of treatment contained in a bucket or sterile container. The temperatures of these immersion baths must be maintained (cold at 50° to 60° F, hot at 98° to 110° F) by adding ice or warm water. It is generally easier to use a large whirlpool for the warm water application and a bucket for the cold water application. There has been considerable controversy regarding the use of contrast baths to control swelling.[7] Contrast baths are most often indicated when changing the treatment modality from cold to hot to facilitate a mild tissue temperature increase. The use of a contrast bath allows for a transitional period during which a slight rise in tissue temperature may be effective for increasing blood flow to an injured area without causing the accumulation of additional edema. The theory that contrast baths induce a type of pumping action by alternating vasoconstriction with vasodilation has little or no credibility. Contrast baths probably cause only a superficial capillary response, resulting from inability of the larger deep blood vessels to constrict and dilate in response to superficial heating.

Thus it is recommended that during the initial stages of contrast bath treatment the ratio of hot to cold treatment begins with a relatively brief period in the hot bath, gradually increasing the length of time in the hot bath during subsequent treatments. Recommendations as to specific lengths of time are extremely variable. However, it would appear that a 3:1 ratio (3 minutes in hot, 1 minute in cold) or 4:1 ratio for 19 to 20 minutes is fairly well accepted. Whether the treatment is ended with cold or hot depends to some extent on the degree of tissue temperature increase desired. Other sports therapists prefer to use the same ratios of 3:1 or 4:1 beginning with cold. The technique may certainly be modified to meet specific needs. Since the extremity is in the gravity-dependent position, once the injured part is removed from the contrast bath, skin sensation and the amount of edema accumulation should be assessed to make sure that the treatment has not actually increased the amount of edema.

Ice Immersion

Ice buckets allow ease of application for the sports therapist. Again, a wet area should be selected (where spilled water is not a concern), with the patient positioned for comfort. The immersion, like the contrast bath, should be maintained until desired results are reached. If cryokinetics are part of the treatment, then the container should be large enough to allow for the movement of the body segment. Ice immersion is similar to cold whirlpool in that the body segment may be subject to gravity-dependent positions.

Cryokinetics

Cryokinetics is a technique that combines cryotherapy or the application of cold with exercise.[26] The goal of cryokinetics is to numb the injured part to the point of analgesia and then work toward achieving normal range of motion through progressive active exercise.

The technique begins by numbing the body part via ice immersion, cold packs, or ice massage. Most athletes will report a feeling of numbness within 12 to 20 minutes. If numbness is not perceived within 20 minutes, the therapist should proceed with exercise regardless. The numbness usually will last for 3 to 5 minutes, at which point ice should be reapplied for an additional 3 to 5 minutes until numbness returns. This sequence should be repeated five times.

Exercises are performed during the periods of numbness. The exercises selected should be pain free and progressive in intensity, concentrating on both flexibility and strength. Changes in the intensity of the activity should be limited by both the nature of the healing process and by individual patient differences in perception of pain. However, progression always should be encouraged within the framework of those limiting factors, the ultimate goal being a return to full athletic activities.[24]

THERMOTHERAPY TECHNIQUES

Heat is still used as a universal treatment for pain and discomfort. Much of the benefit is derived from the treatment simply feeling good. However, in the early stages after injury, heat causes increased capillary blood pressure and increased cellular permeability; this results in additional swelling or edema accumulation.[2,8,17,27,52] *No athlete with edema should be treated with any heat modality until the reasons for the edema are determined.* It is in the best interest of the sports therapist to use cryotherapy techniques to reduce the edema before applying heat. Superficial heat applications seem to feel more comfortable for complaints of the neck, back, low back, and pelvic areas and may be most appropriate for the athlete who exhibits some allergic response to cold applications. However, the tissues in these areas are absolutely no different from those in the extremities. Thus the same physiologic responses to the use of heat or cold will be elicited in all areas of the body.

Primary goals of thermotherapy include increased blood flow and increased muscle temperature to stimulate analgesia, increased nutrition to the cellular level, reduction of edema, and removal of metabolites and other products of the inflammatory process.

Warm Whirlpool

EQUIPMENT NEEDED

A. Whirlpool. The whirlpool must be the correct size for the body segment to be treated.

B. Towels. These are to be used for padding and drying off.

C. Chair.

D. Padding. This is to be placed on the side of the whirlpool.

TREATMENT

A. The athlete should be positioned comfortably, allowing the injured part to be immersed in the whirlpool.
B. Direct flow should be 6 to 8 inches from the body segment.
C. Temperature should be 98° to 110° F (37° to 45° C) for treatment of the arm and hand. For treatment of the leg, the temperature should be 98° to 104° F (37° to 40° C), and for full body treatment, the temperature should be 98° to 102° F (37° to 39° C).
D. Time of application should be 15 to 20 minutes.

CONSIDERATIONS

A. Athlete positioning should allow for exercise of the injured part.
B. The size of the body segment to be treated will determine whether an upper extremity, lower extremity, or full body whirlpool should be used.
C. Frequency.

APPLICATION (FIGURE 9-8). The temperature range of a warm whirlpool is 100° to 110° F (39° to 45° C). It is similar in set-up to a cold whirlpool. The athlete must be positioned in the whirlpool, with appropriate padding provided for the athlete's comfort. The unit should be turned on after it has been ascertained that the GFI is functioning. The timer should be set for the amount of time desired, depending on the size of the body part to be treated (10 to 30 minutes). Treatment time should be long enough to stimulate vasodilation and reduce muscle spasm (approximately 20 minutes). Again, caution is indicated in the gravity-dependent position in subacute

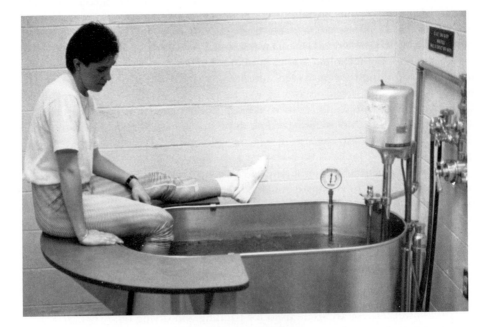

Fig. 9-8. Warm whirlpool.

athletic injuries. If some pitting edema exists (i.e., finger pressure on the skin leaves an indentation), cold or contrast baths are better indicated. In addition to increased circulation and reduction of spasm, benefits of the warm whirlpool include the massaging and vibrating effects of the water movement. On removal of the body segment from the whirlpool, it is necessary to review the skin surface and limb girth to see if the warm whirlpool increased swelling; this step is indicated even if the athlete is past the subacute stage. After allowing the body segment to cool down, the athlete can have appropriate preventive strapping or padding placed on the body segment. If the athlete receives the treatment before exercising, it is recommended that he or she gently do range-of-motion exercises to reduce congestion and increase proprioception (sense of position) in all joints. If the athlete is complaining of muscle soreness, it would be more appropriate to recommend swimming pool exercises. The whirlpool provides a sedative effect. It is recommended that the athlete shower or clean the body surface before using a whirlpool. Random access to the whirlpool is not warranted.

The warm whirlpool is an excellent postsurgical modality to increase systemic blood flow and mobilization of the affected body part. The appropriateness of whirlpool therapy needs to be addressed by the sports therapist because it is the most commonly abused physical therapy modality. An example of this abuse is the common practice of placing an individual in the whirlpool without taking the time to assess the specific physiologic responses desired (such as reflex vasodilation or reduction of inflammatory deposits). However, it is an excellent adjunctive modality when used appropriately in the sports-medicine setting.

Whirlpools should be cleaned frequently to prevent the bacterial growth. When a patient with any open or infected lesion uses the whirlpool, it must be drained and cleaned immediately. Cleaning should be done using both a disinfecting and antibacterial agent. Particular attention should be paid to cleaning the turbine by placing the intake valves in a bucket containing the disinfecting solution and turning the power on. Bacterial cultures should be monitored periodically from the tank, drain, and jets.

Commercial (Warm) Hydrocollator Packs (Figure 9-9)
EQUIPMENT NEEDED
A. Unit heat packs. These are canvas pouches of petroleum distillate. A thermostat maintains the high temperature (170° F) and helps prevent burns. Unit heat packs come in three sizes: (1) regular size is 12 × 12 inches for most body segments, (2) double size is 24 × 24 inches, for the back, low back, and buttocks, (3) cervical is 6 × 18 inches for the cervical spine. Packs are removed by tongs or scissor handles.
B. Towels. Regular bath towels and commercial double pad towels are required. Commercial double pad toweling has a pouch for pack placement and 1-inch thick toweling to be placed in cross fashion, tags on the edge of packs folded in, toweling overlapped on one side and four layers on the opposite side. Six layers equal 1 inch of toweling. Additional toweling may be needed depending on total body surface covered.

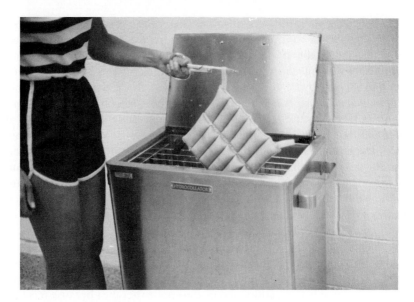

Fig. 9-9. Hydrocollator packs stored in tank.

TREATMENT
A. Position six layers of toweling as described in (Figure 9-10).
B. Sufficient toweling should be provided to protect the patient from burns.
C. Athlete position should be comfortable.
D. Treatment time should be 15 to 20 minutes.

PHYSIOLOGIC RESPONSES
A. Circulation is increased.
B. Muscle temperature is increased.
C. Tissue temperature is increased.
D. Spasms are relaxed.

CONSIDERATIONS
A. The size of the body segment to be treated should determine how many packs are needed.
B. Athlete comfort is always a consideration.
C. Time of application should be 15 to 20 minutes.

APPLICATION. Appropriate toweling and positioning of the athlete is necessary for a comfortable treatment. The moist heat pack tends to stimulate the circulatory response. Dry heat, as discussed in the infrared section, has a tendency to force blood away from the cutaneous capillary bed, thus increasing the possibility of a burn with the skin's inability to dissipate heat. The patient must not be allowed to lie on the packs because this will force the silicate gel out through the seams of the fabric sleeves. If the patient cannot tolerate the weight of the moist heat pack, alternate methods, such as placing the patient sidelying with the majority of the weight of the hot pack on the side

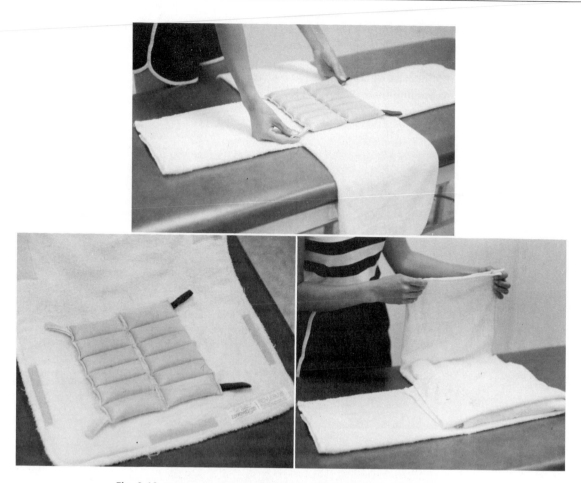

Fig. 9-10. Techniques for wrapping hydrocollator packs.

of the pack and the pack held in place by additional towels or sheets wrapped around the patient, can be used. The most common indications are for muscular spasm, back pain, or as a preliminary treatment to other modalities.

Paraffin Bath

Paraffin bath is a simple and efficient, though somewhat messy, technique for applying a fairly high degree of localized heat. Paraffin treatments provide six times the amount of heat available in water because the mineral oil in the paraffin lowers the melting point of the paraffin. The combination of paraffin and mineral oil has a low specific heat, which enhances the patient's ability to tolerate heat from paraffin better than from water of the same temperature.

The risk of a burn with paraffin is substantial. The sports therapist should weigh heavily the considerations between a paraffin bath and warm whirlpool bath in the athletic setting. The majority of paraffin baths are used for chronic arthritis patients' hands and feet. If the patient-athlete has a chronic hand or foot problem, the use of paraffin instead of water usually gives longer lasting pain relief.[6,27]

EQUIPMENT NEEDED
A. Paraffin bath (Figure 9-11, *A*).
B. Plastic bags and paper towels.
C. Towels.

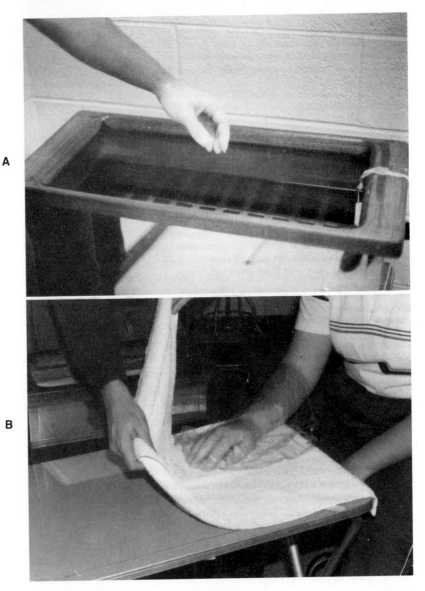

Fig. 9-11. A, Hand being dipped in paraffin bath. **B,** After being dipped in paraffin, the hand should be wrapped in plastic bags and toweling.

TREATMENT

A. Dipping. The extremity should be dipped into the paraffin for a couple of seconds, then removed to allow the paraffin to harden slightly for a few seconds. This procedure is repeated until 10 layers have accumulated on the part to be treated.

B. Wrapping. The paraffin-coated extremity should be wrapped in a plastic bag with several layers of toweling around it to act as insulation (Figure 9-11, *B*).

C. Treatment time should be 20 to 30 minutes.

PHYSIOLOGIC RESPONSES

A. There is an increase in tissue temperature.

B. Pain relief occurs.

C. Thermal hyperthermia occurs.

CONSIDERATIONS

A. Some units are equipped with thermostats that may elevate the temperature to 212° F, thus killing any bacteria that may grow in the paraffin. Otherwise the temperature should be set at 126° F.

B. If the paraffin becomes soiled, it should be dumped and replaced at no longer than 6-month intervals.

APPLICATION. The purchase of a paraffin bath for the training room requires that the bath have a built-in thermostat. Before treatment, the athlete's body segment should be cleaned thoroughly with soap, water, and finally alcohol to remove any soap residue. This will prevent bacterial build-up in the bottom of the paraffin bath, which is an excellent medium for culture growth.

The mixture ratio of paraffin to mineral oil is 1 gallon of mineral oil to 2 pounds of paraffin. The mineral oil reduces the ambient temperature of the paraffin, which is 126° F (at which temperature a burn could occur). It is important to build six layers of paraffin, with the first layer highest on the body segment and each successive layer lower than the previous one. This is important because when dipping the extremity in the paraffin, if the second layer of paraffin is allowed to get between the skin and the first layer of paraffin, the heat will not dissipate and the athlete could be burned. Because heat is retained in the body and is also radiated from the paraffin, there is an increase in capillary dilation and blood supply in the treated segment. The sports therapist should place the athlete in a comfortable position and enclose the paraffin in paper towels, plastic bags, and toweling to maintain the heat. Treatment is applied for approximately 20 to 30 minutes. Removal of the paraffin calls for extra care not to contaminate the used portion so that it does not contaminate the entire bath when it is returned.

Removal of paraffin involves removing towels, plastic bag, and paper towels, then using a tongue depressor to split the paraffin to allow easy removal. If the paraffin has not touched the floor, remove the paraffin cast over the open paraffin bath. It will dissolve on returning to the remaining liquid paraffin. Clean the body segment with soap and water or, if a postsurgical patient is being treated, give a massage, since the mineral oil will make the skin moist and supple. When cleaning the skin, the therapist must examine the surface for burns or mottling. The thermostat will raise the temperature of the paraffin to 212° F, destroy any bacteria, and maintain a sterile contact medium. Paraffin baths require a large amount of supervision to prevent contamination, but they do provide a special type of treatment that is well adapted to the athletic patient with injuries of the hands and feet.

Infrared Lamps

When talking about infrared modalities, the sports therapist most typically thinks of the infrared lamp. The biggest advantages of an infrared lamp are that superficial tissue temperature rises that the unit does not touch the patient. However, radiant heat is seldom used because it is limited in depth of skin penetration to less than 1 mm. Dry heat from an infrared lamp tends to elevate superficial skin temperatures more than moist heat; however, moist heat probably has a greater depth of penetration.

Superficial skin burns occasionally occur because of intense infrared radiation and the reflector becoming extremely hot (4000° F). It is recommended that a warm moist towel be placed over the body segment to be treated to enhance the heating effects. Dry towels should cover the remainder of the body not being treated. This will allow a greater blood/tissue exchange by trapping the heat build-up in the moist towel and reducing the stagnant air over the body segment. Caution should be used, and the skin should be checked every few minutes for mottling.

Infrared generators may be divided into two categories: luminous and nonluminous. Nonluminous generators consist of a spiral coil of resistant metal wire wound around a cone-shaped piece of nonconducting material. The resistance of the wire to the electric flow produces heat and a dull red glow. A properly shaped reflector then radiates the heat to the body. All incandescent bodies and tungsten and carbon filament lamps are in the category of luminous generators. No nonluminous lamps are currently being manufactured since infrared at a wavelength of 12,000 Å will penetrate slightly more deeply than either longer or shorter waves, due to a certain unique characteristic of human skin. Tungsten filament and special quartz red sources produce significant amounts of infrared heat at 12,000 Å. Flare as a result of reflection off the skin can be a real problem.

EQUIPMENT NEEDED
A. Infrared lamp.
B. Dry toweling. This is to be used for draping the parts of the body not being treated.
C. Moist toweling. Moist towels are used to cover the area to be treated.
D. A GFI should be used with an infrared lamp.

TREATMENT
A. The athlete should be positioned 20 inches from the source.
B. Protective toweling should be put in place.
C. Treatment time should be 15 to 20 minutes.
D. Skin should be checked every few minutes for mottling.
E. Areas that are not to be treated must be protected.

PHYSIOLOGIC RESPONSES

A. A superficial rise in tissue temperature occurs.
B. There is some decrease in pain.
C. Moisture and sweat appear on the skin surface.

CONSIDERATIONS

A. To avoid a generalized temperature rise, only the portion that is injured should be treated.
B. The infrared lamp should be used primarily when a patient cannot tolerate pressure from another type of modality (e.g., hydrocollator packs).
C. Caution must be exercised to avoid burns.

APPLICATION (FIGURE 9-12). The athlete should be placed in a comfortable position. Moist heat should be used to stimulate blood flow. It is recommended to prevent blood from being forced away from the area as with dry heat. A moist, warm towel should be applied to the area to be treated. A squirt bottle is needed to keep the towel moist. All areas not to be treated should be draped. The distance from the area to be treated to the lamp should be adjusted according to treatment time: the standard formula is 20 inches distance = 20 minutes treatment time. After treatment, the skin surface should be assessed. This type of treatment tends to force the blood away from the capillary bed and should be used only in superficial skin complaints related to dry heat requirements.

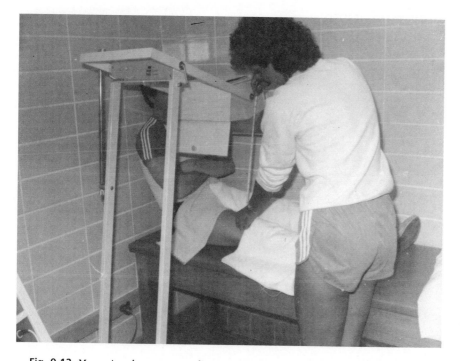

Fig. 9-12. Measuring the treatment distance with far positioning of the infrared baker.

Fluidotherapy

Fluidotherapy is a unique, multifunctional physical medicine modality. The fluidotherapy unit is a dry heat modality that uses a suspended air stream, which has the properties of a liquid. Its therapeutic effectiveness in rehabilitation and healing is based on its ability to simultaneously apply heat, massage, sensory stimulation for desensitization, levitation, and pressure oscillations. Unlike water, the dry, natural medium does not irritate the skin or produce thermal shocks. This allows for much higher treatment temperatures than with aqueous or paraffin heat transfer. The pressure oscillations may actually minimize edema, even at very high treatment temperatures. Outstanding clinical success has been reported in treatment of pain, range of motion, wounds, acute injuries, swelling, and blood flow insufficiency. Fluidotherapy treatment of the hand at 115° F (46.2° C) results in a sixfold increase in blood flow and a fourfold increase in metabolic rates in a normal adult.[6] These properties will increase blood flow, sedate, decrease blood pressure, and promote healing by accelerating biochemical reactions.[6]

Counterirritation, through mechanoreceptor and thermoreceptor stimulation, reduces pain sensitivity, thus permitting high temperatures without painful heat sensations. Pronounced hyperthermia accelerates the chemical metabolic processes and stimulates the normal healing process. The high temperatures enhance tissue elasticity and reduce tissue viscosity, which improves musculoskeletal mobility. Vascular responses are stimulated by long-lasting hyperthermia and pressure fluctuations, resulting in increased blood flow to the injured area.

EQUIPMENT NEEDED
A. Fluidotherapy model 104 (Figure 9-13).
B. Toweling.

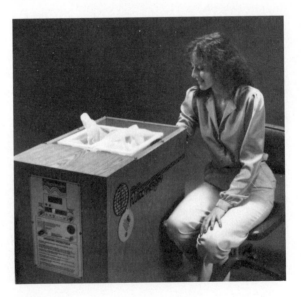

Fig. 9-13. Fluidotherapy treatment
(Photo courtesy of Fluidotherapy Corporation, 6113 Aletha Lane, Houston, TX 77081)

TREATMENT
A. The patient must be positioned for comfort.
B. The patient should place the body segment to be treated (hand or foot) in the fluidotherapy unit.
C. Protective toweling must be placed at the unit interface and body segment.
D. Treatment time should be 15 to 20 minutes.

PHYSIOLOGIC RESPONSES
A. Tissue temperature increases.
B. Pain relief occurs.
C. Thermal hyperthermia occurs.

CONSIDERATIONS
A. Fluidotherapy unit must be kept clean.
B. All knobs must be returned to zero after treatment.

APPLICATION. The patient should be positioned comfortably. The treated body segment should be submerged in the medium before the unit is turned on. There is no thermal shock when heat is applied. Treatments are approximately 20 minutes. Recommended temperature varies by body part and patient tolerance, with a range of 110° to 125° F (43° to 53° C). Maximum temperature rise in the treated part occurs after 15 minutes of treatment. Unless contraindicated, active and passive exercise is encouraged during treatment.

In case of open lesions or infections, a protective dressing is recommended to prevent soiling or contaminating the cloth entry ports. Patients with splints, bandages, tape, orthopedic pins, plastic joint replacement, and artificial tendons may be treated with fluidotherapy. The medium is clean and will not soil clothing. It is not necessary to disrobe to get the full benefit of heat and massage; however, direct contact between skin and the medium is desirable to maximize heat transfer.

In treating the hands, muscles, ankles, and conditions that manifest themselves relatively near the surface of the skin, appreciably higher body temperatures can be achieved using superficial heating modalities.[6] Further, the superficial modalities treat a larger area of the body than ultrasound or microwave diathermies, thus the total amount of heat absorbed will be much higher. Fluidotherapy, hydrotherapy, and paraffin cause about the same amount of temperature increase.[14]

CONCLUSIONS

Infrared sources transmit thermal energy to or from the athlete. In most cases, they are simple, efficient, and inexpensive. Sports therapists who choose to compare modalities and use the most appropriate technique for their athletes will be providing quality care for that athlete. A haphazard approach to the use of infrared modalities will only reflect a disregard for the health care of the athlete.

Questioning, thinking sports therapists will determine which procedure is best and most appropriate clinically. They will take responsibility for seeing that the most appropriate therapeutic modality is applied to enhance the athlete's reconditioning and rehabilitation. This chapter has provided various methods and modalities, their physiologic responses, and special considerations for the sports-medicine practitioner.

Regardless of what infrared modality sports therapists choose, they should be aware of (1) the physiologic implications relative to circulation, (2) the ease of application, and (3) the short- and long-term benefits of treatment.

Additional areas of concern relate to (1) benefits of the infrared modality application, whether cryotherapy or thermotherapy, (2) economy of modality application, and (3) repeatability of applications. Common sense in the application of these modalities will provide optimum injury management and modality usage for tissue healing of athletic trauma.

SUMMARY

1. Any modality that radiates energy with wavelengths and frequencies that fall into the infrared region of the electromagnetic spectrum are referred to as infrared modalities.

2. When infrared modalities are applied to connective tissue or muscle and soft tissue, they will cause either a tissue temperature decrease or tissue temperature increase.

3. The primary physiologic effect of heat is vasodilation of capillaries with increased blood flow, increased metabolic activity, and relaxation of muscle spasm.

4. The primary physiologic effects of cold are vasoconstriction of capillaries with decreased blood flow, decreased metabolic activity, and analgesia with reduction of muscle spasm.

5. The infrared energies have a depth of penetration of less than 1 cm, thus the physiologic effects are primarily superficial and directly affect the cutaneous blood vessels and nerve receptors.

6. Examples of thermotherapy are whirlpools, moist heat packs, infrared lamps, heating pads, and fluidotherapy.

7. Examples of cryotherapy are ice packs, ice massage, commercial ice packs, ice whirlpools, and cold sprays.

GLOSSARY

analgesia Loss of sensibility to pain.

anesthesia Loss of sensation.

conduction Heat loss or gain through direct contact.

congestion Presence of an abnormal amount of blood in the vessels resulting from an increase in blood flow or obstructed venous return.

consensual heat vasodilation Vasodilation and increased blood flow will spread to remote areas, causing increased metabolism in the unheated area.

contrast bath Hot (106° F) and cold (50° F) treatments in a combined sequence to stimulate superficial capillary vasodilation or vasoconstriction.

convection Heat loss or gain through the movement of water molecules across the skin.

conversion Changing from one energy form into another.

cryokinetics The use of cold and exercise in the treatment of pathology or disease.

cryotherapy The use of cold in the treatment of pathology or diseases.

edema Excessive fluid in cells.

erythema Redness of the skin; inflammation. A redness of the skin caused by capillary dilation.

fluidotherapy A modality of dry heat using a finely divided solid suspended in a stream with the properties of liquid.

Hubbard tank An immersion tank for the whole body, it may have vertical depth for walking or supine treatment.

hunting response A reflex vasodilation that occurs in response to cold approximately 15 minutes into the treatment. This has been demonstrated to be only an increase in temperature and not necessarily a change in blood flow.

hydrocollator A synthetic hot (170° F) or cold (0° F) gel used as an adjunctive modality to stimulate a rise or fall in tissue temperature.

hydrotherapy Cryotherapy and thermotherapy techniques that use water as the medium for heat transfer.

hyperemia Presence of an increased amount of blood in part of the body.

indication The reason to prescribe a remedy or procedure.

infrared That portion of the electromagnetic spectrum associated with thermal changes; located adjacent to the red portion of the visible light spectrum. That part of the electromagnetic spectrum dealing with infrared wavelengths.

metabolites Waste products of metabolism or catabolism.

myofascial pain A type of referred pain associated with trigger points.

nutrients Essential or nonessential food substance.

paraffin bath A combined paraffin and mineral oil immersion technique in which the paraffin substance is heated to 126° F for conductive heat gains; commonly used on the hands and feet for distal temperature gains in blood flow and temperature.

radiation The process of emitting energy from some source, in the form of waves. A method of heat transfer through which heat can either be gained or lost.

thermal Pertaining to heat.

thermopane An insulating layer of water next to the skin.

thermotherapy The use of heat in the treatment of pathology or disease.

vasoconstriction Narrowing of the blood vessels.

vasodilation Dilation of the blood vessels.

REFERENCES

1 Abramson DI, Tuck S, Lee SW, et al.: Vascular basis for pain due to cold, *Arch Phys Med Rehabil* 47: 300-305, 1966.

2 Baker RJ, Bell GW: The effect of therapeutic modalities on blood flow in the human calf, *J Orthop Sport Phys Ther* 13: 23, 1991.

3 Basset SW, Lake BM: Use of cold applications in management of spasticity, *Phys Ther* 38(5): 333-334, 1958.

4 Behnke R: Cold therapy, *Athl Train* 9(4): 178-179, 1974.

5 Bierman W, Friedlander M: The penetrative effect of cold, *Arch Phys Med Rehabil* 21: 585-592, 1940.

6 Chambers R: Clinical uses of cryotherapy, *J Am Phys Ther Assoc* 49(3): 145-149, 1969.

7 Clarke DH: Effect of immersion in hot and cold water upon recovery of muscular strength following fatiguing isometric exercise, *Arch Phys Med Rehabil* 44: 565-568, 1963.

8 Clarke DH, Stelmach GE: Muscle fatigue and recovery curve parameters at various temperatures *Res Q* 37(4): 468-479, 1966.

9 Clarke RSJ, Hellon RE, Lind AR: Vascular reactions of the human forearm to cold, *Clin Sci* 17: 165-179, 1958.

10 Cote D, Prentice WE, Hooker D: A comparison of three treatment procedures for minimizing ankle edema, *Phys Ther* 68(7): 1072-1076, 1988.

11 DeJong RH, Hershey WM, Wagman IH: Nerve conduction velocity during hypothermia in man, *Anes* 27: 805-810, 1966.

12 Dontigny R, Sheldon K: Simultaneous use of heat and cold in treatment of muscle spasm, *Arch Phys Med Rehabil* 43: 235-237, 1962.

13 Downer AH: *Physical therapy procedures,* ed 3, Springfield, Ill, 1978, Charles C. Thomas.

14 Downey JA: Physiological effects of heat and cold, *J Am Phys Ther Assoc* 44(8): 713-717, 1964.

15 Eldred E, Lindsley DF, Buchwald JS: The effect of cooling on mammalian muscle spindles, *Exp Neurol* 2: 144-157, 1960.

16 Fischer E, Soloman S: *Physiologic responses to heat and cold.* In Licht S, editor: *Therapeutic heat,* New Haven, Conn, 1965, Elizabeth Licht.

17 Grant AE: Massage with ice (cryokinetics) in the treatment of painful conditions of the musculoskeletal system, *Arch Phys Med Rehabil* 45: 233-238, 1964.

18 Griffin JE, Karselis TC: *Physical agents for physical therapists,* ed 2, Springfield, Ill, 1988, Charles C. Thomas.

19 Guyton AC: *Medical physiology,* ed 6, Philadelphia, WB Saunders.

20 Hayden C: Cryokinetics in an early treatment program, *J Am Phys Ther Assoc* 44: 11, 1964.

21 Hedenberg L: Functional improvement of the spastic hemiplegic arm after cooling, *Scand J Rehabil Med* 2: 154-158, 1970.

22 Hocutt JE Jr, Jaffe R, Rylander CR, et al.: Cryotherapy in ankle sprains, *Am J Sports Med* 10(3): 316-319, 1992.

23 Knight KL: Effects of hypothermia on inflammation and swelling, *Ath Train* 11: 7-10, 1976.

24 Knight KL: *Cryotherapy in sports medicine.* In Scribner K, Burke EJ, editors: *Relevant topics in athletic training,* New York, 1978, Movement Publications.

25 Knight KL: Ice for immediate care of injuries, *Phys Sportsmed* 10(2): 137, 1982.

26 Knight KL: *Cryotherapy: theory, technique and physiology,* Chattanooga, 1985, Chattanooga Corporation.

27 Knight KL, Aquino J, Johannes SM, et al.: A reexamination of Lewis' cold induced vasodilation in the finger and the ankle, *Ath Train* 15: 248-250, 1980.

28 Knight KL, Londeree BR: Comparison of blood flow in the ankle of uninjured subjects during therapeutic applications of heat, cold, and exercise, *Med Sci Sports Exerc* 12(1): 76-80, 1980.

29 Knott M, Barufaldi D: Treatment of whiplash injuries, *Phys Ther* 41: 8, 1961.

30 Knutsson E: Topical cryotherapy in spasticity, *Scand J Rehab Med* 2: 159-163, 1970.

31 Knutsson E, Mattson E: Effects of local cooling on monosynaptic reflexes in man, *Scand J Rehabil Med* 1: 126-132, 1969.

32 Kolb P, Denegar C: Traumatic edema and the lymphatic system, *Ath Train* 18: 339-341, 1983.

33 Lehman JF: *Therapeutic heat and cold,* ed 3, Baltimore, 1982, Williams & Wilkins.

34 Lewis T: Observations upon the reactions of the vessels of the human skin to cold, *Heart* 15: 177-208, 1930.

35 Licht S: *Therapeutic heat and cold,* New Haven, Conn, 1965, Elizabeth Licht.

36 Lippold OCJ, Nicholls JG, Redfearn JWT: A study of the afferent discharge produced by cooling a mammalian muscle spindle, *J Physiol* 153: 218-231, 1960.

37 Lowdon BJ, Moore RJ: Determinants and nature of intramuscular temperature changes during cold therapy, *Am J Phys Med* 54(5): 223-233, 1975.

38 Mancuso D, Knight KL: Effects of prior skin surface temperature response of the ankle during and after a 30-minute ice pack application, *J Ath Train* 27: 242-249, 1992.

39 McMaster WC: A literary review on ice therapy in injuries, *Am J Sports Med* 5(3): 124-126, 1977.

40 Merrick M, Knight KL, Ingersoll C, et al.: The effects of ice and compression wraps on intramuscular temperatures at various depths, *J Ath Train* 28(3): 236-245, 1993.

41 Miglietta O: Electromyographic characteristics of clonus and influence of cold, *Arch Phys Med Rehabil* 45: 508, 1964.

42 Moore R: *Uses of cold therapy in the rehabilitation of athletes: recent advances,* Proceedings 19th American Medical Association National Conference on the medical aspects of sports, San Francisco, June 1977.

43 Moore R, Nicolette R, Behnke R: The therapeutic use of cold (cryotherapy) in the care of athletic injuries, *Ath Train* 2: 613, 1967.

44 Murphy AJ: The physiological effects of cold application, *Phys Ther* 40(2): 112-115, 1960.

45 Olson JE, Stravino V: A review of cryotherapy, *Phys Ther* 62(8): 840-853, 1972.

46 Prentice WE: An electromyographic analysis of the effectiveness of heat or cold and stretching for inducing relaxation in injured muscle *Orthop Sports Phys Ther* 3(3): 133-146, 1982.

47 Rocks A: Intrinsic shoulder pain syndrome, *Phys Ther* 59(2): 153-159, 1979.

48 Stillwell K: *Therapeutic heat and cold.* In Krusen F, Kootke F, Ellwood P, editors: *Handbook of physical medicine and rehabilitation,* Philadelphia, 1971, WB Saunders.

49 Travell J: Rapid relief of acute "stiff neck" by ethyl chloride spray, *Am Med Wom Assoc* 4(3): 89-95, 1949.

50 Travell J: Ethyl chloride spray for painful muscle spasm, *Arch Phys Med Rehabil* 32: 291-298, 1952.

51 Travell J, Simons D: *Myofascial pain and dysfunction: the trigger point manual,* Baltimore, 1983, Williams & Wilkins.

52 Zankel H: Effect of physical agents on motor conduction velocity of the ulnar nerve, *Arch Phys Med Rehabil* 47(12): 787-792, 1966.

SUGGESTED READINGS

Abraham E: Whirlpool therapy for treatment of soft tissue wounds complicated by extremity fractures, *J Trauma* 4: 222, 1974.

Abraham WM: Heat vs. cold therapy for the treatment of muscle injuries, *Ath Train* 9(4): 177, 1974.

Abramson DI, Bell B, Tuck S, et al.: Changes in blood flow, oxygen uptake and tissue temperatures produced by therapeutic physical agents, Effect of indirect or reflex vasodilation, *Am J Phys Med* 40: 5-13, 1961.

Abramson DI, Mitchell RE, Tuck S, et al.: Changes in blood flow, oxygen uptake and tissue temperatures produced by a topical application of wet heat, *Arch Phys Med Rehabil* 42: 305, 1961.

Abramson DI, Tuck S, Zayas AM, et al.: The effect of altering limb position on blood flow, oxygen uptake and skin temperature, *J Appl Physiol* 17: 191, 1962.

Abramson DI, Tuck S, Chu LS, et al.: Effect of paraffin bath and hot fomentation on local tissue temperature, *Arch Phys Med Rehabil* 45: 87, 1964.

Abramson DI, Tuck S, Chu LS, et al.: Indirect vasodilation in thermotherapy, *Arch Phys Med Rehabil* 46: 412, 1965.

Abramson DI: Physiologic basis for the use of physical agents in peripheral vascular disorders, *Arch Phys Med Rehabil* 46: 216, 1965.

Abramson DI, Chu LS, Tuck S, et al.: Effect of tissue temperatures and blood flow on motor nerve conduction velocity, *JAMA* 198: 1082, 1966.

Abramson DI, Tuck S, Lee SW, et al.: Comparison of wet and dry heat in raising temperature of tissues, *Arch Phys Med Rehabil* 48: 654, 1967.

Airhihenbuwa CO, St. Pierre RW, Winchell D: Cold vs. heat therapy: a physician's recommendations for first aid treatment of strain, *Emergency* 19(1): 40-43, 1987.

Arnheim D, Prentice WE: *Principles of athletic training,* ed 8, St Louis, 1993, Mosby.

Ascenzi J: *The need for decontamination and disinfection of hydrotherapy equipment,* vol 1, Surgikos Inc, 1980, Asepsis Monograph.

Austin KF: *Diseases of immediate type hypersensitivity.* In Isselbacher KJ, Adams RD, Braumwald E, et al., editors: *Harrison's principles of internal medicine,* ed 9, New York, 1980, McGraw-Hill.

Barnes L: Cryotherapy: putting injury on ice, *Phys Sportsmed* 7(6): 130-136, 1979.

Basur R, Shephard E, Mouzos G: A cooling method in the treatment of ankle sprains, *Practitioner* 216: 708, 1976.

Beasley R, Kester N: Principles of medical-surgical rehabilitation of the hand, *Med Clin North Am* 53: 645, 1969.

Belitsky RB, Odam SJ, Humbley-Kozey C: Evaluation of the effectiveness of wet ice, dry ice, and cryogen packs in reducing skin temperature, *Phys Ther* 67: 1080, 1987.

Benson TB, Copp EP: The effects of therapeutic forms of heat and ice on the pain threshold of the normal shoulder, *Rheumatol Rehabil* 13: 101, 1974.

Berne R, Levy MN: *Cardiovascular physiology,* ed 4, St Louis, 1981, Mosby.

Bickle R: Swimming pool management, *Physiotherapy* 57: 475, 1971.

Bierman W: Therapeutic use of cold, *JAMA* 157: 1189-1192, 1955.

Bocobo C: The effect of ice on intra-articular temperature in the knee of the dog, *Am J Phys Med Rehab* 70: 181, 1991.

Boes MC: Reduction of spasticity by cold, *J Am Phys Ther Assoc* 42(1): 29-32, 1962.

Boland AL: *Rehabilitation of the injured athlete.* In Strauss RA, editor: *Physiology,* Philadelphia, 1979, WB Saunders.

Borrell RM, Henley ES, Purvis H, et al.: Fluidotherapy: evaluation of a new heat modality, *Arch Phys Med Rehabil* 58: 69, 1977.

Borrell RM, Parker R, Henley E, et al.: Comparison of in vivo temperatures produced by hydrotherapy, paraffin wax treatment, and fluidotherapy, *Phys Ther* 60(10): 1273-1276, 1980.

Boyer T, Fraser, RE, Doyle AE: The haemodynamic effects of cold immersion, *Clin Sci* 19: 539, 1980.

Boyle RW, Balisteri F, Osborne F: The value of the Hubbard tank as a diuretic agent, *Arch Phys Med Rehabil* 45: 505, 1964.

Chastain PB: The effect of deep heat on isometric strength, *Phys Ther* 58: 543, 1978.

Clarke K, editor: *Fundamentals of athletic training: physical therapy procedures,* Chicago, 1971, AMA Press.

Claus-Walker J, et al.: Physiological responses to cold stress in healthy subjects and in subjects with cervical cord injuries, *Arch Phys Med Rehabil* 55: 485, 1974.

Clendenin MA, Szumski, A: Influence of cutaneous ice application on single motor units in humans, *Phys Ther* 51(2): 166-175, 1971.

Cobb CR, deVries H, Urban R, et al.: Electrical activity in muscle pain, *Am J Phys Med* 54: 80, 1975.

Cobbold AF, Lewis OJ: Blood flow to the knee joint of the dog: effect of heating, cooling and adrenaline, *J Physiol* 132: 379, 1956.

Cohen A, Martin G, Waldin K: The effect of whirlpool bath with and without agitation on the circulation in normal and diseased extremities, *Arch Phys Med Rehabil* 30: 212, 1949.

Conolly WB, Paltos N, Tooth RM: Cold therapy: an improved method, *Med J Aust* 2: 424, 1972.

Cordray YM, Krusen EM: Use of hydrocollator packs in the treatment of neck and shoulder pains, *Arch Phys Med Rehabil* 39: 105, 1959.

Covington DB, Bassett FH: When cryotherapy injures, *Phys Sportsmed* 21(3): 78-79, 1993.

Crockford GW, Hellon RF: Vascular responses of human skin to infrared radiation, *J Physiol* 149: 424, 1959.

Crockford GW, Hellon RF, Parkhouse J: Thermal vasomotor response in human skin mediated by local mechanism, *J Physiol* 161: 10, 1962.

Currier DP, Kramer JF: Sensory nerve conduction: heating effects of ultrasound and infrared, *Physiother Can* 34: 241, 1982.

Dawson WJ, Kottke FJ, Kubicek WG, et al.: Evaluation of cardiac output, cardiac work, and metabolic rate during hydrotherapy exercise in normal subjects, *Arch Phys Med Rehabil* 46: 605, 1965.

Day MJ: Hypersensitive response to ice massage: report of a case, *Phys Ther* 54: 592, 1974.

DeLateur BJ, Lehmann JF: *Cryotherapy.* In Lehmann JF, editor: *Therapeutic heat and cold,* ed 3, Baltimore, 1982, Williams & Wilkins.

deVries H: Quantitative electromyographic investigation of the spasms theory of muscle pain, *Am J Phys Med* 45: 119, 1966.

Drez D: *Therapeutic modalities for sports injuries,* Chicago, 1989, Yearbook.

Drez D, Faust DC, Evans JP: Cryotherapy and nerve palsy, *Am J Sports Med* 9: 256, 1981.

Edwards HT, Harris RC, Hultman E, et al.: Effect of temperature on muscle energy metabolism and endurance during successive isometric contractions, sustained to fatigue, of the quadriceps muscle in man, *J Physiol* 220: 335, 1972.

Epstein M: Water immersion: modern researchers discover the secrets of an old folk remedy, *Sciences* 205: 12, 1979.

Eyring EJ, Murray WR: The effect of joint position on the pressure of intra-articular effusion, *J Bone Joint Surg* 46[A](6): 1235, 1964.

Farry PJ, Prentice NG: Ice treatment of injured ligaments: an experimental model, *NZ Med J* 9: 12, 1950.

Folkow B, Fox RH, Krog J, et al.: Studies on the reactions of the cutaneous vessels to cold exposure, *Acta Physiol Scand* 58: 342, 1963.

Fountain FP, Gersten JW, Senger O: Decrease in muscle spasm produced by ultrasound, hot packs and IR, *Arch Phys Med Rehabil* 41: 293, 1960.

Fox RH: Local cooling in man, *Br Med Bull* 17(1): 14-18, 1961.

Fox RH, Wyatt HT: Cold induced vasodilation in various areas of the body surface in man, *J Physiol* 162: 259, 1962.

Gammon GD, Starr I: Studies on the relief of pain by counterirritation, *J Clin Invest* 20: 13, 1941.

Gerig BK: The effects of cryotherapy upon ankle proprioception (abstract), *Ath Train* 25: 119, 1990.

Gieck J: Precautions for hydrotherapeutic devices, *Clin Manage* 3: 44, 1953.

Golland A: Basic hydrotherapy, *Physiotherapy* 67: 258, 1951.

Green GA, Zachazewski JE, Jordan SE: A case conference: peroneal nerve palsy induced by cryotherapy, *Phys Sportsmedi* 17: 63, 1989.

Greenberg RS: The effects of hot packs and exercise on local blood flow, *Phys Ther* 52: 273, 1972.

Halkovich IR, Personius WJ, Clamann HP, et al.: Effect of fluorimethane spray on passive hip flexion, *Phys Ther* 61: 185, 1981.

Halvorson GA: Therapeutic heat and cold for athletic injuries, *Phys Sportsmed* 18: 87, 1990.

Harrison RA: Tolerance of pool therapy by ankylosing spondylitis patients with low vital capacity, *Physiotherapy* 67: 296, 1981.

Head MD, Helms PA: Paraffin and sustained stretching in the treatment of burn contractures, *Burns* 4: 136, 1977.

Hellerbrand T, Holutz S, Eubarik I: Measurement of whirlpool temperature, pressure and turbulence, *Arch Phys Med Rehabil* 32: 17, 1950.

Hendler E, Crosbie R, Hardy JD: Measurement of heating of the skin during exposure to infrared radiation *J Appl Physiol* 12: 177, 1958.

Henrickson AS, Fredricksson K, Persson I, et al.: The effect of heat and stretching on the range of hip motion, *J Ortho Sports Phys Ther* 6: 110, 1984.

Hocutt JE, Jaffe R, Rylander R, et al.: Cryotherapy in ankle sprains, *Am J Sports Med* 10: 316, 1982.

Holmes G: Hydrotherapy as a means of rehabilitation, *Br J Phys Med* 5: 93, 1942.

Horton BT, Brown GE, Roth GM: Hypersensitiveness to cold with local and systemic manifestations of a histamine-like character: its amenability to treatment, *JAMA* 107: 1263, 1936.

Horvath SM, Hollander JL: Intra-articular temperature as a measure of joint reaction, *J Clin Invest* 28: 469, 1949.

Hunter J, Mackin E: *Edema and bandaging.* In Hunter J, editors: *Rehabilitation of the hand,* ed 1, St Louis, 1978, Mosby.

Ingersoll CD, Mangus B: Sensations of cold reexamined: a study using the McGill pain questionnaire, *Ath Train* 26: 240, 1991.

Ingersoll CD, Mangus B, Wolf S: Cold-induced pain: habituation to cold immersion (abstract), *Ath Train* 25: 126, 1990.

Jessup GT: Muscle soreness: temporary distress of injury? *Ath Train* 15(4): 260, 1950.

Jezdirisky J, Marek J, Ochonsky P: Effects of local cold and heat therapy on traumatic oedema of the rat hind paw. I. Effects of cooling on the course of traumatic oedema, *Acta Universitatis Palackianae Olomucensis Facultatis Medicae* 66: 155, 1973.

Johnson DJ: Effect of cold submersion on intramuscular temperature of the gastrocnemius muscle, *Phys Ther* 59: 1238, 1979.

Johnson J, Leider FE: Influence of cold bath on maximum handgrip strength, *Percept Mot Skills* 44: 323, 1977.

Kaempffe FA: Skin surface temperature after cryotherapy to a casted extremity, *J Orthop Sports Phys Ther* 10(11): 448-450, 1989.

Kessler RM, Hertling D: *Management of common musculoskeletal disorders,* Philadelphia, 1953, Harper & Row.

Knight KL: Ankle rehabilitation with cryotherapy, *Phys Sportsmed* 7(11): 133, 1979.

Kowal MA: Review of physiological effects of cryotherapy, *J Orthop Sports Phys Ther* 6(2): 66-73, 1953.

Kramer JF, Mendryk SW: Cold in the initial treatment of injuries sustained in physical activity programs, *Can Assoc Health Phys Ed Rec J* 45(4): 27-29, 38-40, 1979.

Krusen EM, et al.: Effects of hot packs on peripheral circulation, *Arch Phys Med Rehabil* 31: 145, 1950.

Landen BR: Heat or cold for the relief of low back pain? *Phys Ther* 47: 1126, 1967.

Lane LE: Localized hypothermia for the relief of pain in musculoskeletal injuries, *Phys Ther* 51: 182, 1971.

Lee JM, Warren MP, Mason SM: Effects of ice on nerve conduction velocity, *Physiotherapy* 64: 2, 1978.

Lehmann JF: Effect of therapeutic temperatures on tendon extensibility, *Arch Phys Med Rehabil* 51: 481, 1970.

Lehmann JF, Brurmer GD, Stow RW: Pain threshold measurements after therapeutic application of ultrasound, microwaves and infrared, *Arch Phys Med Rehabil* 39: 560, 1958.

Lehmann JF, Silverman JF, Baum BA, et al.: Temperature distributions in the human thigh produced by infrared, hot pack and microwave applications, *Arch Phys Med Rehabil* 47: 291, 1966.

Levine MG, Kabat H, Knott M, et al.: Relaxation of spasticity by physiological techniques, *Arch Phys Med Rehabil* 35: 214, 1954.

Lundgren C, Muren A, Zederfeldt B: Effect of cold vasoconstriction on wound healing in the rabbit, *Acta Chir Scand* 118: 1, 1959.

Magness J, Garrett T, Erickson D: Swelling of the upper extremity during whirlpool baths, *Arch Phys Med Rehabil* 51: 297, 1970.

Major TC, Schwingharner JM, Winston S: Cutaneous and skeletal muscle vascular responses to hypothermia, *Am J Physiol* 240 (Heart Circ. Physiol. 9):H868, 1981.

Marek J, Jezdinsky J, Ochonsky P: Effects of local cold and heat therapy on traumatic oedema of the rat hind paw. II. Effects of various kinds of compresses on the course of traumatic oedema. *Acta Universitatis Palackianae Olomucensis Facultatis Medicae* 66: 203, 1973.

Matsen FA, Questad K, Matsen AL: The effect of local cooling on post fracture swelling, *Clin Orthop* 109: 201, 1975.

McGowen HL: Effects of cold application on maximal isometric contraction, *Phys Ther* 47: 185, 1967.

McGray RE, Patton NJ: Pain relief at trigger points: a comparison of moist heat and shortwave diathermy, *J Orthop Sports Phys Ther* 5: 175, 1984.

McMaster WC: Cryotherapy, *Phys Sports Med* 10(11): 112-119, 1982.

McMaster WC, Liddie S: Cryotherapy influence on posttraumatic limb edema, *Clin Orthop* 150: 283-287, 1980.

McMaster WC, Liddie S, Waugh TR: Laboratory evaluation of various cold therapy modalities, *Am J Sports Med* 6(5): 291-294, 1978.

Mense S: Effects of temperature on the discharges of muscle spindles and tendon organs, *Pflugers Arch* 374: 159, 1978.

Mermel JM: The therapeutic use of cold, *J Am Osteopathic Assoc* 74: 1146-1157, 1975.

Michalski WJ, Sequin JJ: The effects of muscle cooling and stretch on muscle spindle secondary endings in the cat, *J Physiol* 253: 341-356, 1975.

Michlovitz SL: *Thermal agents in rehabilitation,* Philadelphia, 1990, FA Davis.

Miglietta O: Action of cold on spasticity, *Am J Phys Med* 52(4): 198-205, 1973.

Newton MJ, Lehnikuhi D: Muscle spindle response to body heating and localized muscle cooling: implications for relief of spasticity, *J Am Phys Ther Assoc* 45(2): 91,105, 1965.

Nylin J: The use of water in therapeutics, *Arch Phys Med Rehabil* 13: 261, 1932.

Oliver RA, Johnson DJ, Wheelhouse WW, et al.: Isometric muscle contraction response during recovery from reduced intramuscular temperature, *Arch Phys Med Rehabil* 60: 126-129, 1979.

Perkins J, Mao-Chih LI, Nicholas CH, et al.: Cooling and contraction of smooth muscle, *Am J Physiol* 163: 14, 1950.

Petajan JH, Watts N: Effects of cooling on the triceps surae reflex, *Am J Phys Med* 42: 240-251, 1962.

Pope C: Physiologic action and therapeutic value of general and local whirlpool baths, *Arch Phys Med Rehabil* 10: 498, 1929.

Price R: Influence of muscle cooling on the vasoelastic response of the human ankle to sinusoidal displacement, *Arch Phys Med Rehabil* 71(10): 745-748, 1990.

Price R, Lehmann JF, Boswell S: Influence of cryotherapy on spasticity at the human ankle, *Arch Phys Med Rehabil* 74(3): 300-304, 1993.

Randall BF, Imig CJ, Hines HM: Effects of some physical therapies on blood flow, *Arch Phys Med Rehabil* 33: 73, 1952.

Randt GA: Hot tub folliculitis, *Phys Sports Med* 11: 75, 1983.

Ritzmann SE, Levin WC: Cryopathies: a review, *Arch Intern Med* 107: 186, 1961.

Roberts P: Hydrotherapy: its history, theory and practice, *Occup Health* 235: 5, 1981.

Schaubel HH: Local use of ice after orthopedic procedures, *Am J Surg* 72: 711, 1946.

Schultz K: *The effect of active exercise during whirlpool on the hand,* unpublished thesis. San Jose, Calif, 1982, San Jose State University.

Shelley WB, Caro WA: Cold erythema: a new hypersensitivity syndrome, *JAMA* 180: 639, 1962.

Simonetti A, Miller R, Gristina J: Efficacy of povidone-iodine in the disinfection of whirlpool baths and hubbard tanks, *Phys Ther* 52: 450, 1972.

Steve L, Goodhart P, Alexander J: Hydrotherapy burn treatment: use of chloramine-T against resistant microorganisms, *Arch Phys Med Rehabil* 60: 301, 1979.

Stewart JB, Basmajian JV: *Exercises in water.* In Basmajian JV, editor: *Therapeutic exercise,* ed 3, Baltimore, 1978, Williams & Wilkins.

Strandness DE: *Vascular diseases of the extremities.* In Isselbacher KJ, Adams RD, Braunwald EL, et al., editors: *Harrison's principles of internal medicine,* ed 9, New York, 1980, McGraw-Hill.

Taber C, Contryman K, Fahrenbach J: Measurement of reactive vasodilation during cold gel pack application to nontraumatized ankles, *Phys Ther* 72: 294, 1992.

Travell JG, Simons DG: *Myofascial pain and dysfunction: the trigger point manual,* Baltimore, 1983, Williams & Wilkins.

Urbscheit N, Johnston R, Bishop B: Effects of cooling on the ankle jerk and H-response in hemiplegic patients, *Phys Ther* 51: 983, 1971.

Wakim KG, Porter AN, Krusen KH: Influence of physical agents and of certain drugs on intra-articular temperature, *Arch Phys Med Rehabil* 32: 714, 1951.

Walsh M: *Relationship of hand edema to upper extremity position and water temperature during* whirlpool treatments in normals, Unpublished thesis. Philadelphia, 1983, Temple University.

Warren GC: *The use of heat and cold in the treatment of common musculoskeletal disorders.* In Kessler RM, Hertling D: *Management of common musculoskeletal disorders,* Philadelphia, 1983, Harper & Row.

Warren GC, Lehmann JF, Koblanski JN: Heat and stretch procedures: an evaluation using rat tail tendon, *Arch Phys Med Rehabil* 57: 122, 1976.

Watkins AL: *A manual of electrotherapy,* ed 3, Philadelphia, 1972, Lea & Febiger.

Waylonis GW: The physiological effect of ice massage, *Arch Phys Med Rehabil* 48: 37-42, 1967.

Weinberger A, Lev A: Temperature elevation of connective tissue by physical modalities, *Crit Rev Phys Rehab Med* 3: 121, 1991.

Wessman MS, Kottke FJ: The effect of indirect heating on peripheral blood flow, pulse rate, blood pressure and temperature, *Arch Phys Med Rehabil* 48: 567, 1967.

Whitney SL: *Physical agents: heat and cold modalities.* In Scully RM, Barnes MR, editors: *Physical therapy,* Philadelphia, 1987, JB Lippencott.

Whyte HM, Reader SR: Effectiveness of different forms of heating, *Ann Rheum Dis* 10: 449, 1951.

Wickstrom R, Polk C: Effect of whirlpool on the strength endurance of the quadriceps muscle in trained male adolescents, *Am J Phys Med* 40: 91, 1961.

Wilkerson GB: Treatment of inversion ankle sprain through synchronous application of focal compression and cold, *Ath Train* 26: 220, 1991.

Wolf SL, Basmajian JV: Intramuscular temperature changes deep to localized cutaneous cold stimulation, *Phys Ther* 53(12): 1284-1288, 1973.

Wolf SL, Letbetter WD: Effect of skin cooling on spontaneous EMG activity in triceps surae of the decerebrate cat, *Brain Res* 91: 151-155, 1975.

Wright V, Johns RJ: Physical factors concerned with the stiffness of normal and diseased joints, *Bull Johns Hopkins Hosp* 106: 215, 1960.

Wyper DJ, McNiven DR: Effects of some physiotherapeutic agents on skeletal muscle blood flow, *Physiotherapy* 62: 83, 1976.

Yackzan L, Adams C, Francis KT: The effects of ice massage in delayed muscle soreness, *Am J Sports Med* 12(2): 159-165, 1984.

Zankel HT: Effect of physical agents on motor conduction velocity of the ulnar nerve, *Arch Phys Med Rehabil* 47: 787, 1966.

Zeiter WJ: Clinical application of the paraffin bath, *Arch Phys Ther* 20: 469, 1939.

Zislis J: *Hydrotherapy.* In Knisen F, editor: *Handbook of physical medicine and rehabilitation,* ed 2, Philadelphia, 1971, WB Saunders.

Low-Power Lasers

10

Ethan Saliba and Susan Foreman

OBJECTIVES

After completion of this chapter, the student will be able to do the following:

- Describe the different types of lasers.

- Understand the physical principles used to produce laser light.

- Describe the characteristics of the helium neon and gallium arsenide low-power lasers.

- Describe the therapeutic applications of lasers in wound and soft tissue healing, edema reduction, inflammation, and pain.

- Understand the application techniques of low-power lasers.

- Describe the classifications of lasers.

- Describe the safety considerations in the use of lasers.

- Describe the precautions and contraindications for low-power lasers.

LASER is an acronym that stands for Light Amplification of Stimulated Emissions of Radiation. Despite the image presented in science-fiction movies, lasers offer valuable applications in the industrial, military, scientific, and medical environments. Einstein in 1916 was the first to postulate the theorems that conceptualized the development of lasers. The first work with amplified electromagnetic radiation dealt with MASERs—microwave amplification of stimulated emissions of radiation. In 1955, Townes and Schawlow showed it was possible to produce stimulated emission of microwaves beyond the optical region of the electromagnetic spectrum. This work with stimulated emission soon extended into the optical region of the electromagnetic spectrum, resulting in the development of devices called optical masers. The first working optical maser was constructed in 1960 by Theodore Maiman when he developed the synthetic ruby laser. Other types of lasers were devised shortly afterward. It was not until 1965 that the term LASER was substituted for optical masers.[27]

Although lasers are relatively new, they have gone through extensive advances and refinements in a very short time. Lasers have been incorporated into numerous everyday applications that range from audio discs and supermarket scanning to communication and medical applications. This chapter will give an overview of lasers but will deal principally with the application of low-power lasers in conservative management of medical conditions.

PHYSICS

Light is a form of electromagnetic energy that has **wavelengths** between 100 and 10,000 nanometers (nm = 10^{-9}) within the electromagnetic spectrum.[27] Visible light ranges from 400 nm (violet) to 700 nm (red). Beyond the red portion of the visual range are the **infrared** and microwave regions, and below the violet end are the ultraviolet, X-ray, gamma, and cosmic ray regions (see Figure 1-2). Light energy is transmitted through space as waves that contain tiny "energy packets" called photons. Each photon contains a definite amount of energy depending on its wavelength (color).

Basics of the atomic theory are used to explain the principles of laser generation. The atom is the smallest particle of an element that retains all of the properties of that element. The atom is divisible into fundamental particles called neutrons, protons, and electrons. Neutrons and positively charged protons are contained in the nucleus of the atom. **Electrons,** which are negatively charged, are equal in number to protons and orbit the nucleus at distinct energy levels.

If an atom gains or loses an electron, it will become a negatively or positively charged ion. The polarity difference between the positively charged nucleus and negatively charged electrons keeps the electrons orbiting the nucleus at these distinct energy levels. Electrons neither absorb nor radiate energy as long as they are maintained in their distinct orbit. An electron will stay in its lowest energy level **(ground stage)** unless it absorbs an adequate amount of energy to move it to one of its higher orbital levels (Figure 10-1). If an electron changes orbit, it will either gain or lose a distinct amount (quanta) of energy; it cannot exist between orbits.

If a photon of adequate energy level collides with an electron of an atom, it will cause the electron to change levels. When this occurs, the atom is said to be in an **excited state.** The atom stays in this excited state only momentarily and releases an identical photon (energy level) to the one it absorbed, which returns it to a ground state. This process is called **spontaneous emission** (Figure 10-2). Energy levels are particular to the type of atom; therefore an electron accepts only the precise amount of energy that will move it from one energy level to another. Another means of exciting atoms other than with photon collision is with an electrical discharge. The energy is generated by collision of electrons that are accelerated in an electrical field.[17]

Stimulated Emissions

The concept of **stimulated emission** was postulated by Einstein and is essential to the working principle of lasers. It states that a photon released from an excited atom would stimulate another similarly excited atom to deexcite itself by releasing an identical

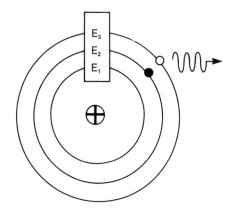

Fig. 10-1. When energy is absorbed by an atom, an orbiting electron can become excited to a higher orbit. As the electron drops back to its original level, energy (photon) is released.

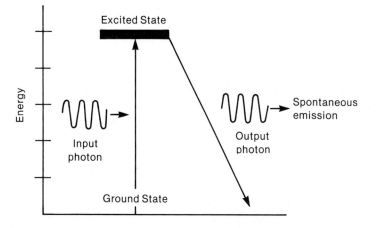

Fig. 10-2. Spontaneous emission occurs when a photon changes energy level.

photon.[27] The triggering photon would continue on its way unchanged, and the subsequent photon released would be identical in frequency, direction, and phase. These two photons would promote the release of additional identical photons as long as other excited atoms were present. A critical factor for this occurrence is having an environment with unlimited excited atoms, which is termed **population inversion.** Population inversion occurs when there are more atoms in an excited state than in a ground state. It is caused by applying an external power source to the lasing medium. The released photons are identical in phase, direction, and frequency. To contain them and to generate more photons, mirrors are placed at both ends of the chamber. One mirror is totally reflective, while the other is semipermeable. The photons are reflected within the chamber, which amplifies the light and stimulates the emission of other photons from excited atoms. Eventually, so many photons are stimulated that the chamber cannot contain the energy. When a specific level of energy is attained, photons of a particular wavelength are ejected through the semipermeable mirror. Thus

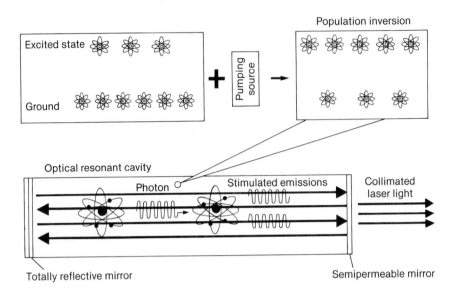

Fig. 10-3. Pumping is a process of elevating an orbiting electron to a higher level, thus creating population diversion that is essential for laser operation.

amplified light through stimulated emissions (LASER) is produced (Figure 10-3).

The laser light is emitted in an organized manner rather than in a random pattern as from a light bulb. Three properties distinguish the laser from incandescent and fluorescent light sources: **coherence, monochromaticity,** and **collimation.**[27]

Coherence means all photons of light emitted from individual gas molecules are the same wavelength and that the individual light waves are in phase with one another. Normal light is composed of many wavelengths that superimpose their phases on one another.

Monochromaticity refers to the specificity of light in a single, defined wavelength; if the specificity is in the visible light spectrum, it is only one color. The laser is one of the few light sources that produces a specific wavelength.

The laser beam is well-collimated, that is, there is minimal divergence of the photons.[1] That means the photons move in a parallel fashion, thus concentrating a beam of light (Figure 10-4).

TYPES OF LASERS

Lasers are classified according to the nature of the material placed between two reflecting surfaces. There are potentially thousands of different types of lasers, each with specific wavelengths and unique characteristics depending on the lasing medium used. The lasing mediums used to create lasers include crystal and glass (solid-state), gas and excimer, semiconductor, liquid dye, and chemical.

- Crystal lasers include the synthetic ruby (aluminum oxide and chromium) and the neodymium, yttrium, aluminum, garnet (Nd:YAG) lasers, among others. Synthetic, rather than natural, materials are used to ensure purity of the medium, which is necessary to generate physical characteristics of lasers.[12]

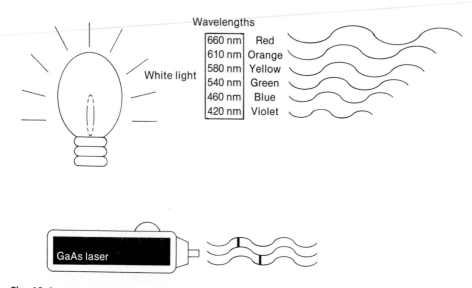

Fig. 10-4. (*Top*), White light contains electromagnetic energy of all wavelengths (colors) that are superimposed on each other. (*Bottom*), Laser light is monochromatic (single wavelength), coherent (in phase), and collimated (minimal divergence).

- Gas lasers were developed in 1961, shortly after the first ruby laser. The gas lasers developed include helium neon (HeNe), argon, and carbon dioxide (CO_2), along with numerous others. The HeNe laser is one type of low-power device under investigation in the United States for application in physical medicine.

- Semiconductor or diode lasers were developed in 1962 after the production of gas (HeNe) lasers. The gallium arsenide (GaAs) laser was the first diode laser developed and is another low-power laser under investigation in the United States for application in physical medicine.

- Liquid lasers are also known as dye lasers because they use organic dyes as the lasing medium. By varying the mixture of the dyes, the wavelengths of the laser can be varied.

- Chemical lasers are usually extremely high powered and frequently used for military purposes.[17]

Lasers can be categorized as either high or low power, depending on the intensity of energy they deliver. High-power lasers are also known as "hot" lasers because of the thermal responses they generate. These are used in the medical realms in numerous areas including surgical cutting and coagulation, ophthalmologic, dermatologic, oncologic and vascular specialties. The use of low-power lasers (also known as "cold" or "soft" lasers) for wound healing and pain management is a relatively new area of application in medicine. These lasers produce a maximal output of less than 1 milliwatt (1 mW = $\frac{1}{1000}$ watt) in the United States and work by causing photochemical, rather than thermal, effects. No tissue warming occurs. The exact distinction of the power output that delineates a low-versus high-power laser varies. Low-power devices are considered any laser that does not generate an appreciable thermal response. This category can include lasers capable of producing up to 500 mW of power (up to a Class IV laser).[6]

Low-power lasers, which have been studied and used in Europe for the past 20 to 25 years, have been investigated in the United States for the past decade. The potential applications for low-power lasers include treatment of tendon and ligament injury, arthritis, edema reduction, soft tissue injury, ulcer and burn care, scar tissue inhibition, and acutherapy.

EQUIPMENT

Lasers require the following components to be operational[17]:

1. Power Supply—Lasers use an electrical power supply that can potentially deliver up to 10,000 volts and hundreds of amps.
2. Lasing Medium—This is the material that generates the laser light. It can include any type of matter: gas, solid, or liquid.
3. Pumping Device—Pumping describes the process of elevating an orbiting electron to a higher, "excited" energy level (see Figure 10-4). This creates the population inversion that is essential for laser operation. The pumping device may be high voltage, photoflash lamps, radio-frequency oscillators, or other lasers. The pumping device is very specific to the type of lasing medium being used.
4. Optical Resonant Cavity—This contains the lasing medium. Once population inversion has occurred, this cavity, which contains the reflecting surfaces, directs the beam propagation.

The helium neon (HeNe) and gallium arsenide (GaAs) lasers are the two principal lasers currently under investigation in the United States for conservative management of medical conditions. The following discussion will concentrate on these two laser types.

Helium Neon Lasers

The helium neon (HeNe) gas laser uses a gas mixture of primarily helium with neon in a pressurized tube. This creates a laser in the red portion of the electromagnetic spectrum with a wavelength of 632.8 nm. The power output of the HeNe laser can vary, but typically runs from 1.0 to 10.0 mW depending on the gas density used. Larger tubes are necessary for higher power outputs, and each requires a precise power drive to operate.[6] Laser output can decrease, depending on the care of the equipment, the number of operating hours, and whether fiberoptics are used. For example, rough handling can jar the reflecting surfaces, and a high number of hours in operation or poor fiberoptic quality can diminish the laser output. The HeNe laser in the United States delivers a power output of 1 mW through a fiber-optic tube in a continuous mode. Although the HeNe laser light is well collimated, the use of fiberoptics causes a divergence of the beam from 18 to 21 degrees.[6] Fiberoptics can decrease the output delivery 50% or more as the light travels from the lasing medium to the tip of the applicator. Fiberoptics are used to make the delivery more convenient because the size of the gas tube would make direct application difficult. HeNe lasers up to 6 mW have been manufactured for clinical use in Canada, which has fewer governmental restrictions. These higher-output lasers, although still considered low power, allow delivery of desired dosages in reduced time.[5]

Gallium Arsenide Lasers

The gallium arsenide (GaAs) lasers use a diode to produce an infrared (invisible) laser at a wavelength of 904 nm. Diode lasers are composed of semiconductor silicone materials that are precisely cut and layered. An electrical source is applied to each side, and lasing action is produced at the junction of the two materials. The cleaved surfaces function as partially reflecting surfaces that will ultimately produce coherent light[12] (Figure 10-5).

Diode lasers produce a beam that is elliptically shaped so that the lasers have a 10 to 35 degree divergence, although no fiberoptics are used.[17] The 904 nm laser is delivered in a pulsed mode because of the heat produced at the junction of the diode chips. The GaAs laser manufactured in the United States has a peak power of 2 W but is delivered in a pulsed mode that decreases the average power to 0.4 mW output if delivered at 1000 Hz (see calculations in dosage section).

The application of additional layers of materials to other types of diodes allows their operation in a continuous mode at room temperature.[17] The continuous mode results in higher average power outputs from the lasers. Higher output diode lasers are manufactured for clinical applications in Canada and include the following:

   780 nm wavelength with a 5 mW output—continuous mode delivery
   810 nm wavelength with a 20 mW output—continuous mode delivery
   830 nm wavelength with a 30 mW output—continuous mode delivery
These diodes are interchangeable in a single base unit.[5]

The laser units available in the United States can deliver both HeNe and GaAs lasers. The same device can both measure electrical impedance and deliver electrical point stimulation. The impedance detector allows hypersensitive or acupuncture points to be located. The point stimulator can be combined with laser application

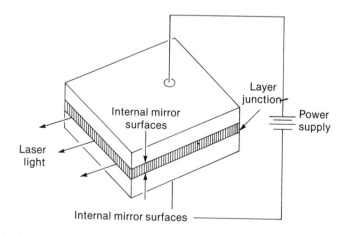

Fig. 10-5. A diode is composed of silicone material that is cleaved and layered. The lasing action occurs at the junction of the layers when an electrical source is applied.

when treating pain. The electrical stimulation is believed to provide spontaneous pain relief, while the laser provides more latent tissue responses.[7]

THERAPEUTIC APPLICATIONS OF LASERS

Since the production of lasers is relatively new, the biologic and physiologic effects of this concentrated light energy are still being explored. The effects of low-power lasers are subtle, primarily occurring at a cellular level. Various in-vitro and animal studies have attempted to elucidate the interaction of photons with the biologic structures. Although there are few controlled clinical studies in the literature, documented case studies and empirical evidence indicate that lasers are effective in reducing pain and aiding wound healing. The exact mechanisms for action are still uncertain, although proposed physiologic effects include an acceleration in collagen synthesis, a decrease in microorganisms, an increase in vascularization, reduction of pain, and an antiinflammatory action.[5]

Low-power lasers are best recognized for increasing the rate of wound and ulcer healing by enhancing cellular metabolism. Results from animal studies have varied as to the benefits on wound healing, perhaps because the types of lasers, dosages, and protocols used have been inconsistent. In humans, improvement of nonhealing wounds indicates promising possibilities for treatment with lasers.

Wound Healing

Early investigations of the effects of low-power laser on biologic tissues were limited to in-vitro experimentation. Although it was known that high power lasers could damage and vaporize tissues, little was known about the effect of small dosages on the viability and stability of cellular structures. Low dosages (less than $10 \, J/cm^2$) of radiation from low-output lasers had a stimulatory action on metabolic processes and cell proliferation compared to incandescent or tungsten light.[2]

Mester et al. conducted numerous in-vitro experiments with two lasers in the red portion of the visual spectrum: the ruby laser—wavelength of 694.3 nm—and the HeNe laser—wavelength 632.8 nm. Human tissue cultures showed significant increases in fibroblastic proliferation after stimulation by either laser tested.[18] Fibroblasts are the precursor cells to connective tissue structures, such as collagen, epithelial cells, and chondrocytes. When the production of fibroblasts is stimulated, one should expect a subsequent increase in the production of connective tissue. Abergel et al. documented that certain dosages of HeNe and GaAs laser—wavelength 904 nm—caused in-vitro human skin fibroblasts to have a threefold increase in procollagen production.[2] This effect was most marked when low-level stimulation (1.94×10^{-7} to $5.84 \times 10^{-6} J/cm^2$ of GaAs and dosages of 0.053 to 1.589 J/cm^2 of HeNe) was repeated over 3 to 4 days versus a single exposure. Samples of tissue showed increases in fibroblast and collagenous structures as well as increases in the intracellular material and swollen mitochondria of cells.[18] Furthermore, cells were undamaged in regard to their morphology and structure after exposure to low-power laser.[3]

Cellular metabolism, with attention to the activity of DNA and RNA, has been analyzed.[2,18,25] Through radioactive markers, it was suggested that laser stimulation enhances the synthesis of nucleic acids and cell division.[8,18] Abergel reported that laser treated cells had significantly greater amounts of procollagen messenger RNA, further confirming that increased collagen production occurs because of modifications at the transcriptional level.[1]

Low-power lasers were used in animal studies further to delineate the beneficial applications of laser light and its potential harm. In an early study by Mester et al., mechanical and burn wounds were made on the backs of mice.[19] Similar wounds on the same animals served as the controls, with the experimental wounds subjected to various doses of ruby laser. Although there were no histologic differences among the wounds, the lased wounds healed significantly faster, especially at a dosage of 1 J/cm^2. It was also demonstrated that repeated laser treatments were more effective than a single exposure.

Other researchers investigated the rate of healing and tensile strength of full-thickness wounds when exposed to laser irradiation.* There were conflicting reports regarding rates of healing, with some studies showing no change in the rate of wound closure[13,16,24] and others showing significantly faster wound healing.[2,14,15] Although the experimental results conflicted, an explanation for the discrepancy may be an indirect systemic effect of laser energy. Mester et al. showed that it was not necessary to irradiate an entire wound to achieve beneficial results, since stimulation of remote areas had similar results.[18] Kana et al. described an increase in the rate of healing of both the irradiated and nonirradiated wounds on the same animal compared to nonirradiated animals.[14] This systemic effect was most marked with the argon laser. Several studies that investigated the rate of healing on living animal tissue used a second, non-treated control wound on the same animal. The rate of healing may have been confounded by this systemic effect. Whether the systemic effect involves a humoral component — a circulating element — producing immunologic effects has yet to be determined or identified. Bacteriocidal and lymphocyte stimulation are proposed mechanisms for this phenomenon.

Tensile Strength

The increased tensile strength of lased wounds was confirmed more often.† Wound contraction, collagen synthesis, and increases in tensile strength are fibroblast mediated functions and were demonstrated most markedly in the early phase of wound healing. Wounds were tested at various stages of healing to determine their breaking point and were compared to a control or nonlased wound. Laser-treated wounds had significantly greater tensile strengths, most commonly in the first 10 to 14 days after injury, although they approached the values of the control after that time.[1,16,24] Hypertrophic scars did not result as tissue responses normalized after a 14-day period. HeNe laser doses ranging from 1.1 to 2.2 J/cm^2 elicited positive results when applied either twice a day or on alternate days. The increased tensile strength corresponds to higher levels of collagen.

---

*References 2, 13, 14, 15, 16, 24.
†References 2, 13, 14, 16, 19, 24.

Immunologic Responses

These early studies led to the hypothesis that laser exposure could enhance healing of skin and connective tissue lesions, but the mechanism was still unclear. Biochemical analysis and radioactive tracers were used to delineate the immunologic effects of laser light on human tissue cultures. The laser irradiation caused increased phagocytosis by leukocytes with dosages of .05 J/cm^2.[18] This led to the possibility of a bacteriocidal effect, which was further demonstrated with laser exposures on cell cultures containing *Escherichia coli,* a common intestinal bacteria in humans. The ruby laser had an increased effect both on cell replication and on the destruction of bacteria via the phagocytosis of leukocytes.[18,19] Mester et al. also concluded that there were immunologic effects with the ruby, HeNe, and argon lasers. Specifically, there was a direct stimulatory influence on the T and B lymphocyte activity, a phenomenon that is specific to laser output and wavelength. HeNe and argon lasers gave the best results, with dosages ranging from 0.5 to 1 J/cm^2.[18] Trelles did similar investigations in-vitro and in-vivo and reported that laser did not have bacteriocidal effects alone, but when used in conjunction with antibiotics, there were significantly higher bacteriocidal effects compared to controls.[25]

With the confidence that they would cause little or no harm and that they could serve a therapeutic purpose, low-power lasers have been used clinically on human subjects since the 1960s. In Hungary, Mester et al. treated non-healing ulcers that did not respond to traditional therapy with HeNe and argon lasers with respective wavelengths of 632.8 and 488 nm.[18] The dosages were varied but had a maximum of 4 J/cm^2. By the time of Mester et al.'s publication, 1125 patients had been treated, of which 875 healed, 160 improved, and 85 did not respond. The wounds, which were categorized by etiology, took an average of 12 to 16 weeks to heal. Trelles also showed promising results clinically using the infrared GaAs and HeNe lasers on the healing of ulcers, non-union fractures, and on herpetic lesions.[25]

Gogia et al., in the United States, treated nonhealing wounds with GaAs lasers pulsed at a frequency of 1000 Hz for 10 seconds/cm^2 with a sweeping technique and the laser held about 5 mm from the wound surface.[11] This protocol was used in conjunction with daily or twice daily sterile whirlpool treatments and produced satisfactory results, although statistical information was not reported. Empirical evidence by these authors suggested faster healing and cleaner wounds when subjected to GaAs laser treatment three times per week.

Inflammation

Biopsies of experimental wounds were examined for prostaglandin activity to delineate the effect of laser stimulation on the inflammatory process. A decrease in prostaglandin (PGE_2) is a proposed mechanism in which laser therapy promotes the reduction of edema. During inflammation, prostaglandins cause vasodilation, which contributes to the flow of plasma into the interstitial tissue. By reducing prostaglandins, the driving force behind edema production is reduced.[5] The prostaglandin E and F contents were examined after treatments with HeNe laser at 1 J/cm^2.[18] In 4 days, both types of prostaglandins accumulated more than the controls. However, at 8 days, the PGE_2 levels decreased, while PGF_{2alpha} increased. There was also an increased capillarization during this phase. These data indicate that prostaglandin production is affected by laser stimulation, and these changes possibly reflect an accelerated resolution of the acute inflammatory process.[18]

Scar Tissue

Macroscopic examination of healed wounds was subjectively described after the laser experiments in most studies. In general, the wounds exposed to laser irradiation had less scar tissue and a better cosmetic appearance. Histologic examination showed greater epithelialization and less exudative material.[15]

Studies that used burn wounds showed more regular alignment of collagen and smaller scars. Trelles lased third-degree burns on the backs of hairless mice with GaAs and HeNe lasers and showed significantly faster healing in the lased animals.[25] The best results were obtained with the GaAs laser because of its greater penetration. Trelles found increased circulation with the production of new blood vessels in the center of the wounds compared to the controls. Edges of the wounds maintained viability and contributed to the epithelialization and closure of the burn. Since there was less contracture associated with irradiated wounds, laser treatment has been suggested for burns and wounds on the hands and neck, where contractures and scarring can severely limit function.

Pain

Lasers have also reduced pain and affected peripheral nerve activity. Rochkind et al. produced crush injuries in rats and treated experimental animals with 10 J/cm^2 of HeNe laser energy transcutaneously along the sciatic nerve projection.[20] The amplitude of electrically stimulated action potentials was measured along the injured nerve and compared with controls up to 1 year later. The amplitude of the action potentials was 43% greater after 20 days, the duration of laser treatment. By 1 year, all lased nerves demonstrated equal or higher amplitudes than before injury. The controls followed an expected course of recovery and did not reach normal levels even after 1 year.

The effect of HeNe irradiation on peripheral sensory nerve latency has been investigated on humans by Snyder-Mackler and Bork.[23] This double-blind study showed that exposure of the superficial radial nerve to low dosages of laser resulted in a significantly decreased sensory nerve conduction velocity, which may provide information about the pain-relieving mechanism of lasers. Other explanations for pain relief may be hastened healing, antiinflammatory action, autonomic nerve influence, and neurohumoral responses (serotonin, norepinephrin) from descending tract inhibition[5,7]

Chronic pain has been treated with GaAs and HeNe lasers, and positive results have been observed empirically and through clinical research. Walker conducted a double-blind study to document analgesia after exposure to HeNe irradiation in chronic pain patients compared with sham treatments.[28] When the superficial sites of the radial, median, and saphenous nerves as well as painful areas were exposed to laser irradiation, there were significant decreases in pain and less reliance on medication for pain control. These preliminary studies suggest positive results, although pain modulation is difficult to measure objectively.

Bone Response

Future uses of laser irradiation include the treatment of other connective tissue structures, such as bone and articular cartilage. Schultz et al. studied various intensities of Nd:YAG laser on the healing of partial thickness articular cartilage lesions in guinea pigs.[21] During the surgical procedure, the lesions were irradiated for 5 seconds, with intensities ranging from 25 to 125 J. After 4 weeks, the low dosage group (25 J) had chondral proliferation, and by 6 weeks the defect had reconstituted to the level of the surface cartilage. Normal basophilia cells were present with staining, indicating normal cellular structures. The higher dosage groups and controls had little or no evidence of restoration of the lesion with cartilage. Bone healing and fracture consolidation have been investigated by Trelles and Mayayo.[26] An adapter was attached to an intramuscular needle so that the laser energy could be directed deeper to the periosteum. Rabbit tibial fractures showed faster consolidation with HeNe treatment of 2.4 J/cm^2 on alternate days. Histologic examination indicated more mature Haversian canals with detached osteocytes in the laser treated bone. There was also a remodeling of the articular line, which is impossible with traditional therapy.[25,26] The use of lasers for the treatment of nonunion fractures has begun in Europe.

Clinical Considerations

There have been no ill effects reported from laser treatments for wound healing.[4] More controlled clinical data are needed to determine efficacy and to establish dosimetry that elicits reproducible responses. The impressions of low-power lasers are that they have a biostimulative effect on impaired tissues unless higher dosages, in excess of 8 to 10 J/cm^2, are administered.[1] This effect does not influence normal tissue. Beyond these ranges a bioinhibitive effect may occur.

The applications of the low-power laser in an athletic training environment are potentially unlimited. Its applications can include wound healing properties on lacerations, abrasions, or infections. Clean procedures should be maintained to prevent cross contamination of the laser tip. Because the depth of penetration of the infrared laser is about 5 cm, other soft tissue injuries can be treated effectively by laser irradiation. Sprains, strains, and contusions have been observed by the authors to have faster healing rates with less pain. Acupuncture and superficial nerve sites also can be lased or combined with electrical stimulation to treat painful conditions.

TECHNIQUES OF APPLICATION

The method of application of laser therapy is relatively simple, but certain principles of dosimetry should be discussed so that the clinician can accurately determine the amount of laser energy delivered to the tissues. For general application, only the treatment time and the pulse rate vary. For research purposes, the investigator should measure the exact energy density emitted from the applicator before the treatments. Dosage is the most important variable in laser therapy and may be difficult to determine because of the variables mentioned previously (e.g., hours of operation or condition of the unit).

The laser energy is emitted from a handheld remote applicator. The GaAs laser houses the semiconductor elements in the tip of the applicator, while the HeNe lasers contain their components inside the unit and deliver the laser light to the target area via a fiberoptic tube. The fiberoptic assembly is fragile and should not be crimped or twisted excessively. The fiberoptics used with the HeNe laser and the elliptical shape of the GaAs laser create beam divergence with both devices. This divergence causes the beam's energy to spread out over a given area so that as the distance from the source increases, the intensity of the beam decreases.

To administer a laser treatment, the tip should be in light contact with the skin and directed perpendicularly to the target tissue while the laser is engaged for the designated time. Commonly, a treatment area is divided into a grid of square centimeters, with each square centimeter stimulated for the specified time. This *gridding technique* is the most frequently used method of application and should be used whenever possible. Lines and points should not be drawn on the patient's skin because this may absorb some of the light energy (Figure 10-6). If open areas are to be treated, a sterilized clear plastic sheet can be placed over the wound to allow surface contact.

An alternative is a *scanning technique* in which there is no contact between the laser tip and the skin. With this technique, the applicator tip should be held 5 to 10 mm from the wound. Since beam divergence occurs, there is a decrease in the amount of energy as the distance from the target increases. The amount of energy lost becomes difficult to quantify accurately if the distance from the target varies. Therefore it is not recommended to treat at distances greater than 1 cm. When using a laser tip of 1 mm with 30 degrees of divergence, the red beam of the HeNe laser should fill an area the size of 1 cm² (Figure 10-7). Although the infrared laser is invisible, the same consideration should be given when using the scanning technique. If the laser tip comes into contact with an open wound, the tip should be cleaned thoroughly with a small amount of bleach or other antiseptic agents to prevent cross contamination.

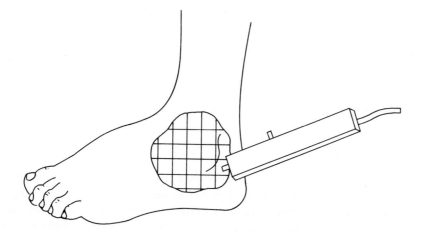

Fig. 10-6. Grid application of laser. Laser aperture should be perpendicular to the surface. Lase each square centimeter of the injured area for the specified time. The aperture should be in light contact with the skin.

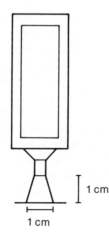

1 cm

1 cm

Fig. 10-7. Scanning technique. When skin contact cannot be maintained, the remote should be held still in the center of the square centimeter grid at a distance of less than 1 cm. If using the HeNe laser, the red beam should fill a 1 cm² grid.

The scanning technique should be differentiated with the *wanding technique*, in which a grid area is bathed with the laser in an oscillating fashion for the designated time. As in the scanning technique, the dosimetry is difficult to calculate if a distance of less than 1 cm cannot be maintained. The wanding technique is not recommended because of irregularities in the dosages.

Dosage

PhysioTechnology Ltd. (Topeka, KS) is the only manufacturer in the United States that currently produces low power HeNe and GaAs lasers (Figure 10-8). Table 10-1 describes the contrasting specifications of these lasers. The HeNe laser has a 1.0 mW average power output at the fiber tip and is delivered in the continuous wave mode. The GaAs laser has an output of 2 W but has only a 0.4 mW average power when pulsed at its maximum rate of 1000 Hz. The frequency of the GaAs is variable, and the clinician may choose a pulse rate of 1 to 1000 Hz, each with a pulse width of 200 nsec (nanosec = 10^{-9}) (Figure 10-9).

The pulsed modes drastically reduce the amount of energy emitted from the laser. For example, a 2 W laser is pulsed at 100 Hz:

$$
\begin{aligned}
\text{Average Power} &= \text{pulse rate} \times \text{peak power} \times \text{pulse width} \\
&= 100 \text{ Hz} \times 2 \text{ W} \times (2\text{x}10^{-7} \text{ sec}) \\
&= 0.04 \text{ mW}
\end{aligned}
$$

This contrasts the power output of 0.4 mW with the 1000 Hz. Therefore adjustment of the pulse rate alters the average power, which significantly affects the treatment time if a specified amount of energy is required. In the past, it was thought that altering the frequency of the laser would increase its benefits. Recent evidence indicates that the total number of Joules is more important; therefore higher pulse rates are recommended to decrease the treatment time required for each stimulation point.[5]

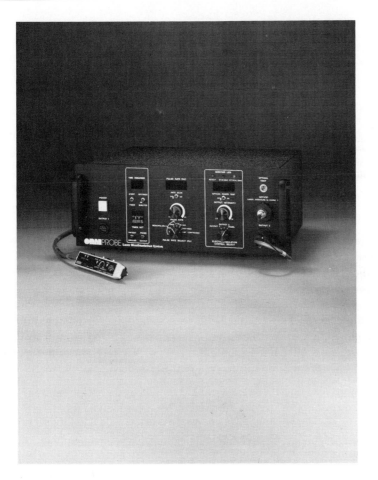

Fig. 10-8. Low-power laser.
(Physio Technology, Ltd. Topeka, KS.)

TABLE 10-1   Parameters of Low-Output Lasers

	Helium Neon (HeNe)	Gallium Arsenide (GaAs)
Laser type	Gas	Semiconductor
Wavelength	632.8 nm	904 nm
Pulse rate	Continuous wave	1-1000 Hz
Pulse width	Continuous wave	200 nsec
Peak power	3 mW	2 W
Average power	1.0 mW	.04-0.4 mW
Beam area	0.01 cm	0.07 cm
FDA class	Class II laser	Class I laser

Copied with permission from Physio Technology.

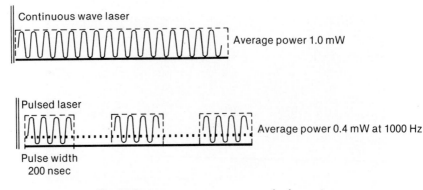

Fig. 10-9. Continuous wave versus pulsed energies.

The dosage or energy density of laser is reported in the literature as J/cm^2. $1J = 1W/sec$. Therefore dosage is dependent on the following:

1. the output of the laser in mW
2. the time of exposure in seconds
3. the beam surface area of the laser in cm^2

Dosage should be accurately calculated to standardize treatments and to establish treatment guidelines for specific injuries. The intention is to deliver a specific number of J/cm^2 or mJ/cm^2. After setting the pulse rate, which determines the average power of the laser, only the treatment time per cm^2 needs to be calculated.[5]

$$T_A = (E/Pav) \times A$$
$$T_A = \text{treatment time for a given area}$$
$$E = \text{mJ of energy per } cm^2$$
$$Pav = \text{Average laser power in mW}$$
$$A = \text{beam area in } cm^2$$

For example: To deliver 1 J/cm^2 with a 0.4 mW average power GaAs laser with a 0.07 cm^2 beam area:

$$T_A = (1 \text{ J/cm}^2/.0004 \text{ W}) \times 0.07 \text{ cm}^2 = 175 \text{ seconds or 2:55 minutes}$$

To deliver 50 mJ/cm^2 with the same laser, it would only take 8.75 seconds of stimulation. Charts are available to assist the clinician in calculating the treatment times for a variety of pulse rates. The GaAs laser can only pulsed up to 1000 Hz, resulting in an average energy of 0.4 mW. Therefore the treatment times may be exceedingly long to deliver the same energy density with a continuous wave laser (Table 10-2).

Depth of Penetration

Any energy applied to the body can be absorbed, reflected, transmitted, and refracted. Biologic effects result only from the absorption of energy, and as more energy is absorbed, there is less available for the deeper and adjacent tissues.

Laser light's depth of penetration depends on the type of laser energy delivered. Absorption of HeNe laser energy occurs rapidly in the superficial structures, especially within the first 2 to 5 mm of soft tissue. The response that occurs from absorption is

TABLE 10-2   **Treatment Times for Low-Output Lasers**

Laser Type	Average Power (mW)	Joules per Centimeter Squared (J/cm^2)						
		0.05	0.1	0.5	1	2	3	4
HeNe (632.8 nm) Continuous wave	1.0	0.5	1.0	5.0	10.0	20.0	30.0	40.0
GaAs (904 nm) Pulsed at 1000 Hz	0.4	8.8	17.7	88.4	176.7	353.4	530.1	706.9

Copied with permission from Physio Technology.

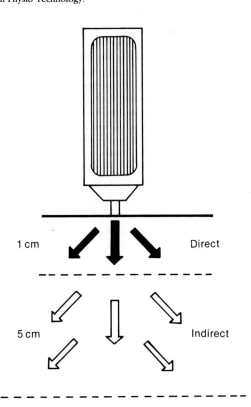

Fig. 10-10. Depth of penetration with the GaAs laser. Direct penetration is up to 1 cm with the GaAs laser. The stimulation causes an indirect effect up to 5 cm. Penetration is greatest with skin contact.

termed the direct effect. The indirect effect is a lessened response that occurs deeper in the tissues. The normal metabolic processes in the deeper tissues are catalyzed from the energy absorption in the superficial structures to produce the indirect effect. HeNe laser has an indirect effect on tissues up to 8 to 10 mm.[5]

The GaAs laser, which has a longer wavelength, is directly absorbed in tissues at depths of 1 to 2 cm and has an indirect effect up to 5 cm (Figure 10-10). Therefore this laser has better potential for the treatment of deeper soft tissue injuries such as strains, sprains, and contusions. The radius of the energy field expands as the nonabsorbed light is reflected, refracted, and transmitted to adjacent cells as the energy penetrates. The clinician should stimulate each square centimeter of a "grid," although there will be an overlap of areas receiving indirect exposure.

SUGGESTED TREATMENT PROTOCOLS

Research suggests some laser densities for treating several clinical models. These range from 0.05 to 0.5 J/cm^2 for acute conditions and from 0.5 to 3 J/cm^2 for more chronic conditions.[5] The responses of the tissues depend on the dosage delivered, although the type of laser used can also influence the effect. The response obtained with different dosages and with different lasers varies considerably among studies, leaving treatment parameters to be determined largely empirically. In the literature, there seems to be little differentiation when comparing the dosages of HeNe and GaAs lasers, although their depths of penetration differ significantly. The laser units produced in the United States have relatively little average power, so the tendency is to administer dosages in milliJoules rather than Joules. Three to six treatments may be required before the effectiveness of laser therapy can be determined.

Although higher laser output is recommended to reduce treatment times, overstimulation should be avoided. The Arndt Schultz principle that states more is not necessarily better is applicable with laser therapy. For this reason, laser should be administered at a maximum of once daily per treatment area. When using large dosages, treatment is recommended on alternate days. If the effects of laser plateau, the frequency of treatments should be reduced or the treatments discontinued for 1 week, at which time the treatment can be reinstated if needed.[25]

Pain

The use of low-power lasers in the treatment of acute and chronic pain can be implemented in various manners. After proper diagnosis of the pain's etiology, the pathology site can be gridded. The entire area of injury should be lased as described previously. Table 10-3 lists some suggested treatment protocols for various clinical conditions. When trigger points are being treated, the probe should be held perpendicular to the skin with light contact. If a specific structure, such as a ligament, is the target tissue, the laser probe should be held in contact with the skin and perpendicular to that structure. When treating a joint, the patient should be positioned so that the joint is open to allow penetration of the energy to the intraarticular areas.

The treatment of acupuncture and trigger points with laser can be augmented with electrical stimulation for pain management. Refer to charts to determine appropriate acupuncture points. The impedance detector in the laser remote enhances the ability to locate these sites. Points should be treated from distal to proximal for best results.

Occasionally, patients may experience an increase in pain after a laser treatment. This phenomenon is believed to initiate the body's normal responses to pain that have become dormant.[6] Laser has helped resolve the condition by enhancing normal physiologic processes needed to resolve the injury. As stated previously, several

TABLE 10-3 **Suggested Treatment Applications**

Application	Laser Type	Energy Density
TRIGGER POINT		
Superficial	HeNe	1-3 J/cm^2
Deep	GaAs	1-2 J/cm^2
EDEMA REDUCTION		
Acute	GaAs	0.1-0.2 J/cm^2
Subacute	GaAs	0.2-0.5 J/cm^2
WOUND HEALING (SUPERFICIAL TISSUES)		
Acute	HeNe	0.5-1 J/cm^2
Chronic	HeNe	4 J/cm^2
WOUND HEALING (DEEP TISSUES)		
Acute	GaAs	0.05-0.1 J/cm^2
Chronic	GaAs	0.5-1 J/cm^2
SCAR TISSUE	GaAs	0.5-1 J/cm^2

Copied with permission from Physio Technology.

treatments should be administered before deeming the modality ineffective in pain management.

Wound Healing

Although ulcerations and open wounds are not common in an athletic training environment, contusions, abrasions, and lacerations can be treated with laser to hasten healing time and decrease infection. The wound should be cleaned appropriately and all debris and eschar removed. Heavy exudate that covers the wound will diminish the laser's penetration; therefore lasing around the periphery of the wound is recommended. The scanning technique should be used over open wounds unless a clear plastic sheet is placed over the wound to allow direct contact. Opaque materials can absorb some of the laser energy and are not recommended. Facial lacerations can be treated with lasers, although care should be taken not to direct the beam into the patient's eyes. Risk of retinal damage from the low-power lasers used in the United States is low.

Scar Tissue

The laser energy affects only what is metabolically diminished and does not change normal tissue. Hypertrophic scars can be treated with lasers because of the bioinhibitive effects. Bioinhibition requires prolonged treatment times and may be clinically impractical because of the low-power output of the lasers used in the United States. Pain and edema associated with pathologic scars have been effectively treated with low-power lasers. Thick scars have varied vascularity, which makes laser transmission irregular. Therefore it is often recommended to treat the periphery of the scar rather than directly over it.

Edema and Inflammation

Laser application for control of edema and inflammation primarily interrupts the formation of intermediate substrates necessary for the production of inflammatory chemical mediators—kinins, histamines, and prostaglandins. Without these chemical mediators, the disruption of the body's homeostatic state is minimized and the extent of pain and edema is diminished. It is also believed that laser energy can optimize cell membrane permeability, which regulates interstitial osmotic–hydrostatic pressures. Therefore, during tissue trauma, the flux of fluid into the intracellular spaces would be reduced. Laser treatment is usually applied by gridding over the involved areas or by treating related acupuncture points if the area of involvement is generalized.

SAFETY

Few safety considerations are necessary with the low-power laser. As the variety of lasers evolved and their uses increased in the United States, it became necessary to develop national guidelines not only for safety but for therapeutic efficacy. The U.S. Food and Drug Administration's Center for Devices and Radiological Health now regulates the manufacture and sale of lasers in the United States.

Laser equipment commonly is grouped into four FDA classes with simplified and well-differentiated safety procedures for each.[22]

Class I, or exempt lasers, are considered nonhazardous to the body. All invisible lasers with average power outputs of 1 mW or less are class I devices. These include the GaAs lasers with wavelengths from 820 to 910 nm.[17] The invisible, infrared lasers should contain an indicator light to identify when the laser is engaged.

Class II, or low-power lasers, are hazardous only if a viewer stares continuously into the source. This class includes visible lasers that emit up to 1 mW average power, such as the HeNe laser.

Class III, or moderate-risk lasers, can cause retinal injury within the natural reaction time. The operator and patient are required to wear protective eyewear. However, these lasers cannot cause serious skin injury nor produce hazardous diffuse reflections from metals or other surfaces under normal use.[22]

Class IV, or high-power lasers, present a high risk of injury and can cause combustion of flammable materials. Other dangers are diffuse reflections that may harm the eyes and cause serious skin injury from direct exposure. These high-power lasers seldom are used outside research laboratories and restricted industrial environments.[22]

The low-power lasers used in treating sports injuries are categorized as Class I and II laser devices and Class III medical devices. Class III medical devices include new or modified devices not equivalent to any marketed before May 28, 1976.[9] To use a low-power laser in the United States on human subjects, a research proposal must be approved by an Institutional Review Board (IRB). The IRB can be established through the manufacturer, a university, or a hospital to obtain an Investigational Device Exemption (IDE). By requiring documentation of the results and side effects of lasers, the FDA regulations serve to generate scientific data to determine safety and efficacy of the device in question.

Precautions and Contraindications

Lasers deliver nonionizing radiation, so no mutagenic effects on DNA and no damage to the cells or cell membranes have been found.[5] No deleterious effects have been reported after low-power laser exposure, including carcinogenic responses unless applied to already cancerous cells. Tumorous cells may proliferate when stimulated.[10]

SOME SUGGESTIONS ON LASER USE:

- Laser should not be used over cancerous growths.
- It is better to underexpose than to overexpose. If clinical results plateau, a reduction in dosage or treatment frequency may facilitate results.
- Avoid direct exposure into the eyes because of possible retinal burns. If lasing for extended periods, as with wound healing, safety glasses are recommended to avoid exposure from reflection.
- Although no adverse reactions have been documented, the use of laser during the first trimester of pregnancy is not recommended.
- A low percentage of patients, especially with chronic pain, may experience a syncope episode during the laser treatment. Symptoms usually subside within minutes. If symptoms exceed 5 minutes, no further treatments should be given.

CONCLUSION

The use of low-power lasers appears to have nothing but positive effects: this in itself should create a state of professional caution in deeming it a panacea modality. Currently, with these power outputs, lasers are recognized as nonsignificant risk devices. However, low-power lasers have not been granted recognition by the Food and Drug Administration as being a safe or effective modality. Although many empirical and clinical findings show promising results, more controlled studies are essential to determine the types of lasers and dosages that are required to attain reproducible results.

SUMMARY

1. The first working laser was the ruby laser developed in 1960 and was initially called an optical maser.
2. Visible light wavelengths range from 400 to 700 nanometers. Light is transmitted through space in waves and is comprised of photons emitted at distinct energy levels.
3. An atom is excited when energy is applied and raises an orbiting electron to a higher orbit. When the electron returns to its original orbit, it releases energy in the form of a photon, a process called spontaneous emission.
4. Stimulated emission occurs when the photon is released from an excited atom and promotes the release of an identical photon to be released from a similarly excited atom.

5. For lasers to operate, a medium of excited atoms must be generated. This is termed population inversion and results when an external energy source (pumping device) is applied to the medium.

6. Characteristics of laser light vary from conventional light sources in three manners: laser light is monochromic (single color or wavelength), coherent (in phase), and collimated (minimal divergence).

7. Laser can be thermal (hot) or nonthermal (low power, soft or cold). The categories of lasers include solid state (crystal or glass), gas, semiconductor, dye, or chemical lasers.

8. Helium neon (HeNe) gas and gallium arsenide (GaAs) semiconductor lasers are two low-power lasers being investigated by the FDA for application in physical medicine. These low-power lasers are currently being used in the United States and other countries for wound and soft tissue healing and pain relief.

9. HeNe lasers deliver a characteristic red beam with a wavelength of 632.8 nm. The laser is delivered in a continuous wave and has a direct penetration of 2 to 5 mm and indirect penetration of 10 to 15 mm.

10. GaAs lasers are invisible and have a wavelength of 904 nm. They are delivered in a pulse mode and have an average power output of 0.4 mw. This laser has a direct penetration of 1 to 2 cm and an indirect penetration to 5 cm.

11. The proposed therapeutic applications of lasers in physical medicine include acceleration of collagen synthesis, decrease in microorganisms, increase in vascularization, and reduction of pain and inflammation.

12. Lasers are ideally applied with gentle contact with the skin surface and should be perpendicular to the target surface. Dosage appears to be the critical factor in eliciting the desired response, but exact dosimetry has not been determined. Dosage fluctuates by varying the pulse frequency and the treatment times.

13. The laser is applied by developing an imaginary grid over the target area. The grid is comprised of 1 cm squares, and the laser is applied to each square for a predetermined time. Trigger or acupuncture points are also treated for painful conditions.

14. The FDA considers low-power lasers as low risk investigational devices. For use in the United States, they require an IRB approval and informed consent before their use.

15. Although no deleterious effects have been reported, certain precautions and contraindications exist. Contraindications include lasing over cancerous tissue, directly into the eyes, and during the first trimester of pregnancy. Occasionally, pain may initially increase when laser treatments begin but does not indicate cessation of treatment. A low percentage of patients have experienced a syncope episode during laser treatment, but this is usually self-resolving. If symptoms persist for longer than 5 minutes, future laser treatments are not advised.

16. Future research for determining efficacy and treatment parameters is critically needed to substantiate the application of low-power lasers in physical medicine.

GLOSSARY

coherence Property of identical phase and time relationship. All photons of laser light are the same wavelength.

collimate To make parallel.

continuous wave An uninterrupted beam of laser light as opposed to pulsed.

diode laser A solid-state/semiconductor used as a lasing medium.

divergence The bending of light rays away from each other, the spreading of light.

electron Fundamental particle of matter possessing a negative electrical charge and small mass.

excited state State of an atom that occurs when outside energy causes it to contain more energy than normal.

fiberoptic A solid glass or plastic tube that conducts light along its length.

frequency The number of cycles or pulses per second.

ground state The normal, unexcited state of an atom.

infrared A portion of the electromagnetic spectrum between the visible and microwave regions.

laser A device that concentrates high energies into a narrow beam of coherent, monochromatic light (Light Amplification by the Stimulated Emission of Radiation).

monochromaticity When a light source produces a single color or wavelength.

photon The basic unit of light; a packet or quanta of light energy.

population inversion A condition where more atoms exist in a high energy, excited state than those atoms that are in a normal ground state. This is required for lasing to occur.

spontaneous emission When an atom in a high energy state emits a photon and drops to a more stable ground state.

stimulated emission When a photon interacts with an atom already in a high energy state and decay of the atomic system occurs, releasing two photons.

wavelength The distance from peak to the same point on the next peak of an electromagnetic or acoustic wave.

REFERENCES

1 Abergel RP: *Biochemical mechanisms of wound and tissue healing with lasers,* Second Canadian Low Power Medical Laser Conference, Ontario, Canada, March 1987.

2 Abergel RP, Lyons RF, Castel JC, et al.: Biostimulation of wound healing by lasers: experimental approaches in animal models and in fibroblast cultures, *J Dermatol Surg Oncol* 13: 127-133, 1987.

3 Bostara M, Jucca A, Olliaro P, et al.: In-vitro fibroblast and dermis fibroblast activation by laser irradiation at low energy, *Dermatologica* 168: 157-162, 1984.

4 Castel JC: *Laser biophysics,* Second Canadian Low Power Medical Laser Conference, Ontario, Canada, March 1987.

5 Castel MF: A clinical guide to low power laser therapy, Downsview, Ontario, 1985, PhysioTechnology Ltd.

6 Castel MF: *Personal communication,* MEDELCO, Downsview, Ontario, March 1989.

7 Cheng R: *Combination laser/electrotherapy in pain management,* Second Canadian Low Power Medical Laser Conference, Ontario, Canada, March 1987.

8 Enwemeka CS: Laser biostimulation of healing wounds: specific effects and mechanisms of action, *JOSPT* 9: 333-338, 1988.

9 *Fact sheet: laser biostimulation,* Rockville, MD, 1984, Center of Devices and Radiological Health, FDA.

10 Farnham J: *Personal communication,* Rockville, MD, March 1989, Center of Devices and Radiological Health, FDA.

11 Gogia PP, Hurt BS, Zirn TT: Wound management with whirlpool and infrared cold laser treatment, *Phys Ther* 68: 1239-1242, 1988.

12 Hallmark CL, Horn DT: *Lasers: the light fantastic,* ed 2, Blue Ridge Summit, PA, 1987, TAB Books.

13 Hunter J, Leonard L, Wilson R, et al.: Effects of low energy laser on wound healing in a porcine model, *Lasers Surg Med* 3: 285-290, 1984.

14 Kana JS, Hutschenreiter G, Haina D, et al.: Effect of low power density laser radiation on healing of open skin wounds in rats, *Arch Surg* 116: 293-296, 1981.

15 Longo L, Evangelista S, Tinacci G, et al.: Effect of diode-laser silver arsenide-aluminum (Ga-Al-As) 904 nm on healing of experimental wounds, *Lasers Surg Med* 7: 444-447, 1987.

16 Lyons RF, Abergel RP, White RA, et al.: Biostimulation of wound healing in vivo by a helium neon laser, *Ann Plas Surg* 18: 47-77, 1987.

17 McComb G: *The laser cookbook: 88 practical projects,* Blue Ridge Summit, PA, 1988, TAB Books.

18 Mester E, Mester AF, Mester A: Biomedical effects of laser application, *Lasers Surg Med* 5: 31-39, 1985.

19 Mester E, Spiry T, Szende B, et al.: Effect of laser rays on wound healing, *Am J Surg* 122: 532-535, 1971.

20 Rochkind S, Nissan M, Barr-Nea L, et al.: Response of peripheral nerve to HeNe laser: experimental studies, *Lasers Surg Med* 7: 441-443, 1987.

21 Schultz RJ, Krishnamurthy S, Thelmo W, et al.: Effects of varying intensities of laser energy on articular cartilage: a preliminary study, *Lasers Surg Med* 5: 577-588, 1985.

22 Sliney D, Wolkarsht M: *Safety with lasers and other optical sources: a comprehensive handbook,* New York, 1980, Plenum Press.

23 Snyder-Mackler L, Bork CE: Effect of helium neon laser irradiation on peripheral nerve sensory latency, *Phys Ther* 68: 223-225, 1988.

24 Surinchak JS, Alago ML, Bellamy RF, et al.: Effects of low-level energy lasers on the healing of full-thickness skin defects, *Lasers Surg Med* 2: 267-274, 1983.

25 Trelles M: *Medical applications of laser biostimulation,* Second Canadian Low Power Medical Laser Conference, Ontario, Canada, March 1987.

26 Trelles MA, Mayayo E: Bone fracture consolidates faster with low power laser, *Lasers Surg Med* 7: 36-45, 1987.

27 Van Pelt WF, Stewart HF, Peterson RW, et al.: *Laser fundamentals and experiments,* Rockville, MD, 1970, U.S. Dept. HEW.

28 Walker J: Relief from chronic pain by low power laser irradiation, *Neuroscience Letters* 43: 339-344, 1983.

SUGGESTED READINGS

Abergel RP, Lam T, Meeker C, et al.: Biostimulation of procollagen production by low energy lasers in human skin fibroblast cultures, *J Invest Dermatol* 82: 395, 1984.

Cummings JP: The effect of low energy (HeNe) laser irradiation on healing dermal wounds in an animal model, *Phys Ther* 65: 737, 1985.

Dyson M, Young S: Effects of laser therapy on wound contraction and cellularity in mice, *Lasers Surg Med* 1: 125, 1986.

Lam TS, Abergel RP, Meeker CA, et al.: Biostimulation of human skin fibroblasts: low energy lasers selectively enhance collagen synthesis, *Lasers Surg Med* 3: 328, 1984.

Lam TS, Abergel RP, Meeker CA, et al.: Laser stimulation of collagen synthesis in human fibroblast cultures, *Laser Life Sci* 1: 61-77, 1986.

Lundeberg T, Haker E, Thomas M: Effect of laser versus placebo in tennis elbow, *Scand J Rehabil Med* 19: 135-138, 1987.

Mester E, Jaszsagi-Nagy E: The effects of laser radiation on wound healing and collagen synthesis, *Studia Biophysica* 35(3): 227, 1973.

Saperia D, Glassberg E, Lyons RF, et al.: Demonstration of elevated type I and type III procollagen mRNA levels in cutaneous wounds treated with helium-neon laser, *Biochem Biophys Res Commun* 138: 1123-1128, 1986.

Young S, Bolton P, Dyson, M, et al.: Macrophage responsivity to light therapy, *Lasers Surg Med* 9: 497-505, 1989.

Ultraviolet Therapy

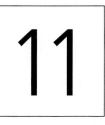

J. Marc Davis

OBJECTIVES

After completion of this chapter, the student will be able to do the following:

- Describe the position of ultraviolet radiation (UVR) in the electromagnetic spectrum and the relationship of UVR to other forms of electromagnetic energy.

- Understand how UVR raises energy levels within irradiated objects.

- Understand the effect of UVR on individual cells and human tissue, and explain the tanning process.

- Describe the effect of long-term exposure to UVR and its effect on the eyes.

- Explain the physical set-up and procedures for operating a UVR device, including safety precautions, the skin test, the inverse square law, and the cosine law.

- Understand various clinical uses of UVR.

U ltraviolet radiation (UVR) is one of the oldest medical modalities. The physicians of ancient Egypt and Greece attributed many healing powers to sunlight, and life itself would be impossible without the interaction of solar UVR and plant photosynthesis. Before this century, the sun was the only satisfactory source of UVR, but now a wide selection of UVR generators is available.

This chapter serves to familiarize the student with the properties of UVR, to explain how UVR affects human tissue, and to explore different UVR treatment apparatus and techniques. Subsequently, the sports therapist should be able to understand why UVR therapy can be effective in treating certain maladies even though it is rarely used in a sports-medicine environment.

UVR is the portion of the electromagnetic spectrum that ranges from 2000 to 4000 Å. It is bordered below 2000 Å by x-ray and above 4000 Å by visible light (see Figure 1-2). The UVR portion of the electromagnetic spectrum is further divided into three sections: UV-A, UV-B, and UV-C. UV-C (also called shortwave UV, extreme UV, and far UV) ranges from 2000 to 2900 Å and is bactericidal.[14,20] UV-B (called middle UV and the sunburn spectrum) ranges from 2900 to 3200 Å and is associated with sunburn and age-related skin changes.[13-19] UV-A (near UV) ranges from 3200 to 4000 Å. Until recently, little or no physiologic effect was attributed to UV-A, but recent research and clinical use of UV-A are showing possible benefits and hazards for UV-A exposure. The UVR apparatus most likely to be encountered in an athletic training or sports-medicine setting would generate UVR in the UV-B or UV-C range.

The beneficial effects of UVR as a treatment modality are mediated by its limited absorption. UVR is absorbed within the first 1 to 2 mm of human skin, and most of the physiologic effects are superficial.[5] Therefore the most effective use of UVR therapy is in the treatment of various skin disorders, such as acne and psoriasis.[8]

EFFECT ON CELLS

UVR is a form of energy. As such, when it contacts any surface, skin included, it must be either reflected or absorbed and transmitted. If UVR strikes the skin at a 90-degree angle, 90% to 95% of the energy will be absorbed. Most energy will be absorbed within the epidermis of the skin (80% to 90%), while the rest will reach the dermis.[5] As the UVR is absorbed within the tissue, it causes the energy level of exposed atoms to increase. These atoms will quickly return to their normal energy state; however, the presence of excess energy causes chemical excitation within the cells of the exposed tissue. This chemical excitation is the cause of the various effects of UVR on living cells and tissue. Even a single exposure to UVR will cause chemical excitation within exposed cells, which leads to physiologic changes within these cells.

These physiologic changes are the result of a photochemical event that is the end product of the UVR-induced chemical excitation. This photochemical event results in an alteration of cell biochemistry and cellular metabolism. The synthesis of **DNA** and **RNA** is affected, leading to alterations in protein and enzyme production. As a consequence, cell protein structure can be altered. This alteration of cellular protein and DNA may leave the cell inactive or dead.[14-19]

Fortunately, defenses have evolved that protect microorganisms and cells that are exposed to a constant barrage of UVR from the sun. The damaged cells may be restored by enzymatic action or by simple deterioration of the damaged portion, the damaged segment may be replaced by normal material, or it may be bypassed when the cell reproduces.[14] DNA synthesis within cells of the human epidermis is suppressed for 24 to 48 hours after exposure to UVR in the range of 2500 to 2700 Å and is then followed by a period of increased DNA synthesis.[14,19]

EFFECT ON NORMAL HUMAN TISSUE
Short-Term Effect On Skin

Normal human skin consists of two layers, the superficial epidermis and the underlying dermis (Figure 11-1). The epidermis is avascular and composed mostly of well-organized layers of **keratinocytes.** These cells produce **keratin,** the fibrous protective protein of the skin. The keratinocytes are produced from cells of the basal layer of the epidermis and then move upward through the epidermis. The dermis is divided into two layers: the papillary layer that contains a rich blood supply, and the reticular layer that is composed of heavy connective tissue and contains fibroblasts, histiocytes, and most cells.

When human skin is exposed to UVR, the individual cells react as previously

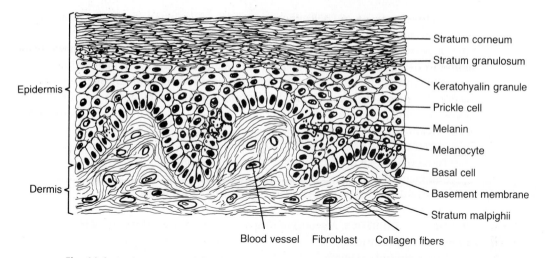

Epidermis

Dermis

Stratum corneum

Stratum granulosum

Keratohyalin granule

Prickle cell

Melanin

Melanocyte

Basal cell

Basement membrane

Stratum malpighii

Blood vessel   Fibroblast   Collagen fibers

Fig. 11-1. A cross section of the skin showing the dermis and epidermis layers.

described. However, the skin is a protective organ, covering the entire human exterior, and will respond in a generalized manner over the entire area that is irradiated. This generalized response culminates in an acute inflammatory reaction. The end results of an active inflammation within the skin are **erythema** (the reddening of the skin associated with sunburn), pigmentation (tanning), and increased epidermal thickness.[5,9,14,19]

Inflammation is the response of any human tissue, skin included, to an irritating or injurious substance or event. In the case of UVR exposure the irritating substances are the end products of the previously described photochemical event and may include damaged DNA, RNA, and cell proteins. The inflammatory process removes these injurious and irritating substances from the skin. Since the appearance of these irritating substances does not occur immediately after UVR exposure, the inflammatory response is delayed. Normally, it begins several hours after irradiation and peaks 8 to 24 hours after exposure.[14]

This inflammatory response is characterized by local vasodilation and increased capillary permeability. Theoretically this is caused by (1) the absorption of UVR by keratinocytes, leading to the release of substances that diffuse to the papillary dermis and cause vasodilation or (2) the absorption of UVR by mast cells in the dermis that in turn release histamine, resulting in vasodilation.[5,9,14] Erythema is caused by this vasodilation and the subsequent increase of blood within the dermis. The increased capillary permeability permits certain proteins to move from the capillaries into the dermis. This results in a change in osmotic pressure; consequently water is drawn into the area and edema occurs. Leukocytes, lymphocytes, and monocytes pass into the dermis and to a small degree into the epidermis. These cells phagocytize (consume or engulf) dead cells and other debris. At 24 hours the inflammatory process is completed, and at 30 hours the rebuilding begins. The reparative process is characterized by increased activity of the keratinocytes and results in a thickening of the epidermis (**hyperplasia**).[14] This is protective; areas covered with a thick epidermis, such as the soles of the feet, do not sunburn.

The acute effects of UVR exposure can be exacerbated if certain chemicals or medications are present on the skin or in the body. Photosensitization is a process in which a person becomes overly sensitive to UVR as a result of the excitation of a chemical by UVR exposure.[5] Any person taking a photosensitizing medication is very susceptible to the effects of UVR and should be treated accordingly. Such an adverse reaction can occur even after limited exposure to natural sunlight. A list of common photosensitizing agents follows:

ANTIBACTERIAL AND MICROBIAL AGENTS
Tetracyclines—a group of broad spectrum antibiotics
Sulfonamides—a group of synthetic antimicrobial drugs
Griseofulvin (Fulvicin, Grifulvin, Grisactin)—an antibiotic with an additional
   antifungal action
THIAZIDE DIURETICS. A group of drugs that act on the kidney to increase sodium and water in the urine
Chlorothiazide (Diuril)
Hydrochlorothiazide (Hydrodiuril, Oretic, Esidrix)
Methychlorothiazide (Enduron)

OTHER MEDICATIONS
Phenothiazines (Thorazine)—widely used tranquilizers
Psoralens—a group of dermal pigmenting agents
Sulfonylureas (Dymelor, Diabinese)
Diphenhydramine (Benadryl)—an antihistamine

MISCELLANEOUS
Sunscreens
Tar
Oral contraceptives
Certain cosmetics[5,13,14]

Tanning

Tanning is the increase of pigmentation within the skin and is a protective mechanism activated by UVR exposure. An increase of **melanin,** the pigment responsible for darkening, within the skin causes the tan (see Figure 11-1). The melanin functions as a biologic filter of UVR by scattering the radiation, absorbing the UVR, and dissipating the absorbed energy as heat.[19] The process of tanning is divided into two phases: immediate tanning and delayed tanning.

Immediate tanning appears most often in darkly pigmented individuals and occurs immediately after UVR exposure. Immediate tanning represents the darkening of melanosomes already present in the skin; it begins to fade 1 hour after exposure and is hardly noticeable 3 to 8 hours later.[14,19] Delayed tanning is the result of the formation of new pigment (melanin) through the process of melanogenesis. The process is initiated by production of erythema (sunburn) within the skin. Melanogenesis occurs within the melanocytes of the basal layer of the epidermis (see Figure 11-1), and the end products of this process are melanosomes, new pigment granules. These melanosomes are transferred from the melanocytes via nerve cells to nearby keratinocytes. As the keratinocytes gradually move outward to the skin's surface, the new pigment also migrates to the periphery. Delayed tanning usually becomes apparent 72 hours after UVR exposure.

Human skin color is a baseline that is influenced by various environmental factors (exposure to solar radiation, occupation, leisure activities) and the genetically determined level of melanin within the skin.[5,20] Individuals of all races have the same number of melanocytes per unit area, but darker individuals are able to produce greater amounts of melanin.[4]

ARTIFICIAL TANNING DEVICES. In the past decade, artificial tanning devices have become popular in the spa and health club industry. These tanning salons, beds, and booths usually consist of an array of long tubes positioned in a frame that allows for exposure of the entire body. The manufacturers claim that these devices produce only UVR in the UV-A spectrum and therefore are safe. However, the production of this type of UV-A generator is largely unregulated, and the effects of long-term exposure to UV-A are unknown. There is no standard of training required for the owners of these machines, and their knowledge of the tanning process and the dangers of UVR might be nil. Caution should be exercised before allowing anyone to be overexposed to UVR, either from sunlight or from an artificial source.

SUNSCREENS.* Sunscreens applied to the skin can help prevent many of the damaging effects of UVR. A sunscreen's effectiveness in absorbing the sunburn-inducing radiation is expressed as the sun protection factor (SPF). An SPF of 6 indicates that you can be exposed to UVR six times longer than without a sunscreen before you will receive a minimal erythemal dose. Higher numbers provide greater protection. However, individuals who have a family or personal history of skin cancer may experience significant damage to the skin even when wearing an SPF 15 sunscreen. Therefore these individuals should wear an SPF 30 sunscreen.

Sunscreen should be worn regularly by anyone who spends time outside. This is particularly true for individuals with fair complexions, light hair, blue eyes, or those whose skin burns easily. People with dark complexions should also wear sunscreens to prevent sun damage. Sunscreens should also be worn by anyone with a personal or family history of skin cancer.

It has been clearly shown that sun exposure causes a premature aging of skin (wrinkling, freckling, prominent blood vessels, coarsing of skin texture), induces the formation of pre-cancerous growths, and increases the risk of developing basal and squamous cell skin cancers. Blistering sunburns in one's youth also increase the risk of developing melanoma, a potentially fatal skin cancer. Since 60% to 80% of our lifetime sun exposure is often obtained by age 20, everyone over 6 months of age should use sunscreens. Sunscreens specifically labeled for children are no different than adult products. Adult sunscreens are not too strong for children's skin. It is estimated that the incidence of skin cancer would be reduced at least 70% if sunscreens were regularly used in childhood. Daily sunscreen use not only decreases or prevents photodamage but promotes repair of sun-damaged skin.

Sunscreens are needed most during March to November but should preferably

---

*Used with permission from Chapel Hill Dermatology, P.A., Chapel Hill, North Carolina.

be used year round. They are needed most between 10 am and 4 pm and should be applied 15 to 30 minutes before sun exposure.

Approximately 80% to 90% of the basal and squamous cell skin cancers occur on the face, neck, ears, and back of the hands. While clothing and hats will provide some protection from the sun, they are not a substitute for sunscreens (a typical white cotton T-shirt provides an SPF of only 5). Reflected sunlight from water, sand, and snow may effectively increase sun exposure and risk of burning.

Long-Term Effect on Skin

The most serious effects of long-term UVR exposure are premature aging of the skin and skin cancer.[10,16,17] Lightly pigmented individuals are more susceptible to these maladies. Premature aging of the skin is characterized by dryness, cracking, and a decrease in the elasticity of the skin. It results from a change in the epidermis called solar elastosis. An alteration in the skin's elastic fibers causes solar elastosis and has been tentatively linked to UVR-induced DNA damage.[14]

Skin cancer is the most common malignant tumor found in humans and has been epidemiologically and clinically associated with solar UVR.[14,16,20] Damage to DNA is suspected as the cause of skin cancer, but the exact cause is yet unknown. The major types of skin cancer are basal cell carcinoma, which rarely metastasizes (spreads to other areas), squamous cell carcinoma, which metastasizes in 5% of all cases, and malignant melanoma, which metastasizes in a majority of cases.[14,16] Fortunately the rate of cure exceeds 95% with early detection and treatment.

EFFECT ON EYES

For centuries it has been known that sunlight can have an adverse effect on vision. Snow blindness, the result of solar UVR being reflected from the snow to the unprotected eyes of winter outdoor enthusiasts, was first described in 375 BC.[19] UVR exposure of the eyes causes an acute inflammation called **photokeratitis.** It is a delayed reaction occurring 6 to 24 hours after exposure, but occasionally it develops within 30 minutes. Conjunctivitis (inflammation of the mucous membrane that lines the inside of the eyelid) develops, accompanied by erythema of adjacent facial skin, and the injured person reports the sensation of a foreign body on the eye. Photophobia, increased tear production, and spasm of the ocular muscles may occur.[14,20] The acute reaction lasts from 6 to 24 hours, and all symptoms will generally clear by 48 hours with few residual effects. The eye, unlike the skin, does not develop a tolerance to UVR. The development of cataracts has been attributed to UVR, especially in wavelengths of greater than 2900 Å.[18,20]

SYSTEMIC EFFECTS

The only systemic effect that can be objectively attributed to UVR (the only positive effect in general for that matter) is the photosynthesis of vitamin D after irradiation of the skin by UVR in the UV-B range.[18] The process is activated when the skin is irradiated by UVR at approximately the 300 Å wavelength. This activates a complicated biochemical pathway that travels from the skin to the liver and kidneys and results in vitamin D being delivered to bones, the intestines, various organs, and muscles. Vitamin D is responsible for regulating calcium and phosphorus, and after UVR exposure the absorption of these elements increases within the intestines and results in increased amounts of calcium and phosphorus within the blood. Consequently UVR can be used to treat disorders of calcium and phosphorus metabolism, such as rickets and tetany. Presently the treatment of choice for such problems is dietary supplementation; however, if this is not effective, UVR is an acceptable alternative.

Although no other systemic effects can be objectively attributed to UVR exposure, there are several psychologic benefits and problems that may result from exposure. Many people relish the immediate sensation of warmth and relaxation that results from resting in the sun on a nice summer day; a general sense of well-being and good health surrounds the individual. Ideally this happy experience is not overindulged, resulting in a painful sunburn. Moderation is the key to preventing damage to the skin; this includes gradually increasing exposure to the sun and prudent use of sunscreens.

Europeans, especially those living in northern latitudes, are probably the world's most active sunbathers. During the spring and summer months, they will congregate in sunny areas and feed on the sunlight that is so unavailable during their dark winters. Artificial UVR for tanning purposes is greatly used in these areas, certainly for the sense of well-being that follows brief UVR exposure and also for medical reasons. The use of artificial UVR to preserve the summer's tan is also on the increase in the United States and can be witnessed in the rapidly increasing number of tanning salons and spas. The apparatus most likely to be used in one of these establishments will produce UVR in the UV-A wavelength, and the management of the salon will be quick to point out that this is a safe alternative to natural sunlight. An individual can certainly achieve tanning from these devices, although not as effectively as from UV-B exposure, but the research is still cloudy on the safety of long-term exposure to UV-A.

Needless to say, the psychologic effect from the extreme skin damage from long-term exposure to UVR can be devastating. The peaches-and-cream complexion of a 20-year-old beauty queen can turn to withered leather at 40 if caution is not used outdoors and in the tanning salon. A diagnosis of skin cancer will surely throw a person's psychologic health into a downward spiral.

APPARATUS

Since the beginning of this century, many types of UVR generators have been developed, including the carbon arc lamp, the fluorescent lamp, the xenon compact arc lamp, and the mercury arc lamp. Of these, mercury arc lamps are the most common and are safe, effective, and easy to operate.

The carbon arc lamp is composed of two carbon electrodes that consist of carbon and certain inorganic salts and metals. Initially the two electrodes are in contact when the current is applied and then are moved slightly apart, causing the current to arc across this small gap. As the salts and metals within the electrodes become heated, UVR is emitted, the majority between 3500 and 4000 Å. The electrode gradually burns, so the lamp will deteriorate and the electrodes must be replaced. This burning is noisy and causes an unpleasant odor, and the device requires a high electrical input.

The xenon compact arc lamp is composed of xenon gas enclosed in a vessel in which it is compressed to 20 times atmospheric pressure. An electric arc is passed through the gas, causing increased temperature. When the gas is heated to 6000° C (10,832° F), the atoms become incandescent and emit infrared, visible, and ultraviolet light waves. Most of the UVR is in the range of 3200 to 4000 Å. Caution must be exercised when using a device with gas under such high pressure, since rupture of the containing vessel could endanger the patient and operator.

The mercury arc lamps are divided into two categories, low-pressure and high-pressure mercury arcs. Both consist of mercury (a heavy metal in a liquid state) contained in a quartz envelope. When an electric arc is passed through the envelope, the mercury becomes vaporized, and at 8000° C (14,432° F) the atoms become incandescent and emit ultraviolet, infrared, and visible light. In the low-pressure lamp, also called the cold quartz lamp, the temperature of the mercury electrons is greater than the mercury vapor. The temperature of the quartz envelope is about 60° C, but it is not dangerous. The UVR spectrum produced by low-pressure lamps is limited to 1849 Å and 2537 Å. The 1849 Å wavelength is blocked by the quartz envelope, or it would combine with oxygen and produce ozone. 95% of the UVR produced by these lamps is the 2537 Å wavelength, which is highly germicidal. The low-pressure mercury arc lamp does not require a warm-up or cool-down period, and it is used mainly where the bactericidal effect of UVR is desired.

A high-pressure mercury arc occurs when the mercury vapor temperature equals the mercury electron temperature and the pressure within the envelope reaches one atmosphere or more.[17] The quartz envelopes of these lamps become quite hot and may be cooled by a water jacket or circulating air; subsequently these are called hot quartz lamps. The UVR spectrum produced peaks at 2537, 2800, 2967, 3025, 3130, and 3660 Å.[5,9,18,19] The 2537 Å wavelength is absorbed by the increased density of the mercury vapor and does not pass from the lamp. Most of the UVR produced falls within the UV-B range. These lamps require a warm-up period before reaching peak efficiency and a cool-down period after the current is stopped before the lamp can be restarted. The high-pressure mercury arc lamps are mainly used to produce erythema and the accompanying photochemical reactions.

The fluorescent ultraviolet lamp or "blacklight" is actually a low-pressure mercury lamp. It consists of a tube of UV-transmitting glass that is coated with phosphors. The phosphors are fluorescing substances that absorb the UVR and then reemit it at a longer wavelength. Most of the UVR emitted ranges from 3000 to 4000 Å, within the high UV-B and entire UV-A range.[18] These lamps are low-powered and generally used in multiples. These lamps are used where exposure of several people simultaneously is desired.

The mercury arc lamps are the most likely kind of UVR lamp to be used in a sports-medicine setting, and generally the lamps will be either a standing model or a hand-held model. The standing model consists of a mercury arc lamp surrounded by a reflector. The opening below the lamp and reflector can be closed by the use of shutters. The lamp, reflector, and shutters are supported by a column with adjustable height. At the base of the column is a housing that contains the electrical controls contained within the configuration of the unit (Figure 11-2). The hand-held unit is used for very local treatments and produces the bactericidal spectral bond of 2536 Å. It is

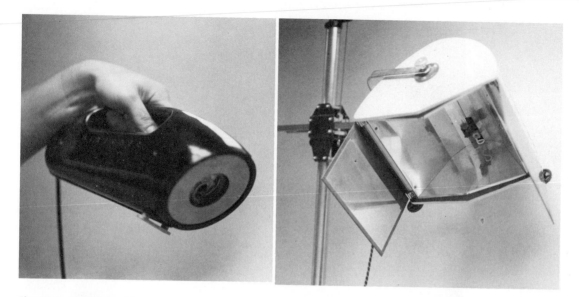

Fig. 11-2. *(Left)* A hand-held cold quartz ultraviolet lamp. *(Right)* A standing hot quartz ultraviolet lamp. Note the open shutters.

very effective for treating local skin infections and, with the addition of a special lens, is used for diagnostic purposes.

TECHNIQUE OF APPLICATION

Before operation of any UVR generator, sports therapists must thoroughly familiarize themselves with the equipment. The operation manual must be understood and available if needed. Faulty operation of the equipment can endanger both the patient and the operator. The lamp and reflector must be kept clean by wiping with gauze and methyl alcohol or by following the manufacturer's instructions. The quality of UVR is greatly diminished by dirty lamps and reflectors. The entire device must be completely inspected before use to ensure safe operation.

The effectiveness of the apparatus must be determined before UVR therapy can begin. The lamps in these devices deteriorate over time, and accumulation of dirt and other residues on the lamp and reflector can also alter the effect of the UVR. Two lamps of the same model may have two different effects, depending on the age of the lamp and its condition. The effectiveness of the lamp is assessed by determining the skin sensitivity to UVR of the patient to be treated. This sensitivity is measured by the **minimal erythemal dose.** The minimal erythemal dose is the exposure time needed to produce a faint erythema of the skin 24 hours after exposure.[5,16] Before testing, the patient should be questioned regarding photosensitizing drugs and the area of skin to be tested should be cleaned. The area of the test should have pigmentation similar to the area to be treated. The forearm is a common choice for the test site.

For the skin test, the patient should be positioned comfortably, and eye protection must be provided to the patient and the operator. The goggles must fit

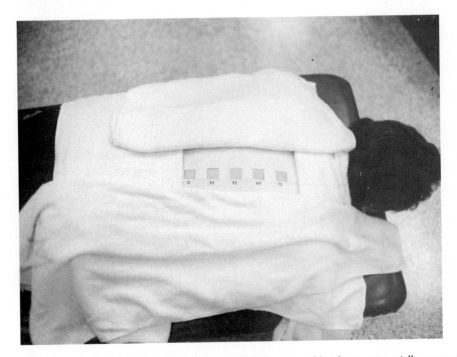

Fig. 11-3. The ultraviolet skin test. The patient's back is draped and has been sequentially exposed to ultraviolet radiation for 15, 30, 45, 60, and 75 seconds.

snugly, since UVR can be reflected behind the lens of ordinary sunglasses. The patient may be instructed to close his or her eyes as an added precaution. The patient is draped except for the test site; a good quality bed sheet or bath towel provides an adequate barrier to UVR. A piece of typing paper with five cutouts 1 inch square and 1 inch apart is placed over the test site (Figure 11-3). If necessary the lamp is warmed up with the protective shutters closed. The lamp is positioned over the patient with care being taken to adjust the height of the lamp to the same distance from the patient as will be used during treatment. With the lamp in position, the shutters are opened and the cutouts covered at 15-second intervals so that the five portions of the skin will be exposed for 15, 30, 45, 60, and 75 seconds. The patient returns in 24 hours, and a visual inspection determines the minimal erythemal dose. This information is used as the basis for determining treatment time.[3]

Areas tested that reveal no erythema 24 hours after testing have received a suberythemal dose, whereas those demonstrating erythema at 24 hours have received the minimal erythemal dose. At 48 hours if erythema is still present, a first-degree erythemal dose has been given, and a second-degree erythemal dose has been given if erythema persists from 48 to 72 hours. If the erythema lasts past 72 hours after testing, then a third-degree erythemal dose has been given. The third-degree erythemal dose is pathologic and causes skin destruction. Second- and third-degree doses are seldom used except in the case of stubborn skin infections, and when they are used, the skin surrounding the area of treatment should be well protected from exposure. First- and second-degree doses can be estimated; first-degree erythemal doses approximately correspond to 2.5 times the minimal erythemal dose, and second-degree doses correspond to 5 times the minimal erythemal dose.[5]

Since human skin adapts to UVR exposure, the minimal erythemal dose will gradually increase with repeated treatments. Therefore it is necessary to gradually increase exposure time to achieve the same reaction. Once the treatment time has been determined, it is increased 5 seconds per treatment with the height of the lamp remaining constant. Conversely, treatment time should be reduced 5 seconds for each day missed, or it should be set back to the original minimal erythemal dose.

To give consistent treatments, the operator needs to be aware of the two laws of physics that apply directly to UVR treatments, the inverse square law and the cosine law. The inverse square law states that the strength of radiation of light from a point source varies inversely with the square of the distance from the source.[5,18] Therefore if the lamp is set closer to the patient than during the skin test, a stronger dose is given; if it is set further away, a weaker dose is given. The distance of the lamp from the patient must be kept constant if the intensity of the treatments is to be equal. The height of the lamp is generally standardized at each clinic, usually ranging from 24 to 40 inches.[10] My preference is to set the height of the lamp at 30 inches.

The cosine law states that for maximum absorption of radiant energy, the source must be perpendicular to the absorbing surface (the patient being the absorbing surface).[5,18] A deviation of 10 degrees causes no major alteration in the amount of energy absorbed. Therefore care should be taken in positioning the lamp and patient during testing and treatment.

Once the minimal erythemal dose has been established, treatment can commence. As with the skin test, the treatment area should be warm and provide maximum privacy, since the patient may be partially or fully disrobed. Goggles, stopwatch, measuring tape, and draping must be readily available. The patient should be carefully draped so that areas not to receive UVR exposure are protected. Besides the eyes, the nipples and genitalia should be protected. UVR can be reflected from white linen and shiny equipment surfaces. If needed, the UVR apparatus should be warmed up with the protective shutter in place. The patient and operator are ready to begin treatment when the patient is comfortable, properly draped, and has his or her eyes protected. The lamp is positioned at proper height and angle, and the operator has his or her goggles in place and stopwatch ready. Treatment commences when the operator simultaneously opens the shutters and activates the stopwatch. At the end of the predetermined treatment time, the shutters are closed, the lamp is extinguished, and the patient is allowed to remove the goggles and dress. Accurate records noting the height of the lamp, time of exposure, and condition of the area treated must be kept. Also, the same lamp should be used for subsequent treatments, since lamp deterioration causes differing intensities from UVR sources of even the same manufacturer's model.

Consistency is crucial if safe and effective UVR treatments are to be given. The set-up of the patient and equipment should not vary without adequate reason. Usually the only variable is the length of treatment (exposure), which is determined by and based on the skin test, the treatment prescription, the lesion to be treated, and the progression of treatment. If the length of treatment is in doubt, it is always best to yield to brevity rather than to endanger a patient.

CLINICAL USE

UVR therapy is used to obtain one or more of the following effects: increased vitamin D production, stimulation of the skin, sterilization, tanning, hyperplasia, and exfoliation (peeling).[18] UVR use is indicated to treat of infectious and noninfectious skin diseases and for the excitation of calcium metabolism.[5] The development of antibiotics and other medications has greatly reduced the clinical use of UVR, since these drugs are very effective and simple to use to treat disease. Today the most common use of UVR is in the treatment of dermatologic conditions, such as psoriasis and acne, and hard to cure infectious skin conditions, such as pressure sores. The protocol for treating certain maladies with UVR follows.

Psoriasis

The Goeckerman technique developed in 1925 is still widely used. This consists of applying a crude tar ointment (2% to 5%) over the patches of psoriasis the night before treatment. The next morning the tar is removed, except for a thin film, and the area is irradiated with a UV-B source at minimal erythemal dosage.[2,5] The exposure time is gradually increased, and the treatment is usually carried out for several weeks. In the past decade, a UV-A source and the photosensitizing drug psoralen have been used to treat psoriasis. Discussion of this technique, called PUVA therapy, follows.

Disturbances of Calcium and Phosphorus Absorption

Conditions such as osteomalacia (rickets) and tetany can be treated with irradiation by a UV-B source. These disturbances of absorption are caused by a vitamin D deficiency. As previously discussed, vitamin D is produced after irradiation of the skin. Whole body irradiation is indicated if diet and oral supplementation of calcium and phosphorus do not produce improvement.[18]

Pressure Sores

Unlike most infectious skin disorders, pressure sores do not respond readily to antibiotic therapy. Irradiation of the lesion by low-pressure mercury or cold quartz lamp, which produces UVR of the bactericidal 2537 Å wavelength, can effectively treat this problem. The hand-held lamps are most useful, since they can be used to produce a very localized reaction. Exposure time should be sufficient to produce a second- or third-degree erythemal dose response.[5,18] Care must be taken to protect the surrounding skin.

PUVA Therapy

PUVA therapy is a treatment for psoriasis that consists of ingestion of oral methoxsalen, a psoralen, and exposure of the affected site to a UV-A light source. The methoxsalen increases the patient's sensitivity to UVR. In the presence of UV-A, it binds with DNA and inhibits DNA synthesis.[6] Unfortunately, several studies point to an increased risk of developing skin cancer after PUVA therapy, and problems with the safety of the UV-A sources have been uncovered.[1,6,7,15] Still, in selected cases PUVA therapy is considered by the American Academy of Dermatology to be safe, but its use should be limited to physicians with training in photochemotherapy.[1]

Sterilization

Bacteria are destroyed when exposed to UVR in the range of 2500 to 2700 Å. This technique has been used to sterilize the air in operating rooms and to sterilize water. The technique is quite safe if human exposure to the UVR source is kept to a minimum.

Diagnosis

A UVR source fitted with a special filter, a Wood's filter, can be used to aid in the diagnosis of certain skin disorders. The filter blocks all the UVR except that in the range of 3600 to 3700 Å. This wavelength is most effective in causing exposed areas to fluoresce. The test is performed in a darkened room, and since all animal tissues fluoresce, the exposure to the filtered UVR will cause the exposed tissue to appear a specific color.[18] However, if an infection is present, the color of the area will correspond to the **fluorescence** of the infecting organism rather than the expected normal color. This abnormal coloration can be evaluated and a tentative diagnosis made.

INDICATIONS

Acne. General body irradiation may help, minimal erythemal dose applied three times per week

Aseptic wounds. Suberythemal dose applied every 3 days[2,5,10,12,16]

Folliculitis. Suberythemal dose applied every 3 days until clear

Pityriasis rosea. General body irradiation, minimal erythemal dose applied three times per week

Tinea capitum. Local first-degree erythemal reaction, repeated when initial response clears

Septic wounds. Local second-degree erythemal response, repeated every 3 days

Sinusitis. General body irradiation

CONTRAINDICATIONS

Porphyrias

Pellagra

Lupus erythematosus

Sarcoidosis

Xeroderma pigmentosum

Acute psoriasis

Acute eczema

Herpes simplex

Renal and hepatic insufficiencies

Diabetes

Hyperthyroidism

Generalized dermatitis

Advanced arteriosclerosis

Active and progressive pulmonary tuberculosis[2,5,10-12,18]

The use of UVR therapy in athletic medicine has been limited. Many indications for its use, such as acne, skin infections, and fungal infections, are adequately treated with medication. Other problems, such as pressure sores and vitamin D deficiency, are seldom found among an athletic population. This does not mean that UVR should be excluded from the clinic; it most certainly has beneficial effects that could be used by sports therapists. Considering the small number of potential patients and the limited budgetary resources most sports therapists have available, UVR equipment will remain a low-priority item.

However, the population of the United States is gradually growing older and more active. Sports medicine is no longer limited to the college football star or the Olympic hopeful. Today, sports-medicine clinics are treating patients ranging from prepubescent marathoners to 70-year-old triathletes. As the number and age of active persons increase, so will the variety of problems to be treated. At present, there is some inconclusive evidence that UVR can aid in the reduction of blood pressure, help to relieve asthma, cause a reduction in blood cholesterol, and aid in reducing the severity of upper respiratory infections.[18] The average patient being seen in a sports-medicine clinic is generally not a world class athlete, but might be a 50-year-old executive who is emerging from 25 years of sedentary living. UVR might be a helpful part of this patient's treatment. As research continues, UVR may become a favored and useful treatment just as it was earlier in this century.

SUMMARY

1. UVR is that portion of the electromagnetic spectrum that ranges from 2000 to 4000 Å.
2. Exposure to UVR causes a photochemical reaction within living cells and can cause alterations of DNA and cell proteins.
3. The irradiation of human skin causes an acute inflammation that is characterized by an erythema, increased pigmentation, and hyperplasia.
4. The effects of long-term exposure to UVR are premature aging of the skin and skin cancer.
5. The eye is extremely sensitive to UVR and will develop photokeratitis after exposure.
6. Many types of equipment are manufactured that produce UVR, but the majority used clinically are of the low- and high-pressure mercury lamp variety.

GLOSSARY

DNA Deoxyribonucleic acid; the substance found in the chromosomes of the cell nucleus that carries the genetic code of the cell.

erythema A redness of the skin caused by capillary dilation.

fluorescence The capacity of certain substances to radiate when illuminated by a source of a given wavelength; a light of a different wavelength (color) than that of the irradiating source when illuminated by a given wavelength.

hyperplasia An increase in the size of a tissue; in the skin, an increased thickness of the epidermis.

keratin The fibrous protein that forms the chemical basis of the epidermis.

keratinocytes A cell that produces keratin.

melanin A group of dark brown or black pigments that occur naturally in the eye, skin, hair, and other animal tissues.

minimal erythemal dose The amount of time of exposure to UVR necessary to cause a faint erythema 24 hours after exposure.

photokeratitis An inflammation of the eyes caused by exposure to UVR.

RNA Ribonucleic acid; an acid found in the cell cytoplasm and nucleolus. It is intimately involved in protein synthesis.

REFERENCES

1 Bickford E., Berger D, Korth R, et al.: Risks associated with the use of UV-A irradiators, *Photochem Photobiol* 30(2): 199-202, 1979.

2 Burdick Corp: *Burdick syllabus,* ed 7, Milton, Wis, 1969.

3 Downer A: *Physical therapy procedures,* ed 3, Springfield, Ill, 1981, Charles C. Thomas.

4 Goldman L: *Introduction to modern phototherapy,* Springfield, Ill, 1978, Charles C. Thomas.

5 Griffin J, Karselis T: *Physical agents for physical therapists,* ed 2, Springfield, Ill, 1982, Charles C. Thomas.

6 Hall L: Current status of oral PUVA therapy for psoriasis, *J Am Acad Dermatol* 1(2): 106-107, 1979.

7 Harbor L: PUVA therapy status, *J Am Acad Dermatol* 1(2): 150, 1979.

8 Kottke F: *Krusen's handbook of physical medicine and rehabilitation,* ed 3, Philadelphia, 1983, WB Saunders.

9 Kovacs R: *Light therapy,* Springfield, Ill, 1950, Charles C. Thomas.

10 Lewis G: *Practical dermatology,* Philadelphia, 1967, WB Saunders.

11 Mayer E: *Clinical application of sunlight and artificial radiation,* Baltimore, 1926, Williams & Wilkins.

12 Mayer E: *The curative value of light,* New York, 1932, D. Appleton.

13 Parish P: *The doctors and patients handbook of medicines and drugs,* New York, 1980, Alfred A. Knopf.

14 Parrish J: *UV-A biological effects of ultraviolet radiation,* New York, 1979, Plenum Publishing.

15 Pittekow M, et al.: Skin cancer in patients with psoriasis treated with coal tar, *Arch Dermatol* 117: 465-468, 1981.

16 Rook A, Wilkinson D, Ebling K, et al.: *Textbook of dermatology,* Oxford, 1979, Blackwell Scientific Publishers.

17 Stewart W: *Dermatology: diagnosis and treatment of cutaneous disorders,* St Louis, 1978, Mosby.

18 Stillwell G: *Therapeutic electricity and ultraviolet radiation,* Baltimore, 1983, Williams & Wilkins.

19 Urbach F: *The biologic effects of ultraviolet radiation,* London, 1969, Pergamon Press.

20 U.S. Department of Health, Education, and Welfare: *Public health service: occupational exposure to ultraviolet radiation,* Washington, D.C., 1972, National Institute for Occupational Safety and Health, HSM73-1 1009.

SUGGESTED READINGS

Bryant BG: Treatment of psoriasis, *Am J Hosp Pharm* 37: 814-820, 1980.

Challner AVJ, Corless D, Davis A, et al.: Personnel monitoring exposure to UV radiation, *Clin Exp Dermatol* 1: 175-179, 1976.

Challner AVJ, Duffey BL: Problems associated with ultraviolet dosimetry in the photochemotherapy of psoriasis, *Br J Dermatol* 97: 643-648, 1977.

Corless D, Gupta, SP: Response of plasma 25 hydroxyvitamin D to ultraviolet irradiation in long stay geriatric patients, *Lancet* 223: 649-651, 1978.

Dietzel F: Effects of non-ionizing electromagnetic radiation on the development and intrauterine implantation of the rat. In Tyler AE, editor: Biological effects of nonionizing radiation, *Ann NY Acad Sci* 247: 367, 1975.

Everett MA, Olson RL, Sayer RM: Ultraviolet erythema, *Arch Dermatol* 92: 713, 1975.

Fischer T: Comparative treatment of psoriasis with UV-light trioxsalen plus UV-light and coal tar plus UV-light, *Acta Derm Venereol Suppl* 57: 345-350, 1977.

Fitzpatrick TB, Pathak A, Magnus IA, et al.: Abnormal reactions of man to light, *Ann Rev Med* 14: 195, 1963.

Giese A, editor: *Photophysiology,* vol IV, New York, 1968, Academic Press.

Giese A, editor: *Photophysiology,* vol V, New York, 1970, Academic Press.

Giese A, editor: *Photophysiology,* vol VI, New York, 1971, Academic Press.

Giese A, editor: *Photophysiology,* vol VII, New York, 1972, Academic Press.

Gordon M, editor: *Pigment cell biology,* New York, 1959, Academic Press.

Grynbaum B, Bierman W, Kurtin A, et al.: Prevention of ultraviolet induced erythema, *Arch Phys Med Rehabil* 31: 587-592, 1950.

Hardie RA, Hunter, JAA: Psoriasis, *Br J Hosp Med* 20: 13-23, 1978.

Holick MF, Clark MB: The photogenesis and metabolism of Vitamin D, *Fed Proc* 37(12): 2567-2574, 1978.

Hollaender A, editor: *Radiation biology,* vol II, New York, 1955, McGraw-Hill.

Holti G: Measurements of the vascular responses in skin at various time intervals after damage with histamine and ultraviolet radiation, *Clin Sci* 14: 143-155, 1955.

Jarratt M, Knox JM: Photodynamic action: theory and applications, *Prog Dermatol* 8: 1, 1974.

Kelner A: Photoreactivation of ultraviolet irradiated eschericoli with special reference to the dose reduction principal and to ultraviolet induced mutation, *J Bacteriol* 58: 11-22, 1949.

Licht S, editor: *Therapeutic electricity and ultraviolet radiation,* ed 2, New Haven, Conn, 1967, Elizabeth Licht.

Lynch WS: Clinical results of photochemotherapy, *Cutis* 20: 477-480, 1977.

Macleod MA, Blacklock NJ: UVL induced changes in calcium absorption and excretion and in serum vitamin D_3 levels measured in black skinned and caucasian males, *J R Nav Med Serv* 65: 75-78, 1979.

Marisco AR, et al.: Ultraviolet light and tar in the Goeckerman treatment of psoriasis, *Arch Dermatol* 112: 1249-1250, 1976.

Montagna W, Labitz W, editors: *The epidermis,* New York, 1964, Academic Press.

Morison WL: Controlled study of PUVA and adjunctive therapy in the management of psoriasis, *Br J Dermatol* 98: 125-132, 1978.

Ohayashi T, Yoshimoto S, Yasamura M: Effect of wavelength on the photochemical reaction of ergocalciferol (vitamin D_2) irradiated by monochromatic ultraviolet light, *J Nutr Sci Vitaminol* 23: 281-290, 1977 (in English).

Parrish JA, et al.: Photochemotherapy of psoriasis with oral methoxsalen and longwave ultraviolet light, *New Engl J Med* 291: 1207-1222, 1974.

Pathak MA, Harber JC, Seiji M, editors: *Sunlight and man,* Tokyo, 1974, University of Tokyo Press.

Peak M: Inactivation of transforming DNA by ultraviolet light. II. Protection by histidine, *Mutat Res* 20: 137-141, 1973.

Roenig HH: Comparison of phototherapy systems for photochemotherapy, *Cutis* 20: 485-489, 1977.

Rogers S: Effect of PUVA on serum 25-OH vitamin D in psoriatics, *Br Med J* 833: 34, 1979.

Salem L: Theory of photochemical reactions, *Science* 191: 822, 1976.

Sams W, Winkleman R: The effect of ultraviolet light on isolated cutaneous blood vessels, *J Invest Dermatol* 53: 79-83, 1969.

Sauer G, editor: *Manual of skin diseases,* ed 3, Philadelphia, 1973, JB Lippincott.

Segal SA: PUVA: a caution, *Pediatrics* 62: 253, 1978.

Sulzberger W, Wolf J, Witten V: *Dermatology: diagnosis and treatment,* ed 2, Chicago, 1961, Year Book.

Task Force Committee on Photobiology of the National Program for Dermatology, LC Harber, Chairman, Report on ultraviolet light sources, *Arch Dermatol* 109: 833-839, 1974.

Taylor RL: Clinical study of ultraviolet in various skin conditions, *Phys Ther* 52: 279-282, 1972.

Telles, Coakley, and Kluger: *Possible hazards from high intensity discharge mercury vapor and metal halide lamps,* Bureau of Radiological Health. Food and Drug Administration, Nov, 1977.

Thomsen DE: Phototherapy: treatment with light, *Science News* 105: 404, 1974.

Tronnier H: Zur Bedeutung der Hornschicht furr die Lichttreaktionen der menschlichen Haut, *Strahlentherapie* 132: 128-133, 1967.

Urbach F, editor: *Biological effects of ultraviolet radiation,* New York, 1969, Pergamon.

Van Der Leun JC: Theory of ultraviolet erythema, *Photochem Photobiol* 4: 453-458, 1965.

Van Pelt WF, Payne WR, Peterson RW: *A review of selected bioeffects thresholds for various spectral ranges of light,* DHEW Publ. no. (FDA) 74-8010.

Weber G: Combined 8-methoxypsoralen and black light therapy of psoriasis: technique and results, *Br J Dermatol* 90: 317-323, 1974.

Wurtman RJ: The effects of light on the human body, *Sci Am* 233: 69, 1975.

Young P: Turning on light turns off disease, *National Observer,* May 29, 1976.

Therapeutic Ultrasound

12

William E. Prentice

OBJECTIVES

After completion of this chapter, the student will be able to do the following:

- Describe the transmission of acoustic energy in biologic tissues relative to waveforms, frequency, velocity, and attenuation.

- Discuss the basic physics involved in the production of a beam of therapeutic ultrasound.

- Discuss both the thermal and nonthermal physiologic effects of therapeutic ultrasound.

- Discuss specific techniques of application of therapeutic ultrasound and how they may be modified to achieve treatment goals.

- Identify the most appropriate and clinically effective uses for therapeutic ultrasound.

- Discuss the technique and clinical application of phonophoresis.

- Describe the contraindications and precautions that should be observed with therapeutic ultrasound.

In the medical community, ultrasound is a modality that is used for a number of different purposes including diagnosis, destruction of issue, and therapy. Diagnostic ultrasound has been used for more than 30 years to image internal structures. Most typically, diagnostic ultrasound is used to image the fetus during pregnancy. Ultrasound has also been used to produce extreme tissue hyperthermia, which has been demonstrated to have tumoricidal effects in cancer patients.

In addition to superficial heat and cold and electrical stimulating currents, ultrasound is one of the most widely used modalities in the sports-medicine arena. It has been used as a valuable tool in the rehabilitation of many different injuries to stimulate the repair of soft tissue injuries and to relieve pain. [19] It has traditionally been classified as a deep heating modality and used primarily to elevate tissue temperatures.

As discussed in Chapter 1, ultrasound is a form of acoustic rather than electromagnetic energy. Ultrasound is defined as inaudible, acoustic vibrations of high frequency that may produce either thermal or nonthermal physiologic effects.[31] The use of ultrasound as a therapeutic agent may be extremely effective if the sports therapist has an adequate understanding of its effects on biologic tissues and of the physical mechanisms by which these effects are produced.[19]

TRANSMISSION OF ACOUSTIC ENERGY IN BIOLOGIC TISSUES

Unlike electromagnetic energy, which travels most effectively through a vacuum, acoustic energy relies on molecular collision for transmission. Molecules in a conducting medium, when set into vibration, will cause vibration and minimal displacement of other surrounding molecules so that eventually this "wave" of vibration has propagated through the entire medium. Sound waves travel in a manner similar to waves created by a stone thrown into a pool of water. Ultrasound is a mechanical wave in which energy is transmitted by the vibrations of the molecules of the biological medium through which the wave is travelling.[74]

Transverse versus Longitudinal Waves

There are two types of waves that can travel through a solid medium: **longitudinal** and **transverse waves.** In a longitudinal wave, the molecular displacement is along the direction in which the wave travels. Within this longitudinal wave are regions of high molecular density referred to as **compressions** and regions of lower molecular density called **rarefactions** along the pathway (Figure 12-1). In a transverse wave, the molecules are displaced in a direction perpendicular to the direction in which the wave is moving. While longitudinal waves travel both in solids and liquids, transverse waves can travel only in solids. Since soft tissues are more like liquids, ultrasound travels primarily as a longitudinal wave. Transverse waves are found predominately in bone.[74]

Frequency of Wave Transmission

The *frequency* of audible sound ranges between 16 kHz and 20 kHz (kilohertz = 1000 cycles per second). Ultrasound has a frequency above 20 kHz. The frequency range for therapeutic ultrasound is between 0.75 and 3 MHz (Megahertz = 1,000,000 cycles per second). The higher the frequency of the sound waves emitted from a sound source, the less the sound will diverge and thus a more focused sound beam is produced. In biologic tissues, the lower the frequency of the sound waves, the greater the depth of penetration. Higher frequency sound waves are absorbed in the more superficial tissues.

Velocity

The *velocity* at which this vibration or sound wave is propagated through the conducting medium is directly related to the density. Denser and more rigid materials will have a higher velocity of transmission. At a frequency of 1 MHz, sound travels through soft tissue at 1540 m/sec and through compact bone at 4000 m/sec.[84]

Attenuation

As the ultrasound wave is transmitted through the various tissues, there will be **attenuation** or a decrease in energy intensity. This decrease is due to either *absorption*

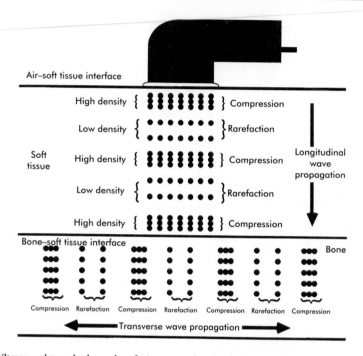

Fig. 12-1 Ultrasound travels through soft tissue as a longitudinal wave alternating regions of high molecular density (compressions) low molecular density (rarefactions). Transverse waves are found primarily in bone.

of energy by the tissues or *dispersion* and *scattering* of the sound wave, which results from reflection or refraction.[74]

The capability of acoustic energy to penetrate or be transmitted to deeper tissues is determined by the frequency of the ultrasound, as well as the characteristics of the tissues through which ultrasound is travelling. Penetration and absorption are inversely related. Absorption increases as the frequency increases, thus less energy is transmitted to the deeper tissues.[47] Tissues that are high in water content have a low rate of absorption, while tissues high in protein content have a high rate of absorption.[20] Fat has a relatively low absorption rate, and muscle absorbs considerably more. Peripheral nerve absorbs at a rate twice that of muscle. Bone, which is relatively superficial, absorbs more ultrasonic energy than any of the other tissues (Table 12-1).

When a sound wave encounters a boundary or an interface between different tissues, some of the energy will scatter due to reflection or refraction. The amount of energy reflected, and conversely the amount of energy that will be transmitted to deeper tissues, is determined by the relative magnitude of the **acoustic impedances** of the two materials on either side of the interface. Acoustic impedance may be determined by multiplying the density of the material by the speed at which sound travels inside it. If the acoustic impedances of the two materials forming the interface are the same, all of the sound will be transmitted and none will be reflected. The larger the difference between the two acoustic impedances, the more energy is reflected and the less that can enter a second medium[79] (Table 12-2).

TABLE 12-1   Relationship Between Penetration and Absorption (1 MHz)

Media	Absorption	Penetration
Water	1	1200
Blood plasma	23	52
Whole blood	60	20
Fat	390	4
Skeletal muscle	663	2
Peripheral nerve	1193	1

From Griffin JE: Physiological effects of ultrasound energy as it is used clinically, *Phys Ther* 46(1): 18-26, 1966. Reprinted with permission of the American Physical Therapy Association.

TABLE 12-2   The Percentage of Incident Energy Reflected at Tissue Interfaces[78]

Interface	Percent Reflection (%)
Soft tissue/air	99.9
Water/soft tissue	0.2
Soft tissue/fat	1.0
Soft tissue/bone	15-40

Sound passing from the transducer to air will be almost completely reflected. Ultrasound is transmitted through fat. It is both reflected and refracted at the muscular interface. At the soft tissue-bone interface, virtually all of the sound is reflected. As the ultrasound energy is reflected at tissue interfaces with different acoustic impedances, the intensity of the energy is increased as the reflected energy meets new energy being transmitted, creating what is referred to as a **standing wave** or a **hot spot.** This increased level of energy has the potential to produce tissue damage. Moving the sound transducer or using pulsed wave ultrasound can help minimize the development of hot spots.[20]

BASIC PHYSICS OF THERAPEUTIC ULTRASOUND
Components of a Therapeutic Ultrasound Generator

An ultrasound generator consists of a high frequency electrical generator connected through an oscillator circuit and a transformer via a coaxial cable to a transducer housed in a type of insulated applicator (Figure 12-2). The oscillator circuit produces a sound beam at a specific frequency that is adjusted by the manufacturer to the frequency requirements of the transducer. The control panel of an ultrasound unit usually has a timer that can be preset, a power meter, an intensity control, a duty cycle control switch, a selector for continuous or pulsed modes and possibly output power in response to tissue loading, and an automatic shut-off in case of overheating of the transducer (Figure 12-3).

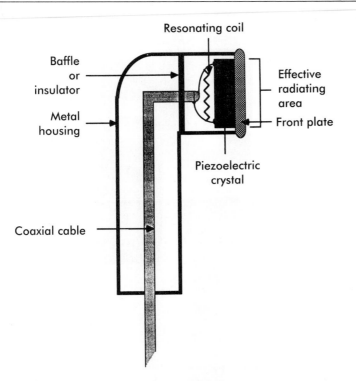

Fig. 12-2 The anatomy of a typical ultrasound transducer.

The transducer, also referred to as an applicator or a sound head, must be matched to particular units that are generally not interchangeable.[15] The transducer consists of some piezoelectric crystal, such as quartz, or synthetic ceramic crystals made of lead zirconate or titanate, barium titanate, or nickle-cobalt ferrite of approximately 2 to 3 mm in thickness. It is the crystal within the transducer that converts electrical energy to acoustic energy through mechanical deformation of the piezoelectric crystal.

Piezoelectric Effect

When an alternating electrical current generated at the same frequency as the crystal resonance is passed through the piezoelectric crystal, the crystal will expand and contract, creating what is referred to as the **piezoelectric effect.** There are two forms of this piezoelectric effect (Figure 12-4, *A* and *B*). A *direct* piezoelectric effect is the generation of a electrical voltage across the crystal when it is compressed or expanded. An *indirect* or *reverse* piezoelectric effect is created when an alternating current moves through the crystal producing compression or expansion. It is this change in voltage polarity that causes the crystal to expand and contract and thus vibrate at the frequency of the electrical oscillation. Thus the reverse piezoelectric effect is used to generate ultrasound at a desired frequency.

Frequency of Therapeutic Ultrasound

Therapeutic ultrasound produced by a piezoelectric transducer has a frequency range between 0.75 and 3.0 MHz. The majority of ultrasound generators are set at a frequency

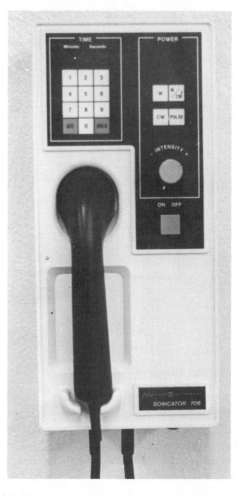

Fig. 12-3 Standard portable ultrasound unit. (Manufactured by Mettler Electronics, Anaheim, CA)

of 1 MHz, although there are ultrasound units that are set at a frequency of 3 MHz. A generator that can be set between 1 and 3 MHz affords the sports therapist the greatest treatment flexibility.

Ultrasound energy generated at 1 MHz is transmitted through the more superficial tissues and absorbed primarily in the deeper tissues at depths of 3 to 5 cm (Figure 12-5). A 1 MHz frequency is most useful in individuals with a high percentage of cutaneous body fat, and whenever the desired effects are in the deeper structures.[31] At 3 MHz the energy is absorbed in the more superficial tissues with a depth of penetration between 1 and 2 cm.[84]

The Ultrasound Beam

If the wavelength of the sound is larger than the source that produced it, then the sound will spread in all directions.[79] Such is the case with audible sound, thus explaining why it is possible for a person behind you to hear your voice almost as well as a person in

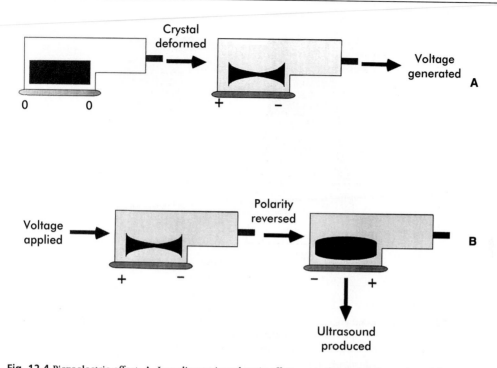

Fig. 12-4 Piezoelectric effect. **A,** In a direct piezoelectric effect, a mechanical deformation of the crystal generates a voltage. **B,** In the reverse piezoelectric effect, as the alternating current reverses polarity the crystal expands and contracts, producing ultrasound energy.

front of you. In the case of therapeutic ultrasound, with a frequency of 1 MHz at a velocity of 1540 m/sec in soft tissue and a wavelength of 1.5 mm, emitted from a transducer that is larger than the wavelength at approximately 25 mm in diameter, the sound is less divergent, thus concentrating energy in a limited area. The portion of the surface of the transducer that actually produces the sound wave is referred to as the **effective radiating area** (see Figure 12-2).[19] The acoustic energy is contained with a focused cylindrical beam that is roughly the same diameter as the transducer (see Figure 12-5).[79] The larger the diameter of the sound head, the more focused or **collimated beam** results. Smaller sound heads produce a more divergent beam. Also, the beam from ultrasound generated at a frequency of 1 MHz is more divergent than ultrasound generated at 3 MHz.

Within this cylindrical beam the distribution of sound energy is highly non-uniform, particularly in an area close to the transducer that is referred to as the near field or near zone (Figure 12-6). The near field is a zone of spatially fluctuating ultrasound strength. The fluctuation occurs because of differences in pressure created by the waves emitted from the transducer. As the beam moves away from the transducer, the waves eventually become indistinguishable, arriving at a certain point simultaneously and thus creating a point of highest acoustic intensity.[79] The point of maximum acoustic intensity can be determined by calculating the distance (L) from the surface of the transducer:

$$L = D^2/4W$$

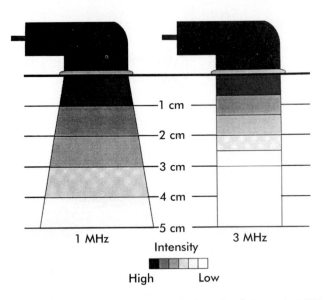

Fig. 12-5 The ultrasound energy attenuates as it travels through soft tissue. At 1 MHz, the energy can penetrate to the deeper tissues although the beam diverges slightly. At 3 MHz, the effects are primarily in the superficial tissues and the beam is less divergent.

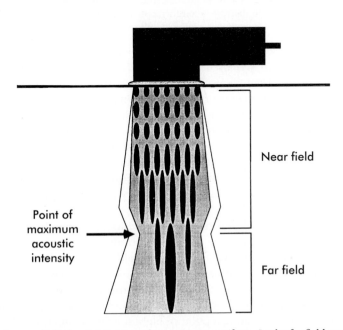

Fig. 12-6 In the near field the distribution of energy is nonuniform. In the far field energy distribution is more uniform, but the beam is more divergent. L represents the point of highest acoustic intensity.

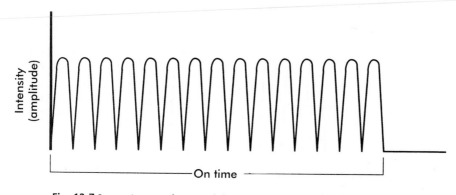

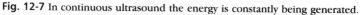

Fig. 12-7 In continuous ultrasound the energy is constantly being generated.

where D is the diameter of the transducer and W is the wavelength.[47] From this point the beam moves into the far field or far zone, where the distribution of energy is much more uniform but the beam becomes more divergent.

The amount of variability of intensity within the ultrasound beam is indicated by the **beam nonuniformity ratio (BNR).** This ratio is determined by the maximal point intensity of the transducer to the average intensity across the transducer surface. Optimally the BNR would be 1:1. Since this is not possible, the BNR should fall between 2 and 6. The lower the BNR, the more uniform the output and therefore the lower the chance of developing hot spots. The Food and Drug Administration requires all ultrasound units to list the BNR, and the sports therapist should be aware of the BNR for that particular unit.[26]

Pulsed versus Continuous Wave Ultrasound

Virtually all therapeutic ultrasound generators can emit either continuous or pulsed ultrasound waves. If **continuous wave ultrasound** is used, the sound intensity remains constant throughout the treatment and the ultrasound energy is being produced all the time (Figure 12-7).

With **pulsed ultrasound** the intensity is periodically interrupted with no ultrasound energy being produced during the off period (Figure 12-8). When using pulsed ultrasound, the average intensity of the output over time is reduced. The percentage of time that ultrasound is being generated (pulse duration) over one pulse period is referred to as the **duty cycle.**

$$\text{Duty cycle} = \frac{\text{Duration of pulse (On time)}}{\text{Pulse Period (On time + Off time)}} \times 100$$

Thus if the pulse duration is 1 msec and the total pulse period is 5 msec, the duty cycle would be 20%. Therefore the total amount of energy being delivered to the tissues would be only 20% of the energy delivered if a continuous wave was being used. The majority of ultrasound generators have duty cycles that are preset at either 20% or 50%. Occasionally the duty cycle is also referred to as the *mark:space* ratio.

Continuous ultrasound is most commonly used when the intent is to produce thermal effects. The use of pulsed ultrasound results in a reduced average heating of the tissues. Pulsed ultrasound or continuous ultrasound at a low intensity will produce nonthermal or mechanical effects that may be associated with soft tissue healing.

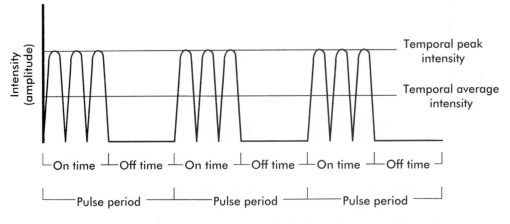

Fig. 12-8 In pulsed ultrasound, energy is generated only during the on time. Duty cycle is determined by the ratio of on time to pulse period.

Amplitude, Power, and Intensity

Amplitude is a term used to describe the magnitude of the vibration in a wave. It is the maximum distance from equilibrium that any particle reaches. Amplitude is used to describe either the movement of particles in the medium through which it travels in units of distance (centimeters or meters) or the variation in pressure found along the path of the wave in units of pressure (Newtons/meter^2).[15]

Power is the total amount of ultrasound energy in the beam and is expressed in watts. **Intensity** is a measure of the rate at which energy is being delivered per unit area. Since power and intensity are unevenly distributed in the beam, several varying types of intensities must be defined.

Spatial-averaged intensity is the intensity of the ultrasound beam averaged over the area of the transducer. It may be calculated by dividing the power output in watts by the total effective radiating area of the sound head in cm^2 and is indicated in watts per square centimeter (W/cm^2). If ultrasound is being produced at a power of 6 watts and the effective radiating area of the transducer is 4 cm^2, the spatial-averaged intensity would be 1.5 W/cm^2. On many ultrasound units, both the power in watts and the spatial-averaged intensity in W/cm^2 may be displayed. If the power output is constant, increasing the size of the transducer will decrease the spatial-averaged intensity.

Spatial peak intensity is the highest value occurring within the beam over time. With therapeutic ultrasound, maximum intensities can range between 0.25 and 3.0 W/cm^2.

Temporal peak intensity, sometimes also referred to as *pulse averaged intensity*, is the maximum intensity during the on period with pulsed ultrasound. It is indicated in W/cm^2 (see Figure 12-8).

Temporal-averaged intensity is important only with pulsed ultrasound and is calculated by averaging the power during both the on and off periods. For a pulsed sound beam with a duty cycle of 20% with a temporal peak intensity of 2.0 W/cm^2, temporal-averaged intensity would be 0.4 W/cm^2. On some machines the intensity setting indicates the temporal peak intensity or on time, while on others it shows the temporal-averaged intensity or the mean of the on-off intensity[58] (see Figure 12-8).

Spatial-averaged temporal peak intensity (SATP) is the maximum intensity occurring during the spatially-averaged intensity. The SATP intensity is simply the spatial average during a single pulse.

There are no definitive rules that govern selection of specific ultrasound intensities during treatment. Perhaps the best recommendation is that the lowest intensity of ultrasound energy at the highest frequency that will transmit the energy to a specific tissue should be used to achieve a desired therapeutic effect.[58] Using too much may likely damage tissues and exacerbate the condition.[79]

A general guideline to follow relative to intensity is that the patient should feel nothing more than the movement of the transducer over the treatment area. Some sports therapists feel that when thermal effects are desired, the intensity should be set so that the patient feels mild warmth. The treatment should never produce reports of pain. If the patient reports that the transducer feels hot at the skin surface, it is likely that the coupling medium is inadequate and possible that the piezoelectric crystal has been damaged and the transducer is overheating.

Some guidance for selecting intensities may come from published reports from those who have obtained successful clinical outcomes. Table 12-3 provides a summary of various studies from the literature that have made recommendations regarding intensity frequencies and treatment modes.[58]

PHYSIOLOGIC EFFECTS OF ULTRASOUND

Therapeutic ultrasound when applied to biologic tissue may induce clinically significant responses in cells, tissues, and organs through both thermal and nonthermal biophysical effects.* Ultrasound will affect both normal and damaged biologic tissues. It has been suggested that damaged tissue may be more responsive to ultrasound than normal tissue.[23] When ultrasound is applied for its thermal effects, nonthermal biophysical effects will also occur that may damage normal tissues.[43] However, if appropriate treatment parameters are selected, nonthermal effects can occur with minimal thermal effects.

Thermal Effects

The ultrasound wave attenuates as it travels through the tissue. Attenuation is caused primarily by the conversion of ultrasound energy into heat through absorption and to some extent by scattering and beam deflection. Traditionally, ultrasound has been used primarily to produce a tissue temperature increase.† The clinical effects of using ultrasound to heat the tissues are similar to other forms of heat that may be applied including[50]:

1. Increase in the extensibility of collagen fibers found in tendons and joint capsules.
2. Decrease in joint stiffness.

---

* References 7, 19, 20, 21, 29, 43, 74, 79, 84.
† References 6, 28, 52, 55, 71, 78.

TABLE 12-3   Summary of Research Relating to Ultrasound

Application	Authors	Frequency
SOFT TISSUE LESIONS		
Acute injuries		
Sports injuries	Patrick (1978)	*
Minor fractures		
Recent occupational soft tissue injuries	Middlemast and Chatterjee (1978)	1.5
Subacute		
Acute subacromial bursitis	Bearzy (1953)	1.0
Bursitis shoulder	Newman et al. (1958)	1.0
Painful shoulder	Downing and Weinstein (1986)	1.0
Subacromial bursitis	Munting (1978)	1.5
Chronic arthritis	Griffin et al (1970)	0.89/1.0
Plantar fasciitis	Clarke and Stenner (1976)	0.75/1.5
Rheumatoid nodules		3.0
Phonophoresis		
Arthritis	Griffin et al. (1967)	1.0
Epicondylitis/bursitis	Kleinkort and Wood (1975)	1.0
Wounds		
Episiotomies	Fieldhouse (1979)	*
Episiotomies and surgical wounds	Ferguson (1981)	1.0
Episiotomies	McLaren (1984)	*
Scars		
Contracture after hip fixation	Lehmann et al. (1961)	*
Hand scars	Bierman (1954)	1.0
Dupuytren's contracture	Markham et al. (1980)	1.0/3.0
PAIN		
Low back pain		
Nerve root pain	Patrick (1966)	*
Prolapsed intervertebral disc	Nwuga (1983)	*

3. Reduction of muscle spasm.
4. Modulation of pain.
5. Increase in blood flow.
6. Mild inflammatory response that may help resolve chronic inflammation.

For the majority of these effects to occur the tissue temperature must be raised to a level of 40° to 45° C for a minimum of 5 minutes. Temperatures below this range will be ineffective, and temperatures above 45° may be potentially damaging.[20] Ultrasound at 1 MHz with an intensity of 1 W/cm^2 can raise soft tissue temperature by as much as 0.86° C per minute in tissues with a poor vascular supply.[79]

SATP Intensity	Mode	Regimen	Outcome
*	P	*	
0.5-2.0	P	5 times a week	Significant improvement
2.0-4.0	*	up to 5 min daily × 3 then alternate days	Success with acute only
0.8-3.0	*	5-10 min × 12	Improvement
1.2-1.3	CW	6 min 3 times a week × 4	No significant difference
0.5	CW	3-5 min × 10	Improvement
2.0	*	3 times a week × 3	0.89 MHz more successful
1.0-2.5	CW	5 min × 8-10	Decreased pain
1.05-2.5	CW	5 min × 8-10	Size unchanged; pain decreased
1.5 max	CW	1 time a week × 9 max	Successful
2.0 max	CW	6-9 min	Improvement
0.5-0.8	*	5 min 3 times a week × 6	Improvement
0.5	P1:5	3 min daily × 2-4	Improvement
0.5	*	5 min	Improvement
1.0-2.5	*	5 min daily up to 3 weeks	Significant improvement
1.0-2.0	*	6-8 min, alternate days	Improvement
0.25-0.75	CW	4-10 min 1 time a week	Improvement
	*		
1.0-1.5	P	5 min daily × 10 max	Improvement
1.0-2.0	*	10 min 3 times a week × 4	Significant improvement

p = Pulsed; cw = Continuous wave.

The primary advantage of ultrasound over other nonacoustic heating modalities is that tissues high in collagen, such as tendons, muscles, ligaments, joint capsules, joint menisci, intermuscular interfaces, nerve roots, periosteum, cortical bone, and other deep tissues, may be selectively heated to the therapeutic range without causing a significant tissue temperature increase in skin or fat.[52,75] Ultrasound will penetrate skin and fat with little attenuation.[18]

The thermal effects of ultrasound are related to frequency. As indicated earlier, an inverse relationship exists between depth of penetration and frequency. Most of the energy in a sound wave at 3 MHz will be absorbed in the superficial tissues. At 1 MHz, there will be less attenuation and the energy will penetrate to the deeper tissues, selectively heating them.

Heating will occur with both continuous and pulsed ultrasound, depending on the intensity of the total current being delivered to the patient. Significant thermal effects will be induced whenever the upper end of the available intensity range is used. Regardless of whether ultrasound is pulsed or continuous, if the spatial-averaged temporal-averaged intensity is in the 0.1 to 0.2 W/cm^2 range the intensity is too low to produce a tissue temperature increase and only nonthermal effects will occur.[20]

Unlike the other heating modalities discussed in this text, whenever ultrasound is used to produce thermal changes, nonthermal changes will also occur simultaneously. Therefore an understanding of these nonthermal changes is essential.

Nonthermal Effects

The nonthermal effects of therapeutic ultrasound include **cavitation** and **acoustic microstreaming** (Figure 12-9, *A* and *B*). Cavitation is the formation of gas-filled bubbles that expand and compress due to ultrasonically induced pressure changes in tissue fluids.[20,74] Cavitation may be classified as being either *stable* or *unstable*. In stable cavitation, the bubbles expand and contract in response to regularly repeated pressure changes over many acoustic cycles. In unstable or transient cavitation, there are violent large excursions in bubble volume before implosion and collapse occurs after only a few cycles. Therapeutic benefits are derived only from stable cavitation, while the collapse of bubbles is thought to create increased pressure and high temperatures that may cause local tissue damage. Unstable cavitation should clearly be avoided. It is likely that high intensity, low frequency ultrasound may produce unstable cavitation, particularly if standing waves develop at tissue interfaces.[20]

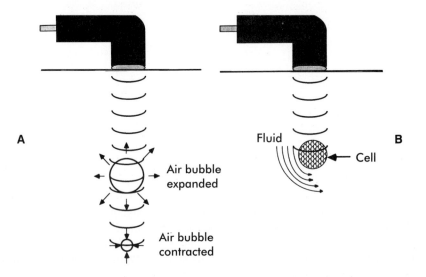

Fig. 12-9 Nonthermal effects of ultrasound. **A,** Cavitation is the formation of gas-filled bubbles that expand and compress because of ultrasonically induced pressure changes in tissue fluids. **B,** Microstreaming is the unidirectional movement of fluids along the boundaries of cell membranes resulting from the mechanical pressure wave in an ultrasonic field.

Cavitation results in an increased flow in the fluid around these vibrating bubbles. Microstreaming is the unidirectional movement of fluids along the boundaries of cell membranes resulting from the mechanical pressure wave in an ultrasonic field.[20,74] Microstreaming produces high viscous stresses, which can alter cell membrane structure and function due to changes in cell membrane permeability to sodium and calcium ions important in the healing process. As long as the cell membrane is not damaged, microstreaming can be of therapeutic value in accelerating the healing process.[20]

It has now been well documented that the nonthermal effects of therapeutic ultrasound in the treatment of injured tissues may be as or more important than the thermal effects. Therapeutically significant nonthermal effects have been identified in soft tissue repair via stimulation of fibroblast activity, which produces an increase in protein synthesis,[23] tissue regeneration,[23] increased blood flow in chronically ischemic tissues,[39] bone healing and repair of nonunion fractures,[67] and in phonophoresis.

The nonthermal effects of cavitation and microstreaming can be maximized while minimizing the thermal effects by using a spatial-averaged temporal-averaged intensity of 0.1 to 0.2 W/cm^2 with continuous ultrasound. This range may also be achieved using a low temporal-averaged intensity by pulsing a higher temporal-peak intensity of 1.0 W/cm^2 at a duty cycle of 20% to give a temporal averaged intensity of 0.2 W/cm^2.

TECHNIQUES OF APPLICATION

The principles and theories of therapeutic ultrasound are well understood and documented. However, specific practical recommendations as to how ultrasound may best be applied therapeutically are quite controversial and are based primarily on the experience of the clinicians who have used it. Even though there are numerous laboratory and clinical reports in the literature, treatment procedures and parameters are highly variable and many contradictory results and conclusions have been presented.[58]

Frequency of Treatment

It is generally accepted that acute conditions require more frequent treatments over a shorter period of time, while more chronic conditions require fewer treatments over a longer period of time.[58] Ultrasound treatments should begin as soon as possible after injury, ideally within hours, but definitely within 48 hours to maximize effects on the healing process.[30,63,65] Acute conditions may be treated using low intensity ultrasound once or even twice daily for 6 to 8 days until acute symptoms, such as pain and swelling, subside. In chronic conditions, when acute symptoms have subsided, treatment may be done on alternating days for a total of 10 to 12 treatments.[73] Ultrasound treatment should continue as long as there is improvement. Assuming the appropriate treatment parameters are chosen and the ultrasound generator is functioning properly, if no improvement is noted after three or four treatments then ultrasound should be discontinued.

It has been recommended that ultrasound be limited to 14 treatments in the majority of conditions, although this has not been documented scientifically. More than 14 treatments can reduce both red and white blood cell counts. After these 14 treatments it may be advisable to avoid treatment with ultrasound for 2 weeks.[31]

Duration of Treatment

The size of the area to be treated usually dictates the length of the treatment. An accepted recommendation is that ultrasound be administered for 1 to 2 minutes for each area 1½ times the size of the transducer. Thus if the diameter of the transducer is 5 cm and the effective treatment area is approximately 10 cm in diameter, the treatment should last between 4 and 8 minutes. Treatment time may be increased by 30-second intervals to a maximum of 3 minutes if the condition is improving.[63] Typically treatments range between 5 and 10 minutes in length.

Coupling Methods

The greatest amount of reflection of ultrasonic energy occurs at the air-tissue interface. To ensure that maximal energy will be transmitted to the patient, the face of the transducer should be parallel with the surface of the skin so that the ultrasound will strike the surface at a 90° angle. If the angle between the transducer face and the skin is greater than 15°, a large percentage of the energy will be reflected and the treatment effects will be minimal.[73]

Reflection at the air-tissue interface can be further reduced by applying the ultrasound via the use of some coupling agent. The purpose of the **coupling medium** is to exclude air from the region between the patient and the transducer so that ultrasound can get to the area to be treated.[79] The acoustic impedance of the coupling medium should match the impedance of the transducer and should be slightly higher than the skin. Also, the medium should have a low coefficient of absorption to minimize attenuation in the coupling medium. The medium must remain free of air bubbles during treatment. The coupling agent should be viscous enough to act as a lubricant while the transducer is moved over the skin surface.[58]

The coupling medium should be applied to the skin surface and the ultrasound transducer should be in contact with the coupling medium before the power is turned on. If the transducer is not in contact with the skin via the coupling medium or if for some reason the transducer is lifted away from the treatment area, the piezoelectric crystal may be damaged and the transducer can overheat.

A number of studies have looked at the efficacy of different coupling media in transmitting ultrasound.[2,20,70] Water, light oils, and various brands of ultrasonic gel have been recommended as coupling agents. The recommendations of these studies have proven to be somewhat contradictory. Essentially it appears that all of these agents have very similar acoustic properties and are effective as coupling agents.[16]

Water is an effective coupling medium, but its low viscosity reduces its suitability in surface application. Light oils, such as mineral oil and glycerol, have relatively higher absorption coefficients and are somewhat difficult to clean up after treatment. Water-soluble gels seem to have the most desirable properties necessary for a good coupling medium.[16] Perhaps the only disadvantage is that the salts in the gel may damage the metal face of the transducer with improper cleaning.

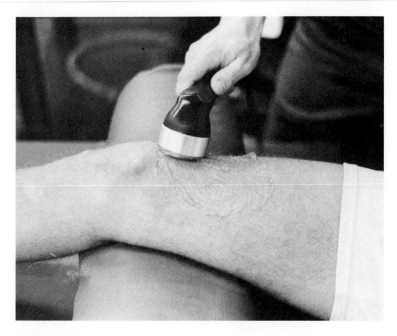

Fig. 12-10 Ultrasound may be applied directly through some gel-like coupling medium.

Exposure Techniques

DIRECT CONTACT. As long as the surface being treated is larger than the diameter of the transducer, a direct exposure technique may be used. If a smaller surface area is to be treated, a smaller transducer should be used so that direct application can still be used. A layer of gel should be applied to the treatment area in sufficient amounts to maintain good contact and lubrication between the transducer and the skin but not so much that air pockets may form from transducer movement. A thin film of gel should be applied directly to the transducer face before transmission begins[58] (Figure 12-10).

Heating the ultrasound gel before treatment has been recommended to improve the thermal effects of ultrasound in deeper tissues. Since ultrasound heats only through conversion of mechanical vibration to heat and not through conduction, heating of the gel will have no effect in the deeper tissues.[31] The only rationale for heating cold ultrasound is patient comfort.

IMMERSION. If the area to be treated is smaller than the diameter of the available transducer, irregular with bony prominences, or very hairy, the spatial-averaged intensity of the exposure is decreased and thus an immersion technique is recommended (Figure 12-11). A plastic, ceramic, or rubber basin should be used. With a metal basin or a whirlpool, some of the ultrasound will reflect from the metal, increasing the intensity near the basin walls. Tap water seems to be just as effective as degassed water as a coupling medium for the immersion technique[30] and less likely to produce surface heating than mineral oil or glycerin.[70] The transducer should be moved parallel to the surface being treated at a distance of 0.5 to 3 cm.[84] If air bubbles accumulate on the transducer or over the treatment area, they may be wiped away quickly during the treatment.

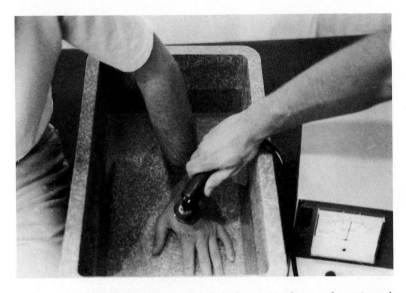

Fig. 12-11 The immersion technique is recommended when using ultrasound over irregular surfaces.

BLADDER TECHNIQUE. If the treatment area cannot be immersed in water, a bladder technique can be used in which a balloon is filled with water and the ultrasound energy is transmitted from the transducer to the treatment surface through this bladder (Figure 12-12). Both sides of the balloon should be coated with gel to ensure better contact. Treatments using a bladder filled with either gel or silicone have also been recommended as effective at higher ultrasound intensities.[2]

Moving the Transducer

In the past, treatment techniques that involved both moving the transducer and holding the transducer stationary were recommended. The stationary technique was most often used when the treatment area was small or when pulsed ultrasound was used at a low temporal-averaged intensity. However, because of the nonuniformity of the ultrasound beam, the energy distribution in the tissue is uneven, thus creating potential tissue damaging hot spots.[84] If the ultrasound beam is stationary, the spatial-peak intensity determines the point of maximal temperature increase. With the moving technique, the spatial-averaged intensity gives the most reasonable measure of the average rate of heating within the treatment area.[79] This stationary technique has been demonstrated to produce disruption of blood flow, platelet aggregation, and damage to the venous system.[82] Therefore the stationary technique is no longer recommended.

Moving the transducer during treatment leads to a more even distribution of energy within the treatment area and can reduce the damaging effects of standing waves, particularly those that are most likely to occur at bone-tissue interfaces. Overlapping circular motions or a longitudinal stroking pattern can be used. The transducer should be moved slowly at approximately 4 cm per second,[46] covering a treatment area 2 to 3 times larger than the diameter of the transducer for every 5

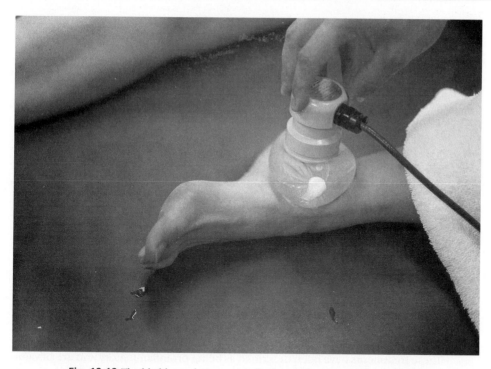

Fig. 12-12 The bladder technique may also be used over irregular surfaces.

minutes of exposure time.[70] Moving the transducer too rapidly decreases the total amount of energy absorbed per unit area. The tranducer should be kept in maximum contact with the skin via some coupling agent throughout the treatment.

Recording Ultrasound Treatments

It is recommended that the sports therapist report or record the specific parameters used in an ultrasound treatment when completing treatment records or progress notes so that the treatment may be reproduced. The parameters that should be recorded include frequency, spatial-averaged temporal peak intensity, whether the beam is pulsed or continuous, the duty factor (if pulsed), effective radiating surface area of the transducer, duration of the treatment, and the number of treatments per week.[58]

A typical treatment might be recorded as 1 MHz, at 1.0 W/cm^2, pulsed at 20% (0.2) duty factor, 5 cm transducer head, 5 minutes, 4 times per week.

CLINICAL USES OF THERAPEUTIC ULTRASOUND

Ultrasound is generally recognized clinically as one of the most effective and widely used modalities in the treatment of many soft tissue and bony lesions that occur with participation in sports activities. However, considering the extensive use of ultrasound in treating sports-related injuries, there is relatively little documented evidence from the sports-medicine community concerning its efficacy. The majority of the decisions as to how ultrasound should be used are empirically based on personal opinion and experience. This section summarizes the various clinical applications of therapeutic ultrasound used in a sports-medicine setting.

Soft-Tissue Healing and Repair

Soft-tissue repair may be accelerated by both the thermal and nonthermal effects of ultrasound.[21] Repair of soft tissues involves three phases of healing: inflammation, proliferation, and remodeling. Ultrasound does not seem to have any antiinflammatory effects; rather it is thought to accelerate the inflammatory phase of healing.

A single treatment with ultrasound can stimulate the release of histamine from mast cells.[38] The mechanism for this may be attributed primarily to nonthermal effects involving cavitation and streaming that increase the transport of calcium ions across the cell membrane, thus stimulating release of histamine by the mast cells.[20] Histamine attracts polymorphonuclear leukocytes that "clean up" debris from the injured area, along with monocytes that primarily release chemotactic agents and growth factors that stimulate fibroblasts and endothelial cells to form a collagen-rich, well-vascularized tissue used to develop new connective tissue essential for rapid repair. Thus ultrasound, if applied after bleeding has stopped but still within the first few hours after injury during the early stages of inflammation, can be effective in facilitating the inflammation process and therefore healing.[20] It has been suggested that this response occurs using pulsed ultrasound at 0.5 W/cm^2 with a duty cycle of 20% for 5 minutes or continuous ultrasound at 0.1 W/cm^2.[19]

These treatments have been described as being proinflammatory and are of value in accelerating repair in short-term or acute inflammation. However, in chronic inflammatory conditions, the proinflammatory effects are of questionable value.[38] If an inflammatory stimulus, such as overuse, remains, the response to therapeutic ultrasound will be poor.[5]

During the proliferative phase of healing, a connective tissue matrix is produced into which new blood vessels will grow. Fibroblasts are mainly responsible for producing this connective tissue. Fibroblasts exposed to therapeutic ultrasound are stimulated to produce more collagen, which gives connective tissue most of its strength.[37] Again, cavitation and streaming alter cell membrane permeability to calcium ions that facilitate increases in collagen synthesis and tensile strength. The intensity levels of therapeutic ultrasound that produce these changes during the proliferative phase are too low to be entirely thermal.

Scar Tissue and Joint Contracture

During remodeling collagen fibers are realigned along lines of tensile stresses and strains, forming scar tissue. This process may continue for months or even years. In scar tissue, collagen never attains the same pattern and remains weaker and less elastic than normal tissue before injury. Scar tissue in tendons, ligaments, and capsules surrounding joints can produce joint contractures that limit range of motion. Increased tissue temperatures increase the elasticity and decrease the viscosity of collagen fibers. Since the deeper tissues that most often restrict range of motion in joints are rich in collagen, ultrasound is the treatment modality of choice.[84]

A number of studies have investigated the effects of ultrasound treatment on scar tissue and joint contracture. Ultrasound has been demonstrated to increase mobility in mature scar.[4] A greater residual increase in tissue length with less potential damage is produced through preheating with ultrasound before stretching.[49] Tissue extensibility increases when continuous ultrasound at 1.0 to 3.0 W/cm^2 is applied, raising temperatures from 30° to 47° C.[31] Thigh periarticular structures and scar tissues become significantly more extensible after treatment with ultrasound involving thermal effects at intensities of 1.2 to 2.0 W/cm^2 for 5 minutes.[49] Scar tissue can be softened if treated with ultrasound at an early stage.[65] If treated early, Dupuytren's contracture shows a beneficial effect on long-standing contracted bands of scar and a decrease in pain when treated with ultrasound.[57]

The majority of the earlier studies attributed the effectiveness of ultrasound to thermal effects and used continuous moderate intensities between 0.5 and 2.0 W/cm^2.

Chronic Inflammations

There are few clinical or experimental studies that discuss the effects of therapeutic ultrasound on chronic inflammations (i.e. tendinitis, bursitis, epicondylitis) commonly seen in sports medicine.

Treatment of bicipital tendinitis with ultrasound decreased pain and tenderness and increased range of motion.[24] While earlier studies have shown ultrasound to be effective in treating pain and increasing range of motion in subacromial bursitis, a more recent study shows no improvement in the general shoulder condition when using continuous ultrasound at 1.0 to 2.0 W/cm^2.[17] Ultrasound applied at an intensity of 1.0 to 2.0 W/cm^2 at a 20% duty cycle significantly enhanced recovery in patients with epicondylitis.[5]

In these chronic inflammatory conditions, ultrasound seems effective in increasing blood flow for healing and for reduction of pain through heating.[84]

Bone Healing

Since bone is a type of connective tissue, damaged bone progresses through the same stages of healing as other soft tissues, the major difference being the deposition of bone salts.[82] Several studies have observed acceleration of fracture repair after ultrasound treatment.[67] The application of ultrasound within the first 2 weeks after fibular fracture during the inflammatory and proliferative stages increases the rate of healing. Treatment parameters were 0.5 W/cm^2 at a duty cycle of 20% for 5 minutes, 4 times per week.[22] Ultrasound was effectively used to stimulate bone repair after osteotomy and fixation of the tibia in rabbits.[8]

Treatment given during the first 2 weeks after injury is sufficient to accelerate bony union. However ultrasound given to an unstable fracture during the cartilage formation phase may cause proliferation of cartilage and consequently delay bony union.[21] It appears that nonthermal mechanisms are most responsible for the accelerated bone healing.[58]

Several studies have looked at the use of ultrasound over growing epiphyses.[13,36] While results have been somewhat inconsistent, some form of damage was observed in each study, including premature closure of the epiphysis, epiphyseal displacement, widening of the epiphysis, fractures, condyle erosion, and shortening of the bones. The degree of destruction appears to be unpredictable.[31] Therefore it is not recommended that ultrasound be applied to growing bone.

No documented evidence exists that ultrasound treatment can cause resorption of calcium deposits. However it has been suggested that ultrasound may help to reduce inflammation surrounding a calcium deposit, thus reducing pain and improving function.[84]

Myositis ossificans is calcification within the muscle after repeated acute trauma. This condition may be exacerbated by applying heat or massaging the area.

ULTRASOUND IN ASSESSING STRESS FRACTURES. The use of ultrasound as a reliable technique for identifying stress fractures has been recommended.[53] Using a continuous beam at 0.75 MHz with a 3 cm transducer and a water-based coupling medium, the sports therapist moves the transducer slowly over the injured area while gradually increasing the intensity from 0 to 2.0 W/cm^2. The ultrasound is turned off when the athlete indicates that he or she feels something. If the athlete reports a feeling of pressure, bruising, or aching, then a stress fracture may be present. Either a radiograph or a bone scan is then necessary to confirm this diagnosis.

Pain Reduction

Many of the studies discussed previously have noted that reduction in pain occurs with ultrasound treatment, even though the treatment was given for other purposes. Several mechanisms have been proposed that might explain this reduction in pain. Ultrasound is thought to elevate the threshold for activation of free nerve endings through thermal effects.[80] Heat produced by ultrasound in large-diameter nerve fibers may reduce pain through the gating mechanism.[12,58] Ultrasound may also increase nerve conduction velocity in normal nerves, creating a counterirritant effect through thermal mechanisms.[44] There is no consensus of opinion in the literature as to the exact mechanism of pain reduction.

Pain reduction after application of ultrasound has been reported in patients with lateral epicondylitis,[4] shoulder pain,[61] plantar fasciitis,[11] surgical wounds,[27] bursitis,[34] prolapsed intervertebral disks,[62] ankle sprains,[56] reflex sympathetic dystrophy,[68] and various other soft tissue injuries.[59]

Plantar Warts

Plantar warts are occasionally seen in the athletic population, occurring on the weightbearing areas of the feet and caused by either a virus or trauma. These lesions contain thrombosed capillaries in a whitish-colored soft core covered by hyperkeratotic epithelial tissue. Among other more conventional techniques, several studies have recommended ultrasound as an effective painless method for eliminating plantar warts.[42,69,77] Intensities average 0.6 W/cm^2 for 7 to 15 minutes.[14]

Placebo Effects

While the physiologic effects of ultrasound have been discussed in detail, it can also have significant therapeutic psychologic effects.[20] A number of studies have demonstrated a placebo effect in patients receiving sham ultrasound.[25,38,54]

PHONOPHORESIS

Phonophoresis is a technique in which ultrasound is used to drive a topical application of a selected medication into the tissues. Perhaps the greatest advantage of phonophoresis is that medication can be delivered via a safe, painless, noninvasive technique.

Medications commonly applied through phonophoresis most often are either antiinflammatories, such as cortisol, salicylates, or dexamethasone, or anagelsics, such as lidocaine. When applying phonophoresis, it is important to select the appropriate drug for the pathology. Since phonophoresis may increase drug penetration, it may also increase the clinical benefits and the risks of topical drug application.[9]

The thermal effects of ultrasound increase tissue permeability, and the acoustic pressure created by the ultrasound beam drives the medication into the tissues.[36] Thus the medication follows the path of the beam. Both pulsed and continuous ultrasound have been used in phonophoresis. Continuous ultrasound at an intensity great enough to produce thermal effects may induce a proinflammatory response.[19] If the goal is to decrease inflammation, pulsed ultrasound with low spatial-averaged temporal peak intensity may be the best choice.[31]

Unlike iontophoresis discussed earlier, phonophoresis drives whole molecules into the tissues as opposed to ions. Consequently, phonophoresis is not as likely to damage or burn skin. Also the depth of penetration with phonophoresis is substantially greater than with iontophoresis.

The most widespread use of the phonophoresis technique in sports medicine has been to deliver hydrocortisone, which has antiinflammatory effects. Several studies have looked at the efficacy of this technique.[40] Using phonophoresis with hydrocortisone was shown to be superior to ultrasound alone in alleviating pain and reducing inflammation in patients with arthritic disorders.[35] It has been used in treating patients with various inflammatory disorders.[45] It has also been used to treat temporomandibular joint dysfunction.[41,81] Typically, either 1% or 10% hydrocortisone cream is used in treatment. The 10% hydrocortisone preparation appears to be superior to the 1% preparation.[45]

Salicylates are compounds that evoke a number of pharmacologic effects, including analgesia and decreased inflammation caused by a reduction in prostaglandins. There are few reports that suggest that phonophoresis using salicylates enhances analgesic or antiinflammatory effects. However, recently it has been reported that salicylate phonophoresis may be used to decrease delayed onset muscle soreness without promoting cellular changes that mimic an inflammatory response.[10]

Lidocaine is a commonly used local anesthetic drug. The use of phonophoresis with lidocaine was found to be effective in treating a series of trigger points.[60]

The efficacy of various coupling media has been discussed previously. The addition of an active ingredient into the coupling medium is common practice. However, topical pharmacologic products are usually not formulated to optimize their efficiency as ultrasound coupling media.[3] For example, 1% or 10% hydrocortisone usually comes in a thick white cream base that is a poor conductor of ultrasound. Clinicians have tried mixing this preparation with ultrasound gel, which is known to be a good transmitter, without improvement in transmission capabilities. The use of topical preparations with poor transmission capabilities may negate the effectiveness of the ultrasound therapy. Unfortunately there are few suitable products available, and there is clearly a need for appropriate active ingredients in gel form. Table 12-4

TABLE 12-4   Ultrasound Transmission by Phonophoresis Media

Product	Transmission Relative to Water (%)
MEDIA THAT TRANSMIT ULTRASOUND WELL	
Lidex® gel, fluocinonide 0.05%[a]	97
Thera-Gesic® cream, methyl salicylate 15%[b]	97
Mineral oil[c]	97
US gel[d]	96
US lotion[e]	90
Betamethasone 0.05% in US gel[d]	88
MEDIA THAT TRANSMIT ULTRASOUND POORLY	
Diprolene® ointment, betamethasone 0.05%[g]	36
Hydrocortisone (HC) powder 1%[b] in US gel[d]	29
HC powder 10%[b] in US gel[d]	7
Cortril® ointment, HC 1%[i]	0
Eucerin® cream[j]	0
HC cream 1%[k]	0
HC cream 10%[k]	0
HC cream 10%[k] mixed with equal weight US gel[d]	0
Myoflex® cream, trolamine salicylate 10%[j]	0
Triamcinolone acetonide cream 0.1%[k]	0
Velva HC cream 10%[b]	0
Velva HC cream 10%[b] with equal weight US gel[d]	0
White petrolatum[m]	0
OTHER	
Chempad-L®[n]	68
Polyethylene wrap[o]	98

[a]Syntex Laboratories Inc, 3401 Hillview Ave, PO Box 10850, Palo Alto, CA 94303.
[b]Missions Pharmacal Co, 1325 E Durango, San Antonio, TX 78210.
[c]Pennex Corp, Eastern Ave at Pennex Dr, Verona, PA 15147.
[d]Ultraphonic®, Pharmaceutical Innovations Inc, 897 Frelinghuysen Dr, Newark, NJ 07114.
[e]Polysonic, Parker Laboratories Inc, 307 Washington St, Orange NJ 07050.
[f]Pharmfair Inc, 110 Kennedy Dr, Hauppauge, NY 11788.
[g]Schering Corp, Galloping Hill Rd, Kenilworth, NJ 07033.
[h]Purepace Pharmaceutical Co, 200 Elmora Ave, Elizabeth, NJ 07207.
[i]Pfizer Labs Division, Pfizer Inc, 253 E 42nd St, New York, NY 10017.
[j]Beiersdorf Inc, PO Box 5529, Norwalk, CT 06856-5529.
[k]E Fougera & Co, 60 Baylis Rd, Melville, NY 11747.
[l]Rorer Consumer Pharmaceuticals, Div of Rhône-Poulenc Rorer Pharmaceuticals Inc, 500 Virginia Dr, Fort Washington, PA 19034.
[m]Universal Cooperatives Inc, 7801 Metro Pkwy, Minneapolis, MN 55420.
[n]Henley International, 104 Industrial Blvd, Sugar Land, TX 77478.
[o]Saran Wrap®, Dow Brands Inc, 9550 Zionsville Rd, Indianapolis, IN 46268.
From Cameron M, Monroe, L: Relative transmission of ultrasound by media customarily used for phonophoresis, *Phys Ther* 72(2): 142-148, 1992. Reprinted with permission from the American Physical Therapy Association.

provides a list of transmission capabilities of various commercially available phonophoresis media.[9]

In phonophoresis, coupling can be either direct or use immersion. The medication in preparation is rubbed directly into the surface of the skin over the treatment area. With the direct technique transmission gel should be applied, and with immersion the area with the preparation applied is simply treated underwater.

USING ULTRASOUND IN COMBINATION WITH OTHER MODALITIES

In a sports-medicine setting, it is not uncommon to combine modalities to accomplish a specific treatment goal. Ultrasound is frequently used with other modalities, including hot packs, cold packs, and electrical stimulating currents. Unfortunately, there is very little documented evidence in the literature to substantiate the effectiveness of these various modality combinations.

Hot packs, like continuous or high intensity ultrasound, are used primarily for their thermal effects. Heat is effective in reducing muscle spasm and muscle guarding. It also has an analgesic effect and is useful in pain reduction. For these reasons, heat and ultrasound used in combination can be effective for accomplishing these treatment goals. Since hot packs produce an increase in blood flow superficially, thus creating a less dense medium for transmission of ultrasound, attenuation may be increased and the depth of penetration of ultrasound reduced.

Cold packs are most often used for analgesia and to decrease acute blood flow after injury. Because cold is such an effective analgesic, caution must be exercised when using ultrasound at higher intensities that produce thermal effects, since the athlete's perception of temperature and pain is diminished. However, in treating acute and post acute injuries, the combination of cold, to reduce blood flow (i.e., swelling) and produce analgesia, and low intensity ultrasound, for its nonthermal effects that promote soft tissue healing, may be the treatment of choice. Since cold produces a decrease in blood flow superficially and thus a more dense medium, superficial attenuation of ultrasound may be decreased, facilitating transmission to deeper tissues.

Ultrasound and electrical stimulating currents are frequently used in combination (Figure 12-13). Electrical stimulating currents are used for analgesia or producing muscle contraction. Ultrasound and electrical stimulating currents in combination have been recommended to treat myofascial trigger points.[33] Both modalities provide analgesic effects, and both are effective in reducing the pain-spasm-pain cycle, although the mechanisms responsible are not clearly understood.

CONTRAINDICATIONS AND PRECAUTIONS

There are a number of contraindications and precautions to the use of therapeutic ultrasound.

The use of continuous ultrasound with a high spatial-averaged temporal peak intensity should be avoided in acute and postacute conditions because of the associated thermal effects.

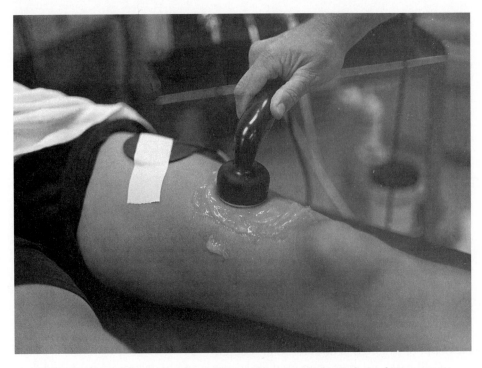

Fig. 12-13 Ultrasound is frequently used in combination with electrical stimulating currents.

Caution should be used when treating areas of decreased sensation, particularly when there is a problem in perceiving pain and temperature.

In areas of decreased circulation, caution must be exercised due to excessive heat build up, which can potentially damage tissues.

Though rare in the athletic population, individuals with vascular problems involving thrombophlebitis should not receive ultrasound because of the possibility of dislodging a clot and creating an embolus.

Ultrasound should not be applied around the eye, since heat is not dissipated well and both the lens and the retina may be damaged.

Ultrasound should not be applied over reproductive organs, especially the testes, since temporary sterility may result. Caution should be used in treating the abdominal region of the female during the reproductive years or immediately after menses.

The use of ultrasound is contraindicated during pregnancy because of potential damage to the fetus.

Some precaution should be used when treating areas around the heart due to potential changes in ECG activity. Ultrasound can certainly interfere with normal function of a pacemaker.

Therapeutic ultrasound should not be used over malignant tissue, since this may cause cell detachment and metastasis.

As previously mentioned, ultrasound should never be used over epiphyseal areas in young children.

Ultrasound may be used safely over metal implants, since there is no increase in temperature of tissue adjacent to the implant because metal has high thermal conductivity and thus heat is removed from the area faster than it can be absorbed. However in cases of total joint replacement, the cement used (methyl methacrylate) absorbs heat rapidly and may be overheated, damaging surrounding soft tissues.

GUIDELINES FOR THE SAFE USE OF ULTRASOUND EQUIPMENT

Currently, ultrasound units are the only therapeutic modality for which Federal Performance Standards exist.[66] Ultrasound units produced since 1979 are required to indicate the magnitudes of ultrasound power and intensity with an accuracy of $\pm 20\%$ and accurately control treatment time. It is recommended that intensity output, pulse regimen accuracy, and timer accuracy be checked at regular intervals by qualified personnel who have access to the appropriate testing equipment. The effective radiating area and the beam nonuniformity ratio of the transducer should be accurately provided by the manufacturer.

SUMMARY

1. Ultrasound is defined as inaudible, acoustic vibrations of high frequency that may produce either thermal or nonthermal physiologic effects.
2. Ultrasound travels through soft tissue as a longitudinal wave at therapeutic frequencies of either 1 or 3 MHz.
3. As the ultrasound wave is transmitted through the various tissues, there will be attenuation, or a decrease in energy intensity, due to either absorption of energy by the tissues or dispersion and scattering of the sound wave.
4. Ultrasound is produced by a piezoelectric crystal within the transducer that converts electrical energy to acoustic energy through mechanical deformation via the piezoelectric effect.
5. Ultrasound energy travels within the tissues as a highly focused collimated beam with a nonuniform intensity distribution.
6. While continuous ultrasound is most commonly used when the intent is to produce thermal effects, pulsed ultrasound or continuous ultrasound at a low intensity will produce nonthermal or mechanical effects.
7. Therapeutic ultrasound, when applied to biologic tissue, may induce clinically significant responses in cells, tissues, and organs through both thermal effects, which produce a tissue temperature increase, and nonthermal effects, such as cavitation and microstreaming.
8. Even though there are numerous laboratory and clinically based reports in the literature, treatment procedures and parameters are highly variable and many contradictory results and conclusions have been presented.
9. Therapeutic ultrasound is most effective when an appropriate coupling medium and technique using either direct contact, immersion, or a bladder is combined with a moving transducer.
10. Even though there is relatively little documented evidence from the sports-medicine community concerning the efficacy of ultrasound, it is most often used for soft-tissue healing and repair, with scar tissue and joint

contracture, for chronic inflammation, for bone healing, with plantar warts, and for placebo effects.

11. Phonophoresis is a technique in which ultrasound is used to drive molecules of a topically applied medication, usually either antiinflammatories or analgesics, into the tissues.

12. In a sports-medicine setting, ultrasound is frequently used in combination with other modalities, including hot packs, cold packs, and electrical stimulating currents, to produce specific treatment effects.

13. Although ultrasound is a relatively safe modality if used appropriately, the sports therapist must be aware of the various contraindications and precautions.

GLOSSARY

acoustic impedance Determines the amount of ultrasound energy reflected at tissue interfaces.

acoustic microstreaming The unidirectional movement of fluids along the boundaries of cell membranes, resulting from the mechanical pressure wave in an ultrasonic field.

amplitude Describes the magnitude of the vibration in a wave. It is the maximum distance from equilibrium that any particle reaches.

attenuation A decrease in energy intensity while the ultrasound wave is transmitted through various tissues caused by scattering and dispersion.

beam nonuniformity ratio (BNR) Indicates the amount of variability of intensity within the ultrasound beam and is determined by the maximal point intensity of the transducer to the average intensity across the transducer surface.

cavitation The formation of gas-filled bubbles that expand and compress because of ultrasonically induced pressure changes in tissue fluids.

collimated beam A focused, less divergent beam of ultrasound energy produced by a large-diameter transducer.

compressions Regions of high molecular density (i.e., a great amount of ultrasound energy) within the longitudinal wave.

continuous wave ultrasound The sound intensity remains constant throughout the treatment and the ultrasound energy is being produced 100% of the time.

coupling medium A substance used to decrease the acoustic impedance at the air-skin interface and thus facilitate the passage of ultrasound energy.

duty cycle The percentage of time that ultrasound is being generated (pulse duration) over one pulse period, which is also referred to as the mark:space ratio.

effective radiating area The total area of the surface of the transducer that actually produces the sound wave.

hot spots Areas at tissue interfaces that may become overheated.

intensity A measure of the rate at which energy is being delivered per unit area.

longitudinal wave The primary waveform in which ultrasound energy travels in soft tissue, with the molecular displacement along the direction in which the wave travels.

phonophoresis A technique in which ultrasound is used to drive a topical application of a selected medication into the tissues.

piezoelectric effect When an alternating electrical current generated at the same frequency as the crystal resonance is passed through the piezoelectric crystal, the crystal will expand and contract or vibrate at the frequency of the electrical oscillation, thus generating ultrasound at a desired frequency.

power The total amount of ultrasound energy in the beam. Power is expressed in watts.

pulsed ultrasound The intensity is periodically interrupted with no ultrasound energy being produced during the off period. When using pulsed ultrasound, the average intensity of the output over time is reduced.

rarefactions Regions of lower molecular density (i.e., a small amount of ultrasound energy) within a longitudinal wave.

standing wave As the ultrasound energy is reflected at tissue interfaces with different acoustic impedances, the intensity of the energy is increased as the reflected energy meets new energy being transmitted, forming waves of high energy that can potentially damage surrounding tissues.

transverse wave Occurring only in bone, the molecules are displaced perpendicular to the direction in which the ultrasound wave is moving.

REFERENCES

1 Antich TJ: Phonophoresis: the principles of the ultrasonic driving force and efficacy in treatment of common orthopedic diagnosis, *J Orthop Sport Phys Ther* 4(2): 99-103, 1982.

2 Balmaseda MT, Fatehi MT, Koozekanani SH: Ultrasound therapy: a comparative study of different coupling medium, *Arch Phys Med Rehabil* 67: 147, 1986.

3 Benson HAE, McElnay IC: Transmission of ultrasound energy through topical pharmaceutical products, *Physiotherapy* 74: 587, 1988.

4 Bierman W: Ultrasound in the treatment of scars, *Arch Phys Med Rehabil* 35: 209, 1954.

5 Binder A, Hodge J, Greenwood T: Is therapeutic ultrasound effective in treating soft tissue lesions? *Br Med J* 290: 512, 1985.

6 Black K, Halvsrson JL, Maierus K, et al.: Alterations in ankle dorsiflexion torque as a result of continuous ultrasound to the anterior tibial compartment, *Phys Ther* 64(6): 910-913, 1984.

7 Bly N, McKenzie A, West J, et al.: Low dose ultrasound effects on wound healing: a controlled study with Yucatan pigs, *Arch Phys Med Rehabil* 73: 656-664, 1992.

8 Brueton RN, Campbell B: The use of geliperm as a sterile coupling agent for therapeutic ultrasound, *Physiotherapy* 73: 653, 1987.

9 Cameron M, Monroe L: Relative transmission of ultrasound by media customarily used for phonophoresis, *Phys Ther* 72(2): 142-148, 1992.

10 Ciccone C, Leggin B, Callamaro J: Effects of ultrasound and trolamine salicylate phonophoresis on delayed-onset muscle soreness, *Phys Ther* 71(9): 666-675, 1991.

11 Clarke GR, Stenner L: Use of therapeutic ultrasound, *Physiotherapy* 62(6): 185-190, 1976.

12 Currier DP, Kramer IF: Sensory nerve conduction: heating effects of ultrasound and infrared, *Physiother Can* 34: 241, 1982.

13 DeForest RE, Henick JF, Janes JM: Effects of ultrasound on growing bone: an experimental study, *Arch Phys Med Rehabil* 34: 21, 1953.

14 Delacerda FG: Ultrasonic techniques for treatment of plantar warts in athletes, *J Orthop Sports Phys Ther* 1: 100, 1979.

15 Docker MF: A review of instrumentation available for therapeutic ultrasound, *Physiotherapy* 73(4): 154, 1987.

16 Docker MF, Foulkes DJ, Patrick MK: Ultrasound couplants for physiotherapy, *Physiotherapy* 68(4): 124-125, 1982.

17 Downing DS, Weinstein A: Ultrasound therapy of subacromial bursitis (abstract), *Phys Ther* 66: 194, 1986.

18 Draper D, Sunderland S: Examination of the law of Grotthus-Draper: does ultrasound penetrate subcutaneous fat in humans? *J Ath Train* 28(3): 246-250, 1993.

19 Dyson M: *Therapeutic application of ultrasound.* In Nyborg WL, Ziskin MC, editor: *Biological effects of ultrasound*, Edinburgh, 1985, Churchill-Livingstone.

20 Dyson M: Mechanisms involved in therapeutic ultrasound, *Physiotherapy* 73(3): 116-120, 1987.

21 Dyson M: *The use of ultrasound in sports physiotherapy.* In Grisogono V, editor: *Sports injuries: international perspectives in physiotherapy*, Edinburgh, 1989, Churchill Livingstone.

22 Dyson M, Brookes M: Stimulation of bone repair by ultrasound (abstract), *Ultrasound Med Biol* 8(Suppl 50): 50, 1982.

23 Dyson M, Luke DA: *Induction of mast cell degranulation in skin by ultrasound,* IEEE Transactions and Ultrasonics, Ferroelectrics, and Frequency Control UFFC-33: 194, 1986.

24 Echternach JL: Ultrasound: an adjunct treatment for shoulder disability, *Phys Ther* 45: 565, 1965.

25 El Hag M, Coghlan K, Christmas P: The anti-inflammatory effects of dexamethasone and therapeutic ultrasound in oral surgery, *Br J Oral Maxillofac Surg* 23: 17, 1985.

26 Ferguson BA: *A practitioners' guide to ultrasonic therapy equipment standard,* U.S. Department of Health and Human Services, Public Health Service, Food and Drug Administration, Rockville, Md, 1985.

27 Ferguson HN: Ultrasound in the treatment of surgical wounds, *Physiotherapy* 67: 12, 1981.

28 Frizell LA, Dunn F: Biophysics of ultrasound and bioeffects of ultrasound. In Lehmann JF, editor: *Therapeutic heat and cold,* ed 3, Baltimore, 1982, Williams & Wilkins.

29 Fyfe MC, Bullock M: Therapeutic ultrasound: some historical background and development in knowledge of its effects on healing, *Aust J Physio,* 31(6): 220-224, 1985.

30 Fyfe MC, Chahl LA: The effect of single or repeated applications of "therapeutic" ultrasound on plasma extravasation during silver nitrate induced inflammation of the rat hindpaw ankle joint, *Ultrasound Med Biol* 11: 273, 1985.

31 Gann N: Ultrasound: current concepts, *Clin Manage* 11(4): 64-69, 1991.

32 Gersten JW: Effect of ultrasound on tendon extensibility, *Am J Phys Med* 34: 662, 1955.

33 Girardi CQ, Seaborne D, Savard-Goulet F: The analgesic effect of high voltage galvanic stimulation combined with ultrasound in the treatment of low back pain: a one group pretest/posttest study, *Physiother Can* 36(6): 327-333, 1984.

34 Gorkiewicz R: Ultrasound for subacromial bursitis, *Phys Ther* 64: 46, 1984.

35 Griffin JE, Echternach JL, Price RE: Patients treated with ultrasonic driven hydrocortisone and ultrasound alone, *Phys Ther* 47: 594-601, 1967.

36 Griffin JE, Karsalis TC: *Physical agents for physical therapists,* Springfield, Ill, 1978, Charles C. Thomas.

37 Harvey W, Dyson M, Pond JB: The simulation of protein synthesis in human fibroblasts by therapeutic ultrasound, *Rheumato Rehab* 14: 237, 1975.

38 Hashish I, Harvey W, Harris M: Anti-inflammatory effects of ultrasound therapy: evidence for a major placebo effect, *Br J Rheumatol* 25: 77, 1986.

39 Hogan RD, Burke KM, Franklin TD: The effect of ultrasound on microvascular hemodynamics in skeletal muscle: effects during ischemia, *Microvasc Res* 23: 370, 1982.

40 Holdsworth LK, Anderson DM: Effectiveness of ultrasound used with hydrocortisone coupling medium or epicondylitis clasp to treat lateral epicondylitis: pilot study, *Physiotherapy* 79(1): 19-25, 1993.

41 Kahn J: Iontophoresis and ultrasound for post-surgical temporo-

mandibular trismus and paresthesia, *Phys Ther* 60(3): 307-308, 1980.

42 Kent H: Plantar wart treatment with ultrasound, *Arch Phys Med Rehabil* 40: 15, 1959.

43 Kitchen S, Partridge C: A review of therapeutic ultrasound. I. Background and physiological effects, *Physiotherapy* 76(10): 593, 1990.

44 Kitchen S, Partridge C: A review of therapeutic ultrasound. II. The efficacy of ultrasound, *Physiotherapy* 76(10): 595-599, 1990.

45 Kleinkort IA, Wood F: Phonophoresis with 1 percent versus 10 percent hydrocortisone, *Phys Ther* 55: 1320, 1975.

46 Kramer JF: Ultrasound: evaluation of its mechanical and thermal effects, *Arch Phys Med Rehabil* 65: 223, 1984.

47 Kremkau F: *Physical considerations*. In Nyborg WL, Ziskin MC, editors: *Biological effects of ultrasound*, Edinburgh, 1985, Churchill-Livingstone.

48 Lehmann JF: Clinical evaluation of a new approach in the treatment of contracture associated with hip fracture after internal fixation, *Arch Phys Med Rehabil* 42: 95, 1961.

49 Lehmann JF: Effect of therapeutic temperatures on tendon extensibility, *Arch Phys Med Rehabil* 51: 481, 1970.

50 Lehmann JF, De Lateur BJ: *Therapeutic heat*. In Lehmann JF, editor: *Therapeutic heat and cold*, ed 4, Baltimore, 1990, Williams & Wilkins.

51 Lehmann JF, De Lateur BJ, Silvermann DR: Selective heating effects of ultrasound in human beings, *Arch Phys Med Rehabil* 46: 331, 1966.

52 Lehmann JF, Guy AW: *Ultrasound therapy*. In Reid J, Sikov MR, editors: *Interaction of ultrasound and biological tissues*, DHEW Pub (FDA) 73-8008, Session 3(8): 141, 1971.

53 Lowden A: Application of ultrasound to assess stress fractures, *Physiotherapy* 72(3): 160-161, 1986.

54 Lundeberg T, Abrahamsson P, Haker E: A comparative study of continuous ultrasound, placebo ultrasound and rest in epicondylalgia, *Scand Rehab Med* 20: 99, 1988.

55 MacDonald BL, Shipster SB: Temperature changes induced by continuous ultrasound, *South African J Physiotherapy* 37(1): 13-15, 1981.

56 Makuloluwe RT, Mouzas GL: Ultrasound in the treatment of sprained ankles, *Practitioner* 218: 586-588, 1977.

57 Markham DE, Wood MR: Ultrasound for Dupuytren's contracture, *Physiotherapy* 66(2): 55-58, 1980.

58 McDiarmid T, Burns PN: Clinical applications of therapeutic ultrasound, *Physiotherapy* 73: 155, 1987.

59 Middlemast S, Chatterjee DS: Comparison of ultrasound and thermotherapy for soft tissue injuries, *Physiotherapy* 64: 331, 1978.

60 Moll MJ: A new approach to pain: lidocaine and decadron with ultrasound, *USAF Medical Service Digest*, May-June: 8, 1977.

61 Munting E: Ultrasonic therapy for painful shoulders, *Physiotherapy* 64: 180, 1978.

62 Nwuga VCB: Ultrasound in treatment of back pain resulting from prolapsed intervertebral disc *Arch Phys Med Rehabil* 64: 88, 1983.

63 Oakley EM: Application of continuous beam ultrasound at therapeutic levels, *Physiotherapy* 64(4): 103-104, 1978.

64 Partridge CJ: Evaluation of the efficacy of ultrasound, *Physiotherapy* 73(4): 166-168, 1987.

65 Patrick MK: Applications of pulsed therapeutic ultrasound, *Physiotherapy* 64(4): 03-104, 1978.

66 Performance Standards for Sonic, Infrasonic, and Ultrasonic Radiation Emitting Products: 21 CFR 1050: 10 *Federal Registar* 43: 7166, 1978.

67 Pilla AA, Figueiredo M, Nasser P, et al.: *Non-invasive low intensity pulsed ultrasound: a potent accelerator of bone repair*, Proceedings of the 36th Annual Meeting, Orthopaedic Research Society, New Orleans, 1990.

68 Portwood MM, Lieberman SS, Taylor RG: Ultrasound treatment of reflex sympathetic dystrophy, *Arch Phys Med Rehabil* 68: 116, 1987.

69 Quade AG, Radzyminski SF: Ultrasound in verruca plantaris, *J Am Podiatric Assoc* 56: 503, 1966.

70 Reid DC, Cummings GE: Factors in selecting the dosage of ultrasound with particular reference to the use of various coupling agents, *Physiother Can* 63: 255, 1973.

71 Sandler V, Feingold P: The thermal effect of pulsed ultrasound, *South African J Physiotherapy* 37(1): 10-12, 1951.

72 Snow CJ, Johnson KA: Effect of therapeutic ultrasound on acute inflammation, *Physiother Can* 40: 162, 1988.

73 Summer W, Patrick MK: *Ultrasonic therapy*, New York, 1964, American Elsevier.

74 ter Haar C: Basic physics of therapeutic ultrasound, *Physiotherapy* 73(3): 110-113, 1987.

75 ter Haar G, Hopewell JW: Ultrasonic heating of mammalian tissue in vivo, *Bri J Cancer* 45 (suppl V): 65-67, 1982.

76 Vaughen IL, Bender LF: Effect of ultrasound on growing bone, *Arch Phys Med Rehabil* 40: 158, 1959.

77 Vaughn DT: Direct method versus underwater method in treatment of plantar warts with ultrasound, *Phys Ther* 53: 396, 1973.

78 Ward AR: *Electricity fields and waves in therapy*, Marrickville, NSW, Australia, 1986, Science Press.

79 Williams AR: Production and transmission of ultrasound, *Physiotherapy* 73(3): 113-116, 1987.

80 Williams AR, McHale I, Bowditch M: Effects of MHz ultrasound on electrical pain threshold perception in humans. *Ultrasound Med Bio* 13: 249, 1987.

81 Wing M: Phonophoresis with hydrocortisone in the treatment of temporomandibular joint dysfunction, *Phys Ther* 62: 32-33, 1982.

82 Woolf N: *Cell, tissue and disease*. ed 2, London, 1986, Bailliere Tindall.

83 Zarod AP, Williams AR: Platelet aggregation in vivo by therapeutic ultrasound, *Lancet* 1: 1266, 1977.

84 Ziskin M, McDiarmid T, Michlovitz S: *Therapeutic ultrasound*. In Michlovitz S, editor: *Thermal agents in rehabilitation*, Philadelphia, 1990, FA Davis.

SUGGESTED READINGS

Abramson DI: Changes in blood flow, oxygen uptake and tissue temperatures produced by therapeutic physical agents. I. Effect of ultrasound, *Am J Phys Med* 39: 51, 1960.

Aldes IH, Grabin S: Ultrasound in the treatment of intervertebral disc syndrome, *Am J Phys Med* 37: 199, 1958.

Allen KGR, Battye CK: Performance of ultrasonic therapy instruments, *Physiotherapy* 64(6): 174-179, 1978.

Antich TJ: Physical therapy treatment of knee extensor mechanism disorders: comparison of four treatment modalities, *J Orthop Sports Phys Ther* 8: 255, 1986.

Aspelin P, Ekberg O, Thorsson O, et al.: Ultrasound examination of soft tissue injury in the lower limb in athletes, *Am J Sports Med* 20(5): 601-603, 1992.

Banties A, Klomp R: Transmission of ultrasound energy through coupling agents, *Physiother Sport* 3: 9-13, 1979.

Bearzy HJ: Clinical applications of ultrasonic energy in the treatment of acute and chronic subacromial bursitis, *Arch Phys Med Rehabil* 34: 228, 1953.

Benson HA, McElnay JC, Harland RL: Use of ultrasound to enhance percutaneous absorption of benzydamine, *Phys Ther* 69(2): 113-118, 1989.

Bickford RH, Duff RS: Influence of ultrasonic irradiation on temperature and blood flow in human skeletal muscle, *Circ Res* 1: 534, 1953.

Bondolo W: Phenylbutazone with ultrasonics in some cases of anhrosynovitis of the knee, *Arch Orthop* 73: 532-540, 1960.

Borrell RM, Parker R, Henley EJ: Comparison of in vitro temperatures produced by hydrotherapy paraffin wax treatment and fluidotherapy, *Phys Ther* 60: 1273-1276, 1984.

Brueton RN, Blookes M, Heatley FW: The effect of ultrasound on the repair of a rabbit's tibial osteotomy held in rigid external fixation, *J Bone Joint Surg* 69: 494, 1987.

Buchan JF: Heat therapy and ultrasonics, *The Practitioner* 208: 130-131, 1972.

Buchtala V: The present state of ultrasonic therapy, *Br J Phys Med* 15: 3, 1952.

Bundt FB: Ultrasound therapy in supraspinatus bursitis, *Phys Ther* 38: 826, 1958.

Burns PN, Pitcher EM: Calibration of physiotherapy ultrasound generators, *Clin Phys Physiol Meas* 5: 37 (abstract), 1984.

Callam MJ, Harper DR, Dale JJ, et al.: A controlled trial of weekly ultrasound therapy in chronic leg ulceration, *Lancet* 2(8552): 204, 1987.

Cerino LE, Ackerman E, Janes JM: Effects of ultrasound on experimental bone tumor, *Surg Forum* 16: 466, 1965.

Chan AK, Siealmann RA, Guy AW: Calculations of therapeutic heat generated by ultrasound in fat-muscle-bone layers, IEEE Transactions on Biomedical Engineering, BME-2t. 280-284, 1973.

Cherup N, Urben J, Bender LF: The treatment of plantar warts with ultrasound, *Arch Phys Med Rehabil* 44: 602, 1963.

Cline PD: Radiographic follow-up of ultrasound therapy in calcific bursitis, *Phys Ther* 43: 16, 1963.

Coakley WT: Biophysical effects of ultrasound at therapeutic intensities, *Physiotherapy* 94(6): 168-169, 1978.

Conger AD, Ziskin MC, Wittels H: Ultrasonic effects on mammalian multicellular tumor spheroids, *Clin Ultrasound* 9: 167, 1981.

Costentino AB, Cross DL, Harrineton RJ: Ultrasound effects on electroneuromyographic measures in sensory fibers of the median nerve, *Phys Ther* 63(11): 1788-1792, 1983.

Creates V: A study of ultrasound treatment to the painful perineum after childbirth, *Physiotherapy* 73: 162, 1987.

Currier DF, Greathouse D, Swift T: Sensory nerve conduction: effect of ultrasound, *Arch Phys Med Rehabil* 59: 181, 1978.

Duarte LR: The stimulation of bone growth by ultrasound, *Arch Orthop Trauma Surg* 101: 153-159, 1983.

Dyson M: The stimulation of tissue regeneration by means of ultrasound, *Clin Sci* 35: 273, 1968.

Dyson M: The production of blood cell stasis and endothelial damage in the blood vessels of chick embryos treated with ultrasound in a stationary wave field, *Ultrasound Med Biol* 11: 133, 1974.

Dyson M, Pond JB: The effect of pulsed ultrasound on tissue regeneration, *Physiotherapy* 56(6): 134-142, 1970.

Dyson M, Suckling J: Stimulation of tissue repair by ultrasound: a survey of mechanisms involved, *Physiotherapy* 64: 105, 1978.

Dyson M, ter Haar GR: *The response of smooth muscle to ultrasound* (abstract), In Proceedings from an International Symposium on Therapeutic Ultrasound, Winnipeg, Manitoba, September 10, 1981.

Dyson M, Woodward B, Pond JB: Flow of red blood cells stopped by ultrasound, *Nature* 232: 572-573, 1971.

Edwards MI: Congenital defects in guinea pigs: prenatal retardation of brain growth of guinea pigs following hyperthermia during gestation, *Teratology* 2: 329, 1969.

Enwemeka CS: The effects of therapeutic ultrasound on tendon healing, *Am J Phys Med Rehabil* 68(6): 283-287, 1989.

Falconer J, Hayes KW, Ghang RW: Therapeutic ultrasound in the treatment of musculoskeletal conditions, *Arth Care Res* 3(2): 85-91, 1990.

Farmer WC: Effect of intensity of ultrasound on conduction of motor axons, *Phys Ther* 48: 1233-1237, 1968.

Faul ED, Imig CJ: Temperature and blood flow studies after ultrasonic irradiation, *Am J Phys Med* 34: 370, 1955.

Fieldhouse C: Ultrasound for relief of painful episiotomy scars, *Physiotherapy* 65: 217, 1979.

Forrest G, Rosen K: Ultrasound: effectiveness of treatments given under water, *Arch Phys Med Rehabil* 70: 28, 1989.

Fountain FP, Gersten JW, Sengu O: Decrease in muscle spasm produced by ultrasound, hot packs and IR, *Arch Phys Med Rehabil* 41: 293, 1960.

Friedar S: A pilot study: the therapeutic effect of ultrasound following partial rupture of Achilles tendons in male rats, *J Orthop Sports Phys Ther* 10: 39, 1988.

Fyfe MC: A study of the effects of different ultrasonic frequencies on experimental oedema, *Aust J Physiother* 25(5): 205-207, 1979.

Fyfe MC, Bullock M: Acoustic output from therapeutic ultrasound units, *Aust J Physiother* 32(1): 13-16, 1986.

Fyfe MC, Chahl LA: The effect of ultrasound on experimental oedema in rats, *Ultrasound Med Biol* 6: 107, 1980.

Gantz S: Increased radicular pain due to therapeutic ultrasound applied to the back, *Arch Phys Med Rehabil* 70: 493-494, 1989.

Garrett AS, Garrett M: Letters: ultrasound for herpes zoster pain, *J Royal College Gen Prac*, Nov: 709, 1982.

Gersten JW: Effect of metallic objects on temperature rises produced in tissues by ultrasound, *Am J Phys Med* 37: 75, 1958.

Goddard DH, Revell PA, Cason J: Ultrasound has no anti-inflammatory effect, *Ann Rheum Dis* 42: 582-584, 1983.

Gracewski SM, Wagg RC, Schenk EA: High-frequency attenuation measurements using an acoustic microscope, *J Acous Soc Am* 83(6): 2405-2409, 1988.

Grant A, Sleep J, McIntosh J, et al.: Ultrasound and pulsed electromagnetic energy treatment for peroneal trauma: a randomised placebo-controlled trial, *Br J Obstet Gynecol* 96: 434-439, 1989.

Grieder A, Vinton P, Cinott W, et al.: An evaluation of ultrasonic therapy for temporomandibular joint dysfunction, *Oral Surg* 31: 25, 1971.

Griffin JE: Patients treated with ultrasonic driven cortisone and with ultrasound alone, *Phys Ther* 47: 594, 1967.

Griffin JE: Transmissiveness of ultrasound through tap water, glycerin, and mineral oil, *Phys Ther* 60: 1010, 1980.

Griffin JE, Touchstone JC: Ultrasonic movement of cortisol into pig tissue. I. Movement into skeletal muscle, *Am J PHys Med* 42: 77-85, 1962.

Griffin JE, Touchstone JC: Low intensity phonophoresis of cortisol in swine, *Phys Ther* 48(10): 1336-1344, 1968.

Griffin JE, Touchstone JC, Liu A: Ultrasonic movement of cortisol into pig tissues. II. Peripheral nerve, *Am J Phys Med* 44: 20, 1965.

Halle JS, Franklin RJ, Karalfa BL: Comparison of four treatment approaches for lateral epicondylitis of the elbow, *J Orthop Sports Phys Ther* 8: 62, 1986.

Halle JS, Scoville CR, Greathouse DG: Ultrasound's effect on the conduction latency of superficial radial nerve in man, *Phys Ther* 61: 345, 1981.

Hamer J, Kirk JA: Physiotherapy and the frozen shoulder: a comparative trial of ice and ultrasound therapy, *NZ Med J* 83(3): 191, 1976.

Hansen TI, Kristensen JH: Effects of massage: shortwave and ultrasound upon 133Xe disappearance rate from muscle and subcutaneous tissue in the human calf, *Scand J Rehab Med* 5: 197, 1973.

Hashish I, Hai HK, Harvey W, et al.: Reduction of post-operative pain and swelling by ultrasound treatment: a placebo effect, *Pain* 33: 303-311, 1988.

Hekkenberg RT, Oosterbaan WA, van Beekum WT: Evaluation of ultrasound therapy devices, *Physiotherapy* 72: 390, 1986.

Hill CR, ter Haar G: *Ultrasound and non-ionising radiation protection.* In Suess MJ, editor: *WHO regional publication,* European Series No. 10, World Health Organization, Copenhagen, 1981.

Hogan RD, Burke KM, Franklin TD: The effect of ultrasound on microvascular hemodynamics in skeletal muscle: effects during ischemia, *Microvasc Res* 23: 370, 1982.

Hone C-Z, Liu HH, Yu J: Ultrasound thermotherapy effect on the recovery of nerve conduction in experimental compression neuropathy, *Arch Phys Med Rehabil* 69: 410-414, 1988.

Hustler JE, Zarod AP, Williams AR: Ultrasonic modification of experimental bruising in the guinea-pig pinna, *Ultrasound* 16: 223-228, 1978.

Imig CJ, Randall BF, Hines HM: Effect of ultrasonic energy on blood flow, *Am J Phys Med* 53: 100-102, 1954.

Inaba MK, Piorkowski M: Ultrasound in treatment of painful shoulder in patients with hemiplegia, *Phys Ther* 52: 737, 1972.

Jones RI: Treatment of acute herpes zoster using ultrasonic therapy, *Physiotherapy* 70: 94, 1984.

Klemp P, Staberg B, Korsgard J, et al.: Reduced blood flow in fibromyotic muscles during ultrasound therapy, *Scand J Rehab Med* 15: 21-23, 1982.

Kramer JF: Effect of ultrasound intensity on sensory nerve conduction velocity, *Physiother Can* 37: 5-10, 1985.

Kramer JF: Effects of therapeutic ultrasound intensity on subcutaneous tissue temperature and ulnar nerve conduction velocity, *Am J Phys Med* 64: 9, 1985.

Kramer JF: Sensory and motor nerve conduction velocities following therapeutic ultrasound, *Aust J Physiother* 33(4): 235-243, 1987.

Kuitert JH: Ultrasonic energy as an adjunct in the management of radiculitis and similar referred pain, *Am J Phys Med* 33: 61, 1954.

Kuitert JH, Harr ET: Introduction to clinical application of ultrasound, *Phys Ther* 35: 19, 1955.

LaBan MM: Collagen tissue: implications of its response to stress in vitro, *Arch Phys Med Rehabil* 43: 461, 1962.

Lehmann JF: Ultrasound effects as demonstrated in live pigs with surgical metallic implants, *Arch Phys Med Rehabil* 40: 483, 1959.

Lehmann JF: Heating produced by ultrasound in bone and soft tissue, *Arch Phys Med Rehabil* 48: 397, 1967.

Lehmann JF: Therapeutic temperature distribution produced by ultrasound as modified by dosage and volume of tissue exposed, *Arch Phys Med Rehabil* 48: 662, 1967.

Lehmann JF: Heating of joint structures by ultrasound, *Arch Phys Med Rehabil* 49: 28, 1968.

Lehmann JF, Biegler R: Changes of potentials and temperature gradients in membranes caused by ultrasound, *Arch Phys Med Rehabil* 35: 287, 1954.

Lehmann JF, Brunner GD, Stow RW: Pain threshold measurements after therapeutic application of ultrasound, microwaves and infrared, *Arch Phys Med Rehabil* 39: 560, 1958.

Lehmann JF, Erickson DJ, Martin GM: Comparative study of the efficiency of shortwave, microwave and ultrasonic diathermy in heating the hip joint, *Arch Phys Med Rehabil* 40: 510, 1959.

Lehmann JR, Henrick JF: Biologic reactions to cavitation: a consideration for ultrasonic therapy, *Arch Phys Med Rehabil* 34: 86, 1953.

Lehmann JF, Stonebridge JB, de Lateur BJ, et al.: Temperatures in human thighs after hot pack treatment followed by ultrasound, *Arch Phys Med Rehabil* 59: 472-475, 1978.

Lehmann JF, Warren CC, Scham SM: Therapeutic heat and cold, *Clin Orthop* 99: 207-245, 1974.

Levenson JL, Weissberg MP: Ultrasound abuse: a case report, *Arch Phys Med Rehabil* 64: 90-91, 1983.

Lloyd JJ, Evans JA: A calibration survey of physiotherapy equipment in North Wales, *Physiotherapy* 74(2): 56-61, 1988.

Lota MI, Darling RC: Change in permeability of the red blood cell membrane in a homogenous ultrasonic field, *Arch Phys Med Rehabil* 36: 282, 1955.

Lyons ME, Parker KJ: Absorption and attenuation in soft tissues. II. Experimental results, *IEEE Transactions on Ultrasonics, Ferroelectrics and Frequency Control* 35: 4, 1988.

Madsen PW, Gersten JW: Effect of ultrasound on conduction velocity of peripheral nerves, *Arch Phys Med Rehabil* 42: 645-649, 1963.

Maxwell L: Therapeutic ultrasound: its effects on the cellular and molecular mechanisms of inflammation and repair, *Physiotherapy* 78(6): 421-425, 1992.

McDiarmid T, Burns PN, Lewith GT: Ultrasound and the treatment of pressure sores, *Physiotherapy* 71: 661, 1985.

McLaren J: Randomised controlled trial of ultrasound therapy for the damaged perineum, abstract, *Clin Phys Physiol Meas* 5: 40, 1984.

Michlovitz SL, Lynch PR, Tuma, RF: Therapeutic ultrasound: its effects on vascular permeability (abstract), *Fed Proc* 41: 1761, 1982.

Miller DL: A review of the ultrasonic bioeffects of microsonation, gas body activation and related cavitation-like phenomena, *Ultrasound Med Biol* 13(8): 443-470, 1987.

Mortimer AJ, Dyson M: The effect of therapeutic ultrasound on calcium uptake in fibroblasts, *Ultrasound Med Biol* 14: 499-508, 1988.

Mummery CL: *The effect of ultrasound on fibroblasts in vitro*, PhD thesis, London University, 1978.

National Council on Radiation Protection and Measurements (NCRP) Report No 74: Biological effects of ultrasound, Mechanisms and clinical applications, NCRP, Bethesda, Maryland.

Newman MK, Kill M, Frampton G: Effects of ultrasound alone and combined with hydrocortisone injections by needle or hydrospray, *Am J Phys Med* 37: 206, 1958.

Novak EJ: Experimental transmission of lidocaine through intact skin by ultrasound, *Arch Phys Med Rehabil* 45: 231, 1964.

Oakley EM: Evidence for effectiveness of ultrasound treatment in physical medicine, *Br J Cancer* 45 (suppl V): 233-237, 1982.

Paaske WP, Hovind H, Seyerson P: Influence of therapeutic ultrasonic irradiation on blood flow in human cutaneous, subcutaneous and muscular tissues, *Scan J Clin Lab Invest* 31: 389, 1973.

Paul B: Use of ultrasound in the treatment of pressure sores in patients with spinal cord injury, *Arch Phys Med Rehabil* 41: 438, 1960.

Payne C: Ultrasound for post-herpetic neuralgia. *Physiotherapy* 70: 96, 1984.

Popspisilova L, Rottova A: Ultrasonic effect on collagen synthesis and deposition in differently localised experimental granulomas, *Acta Chir Plast* 19: 148-157, 1977.

Reid DC: *Possible contra-indications and precautions associated with ultrasound therapy*. In Mortimer A, Lee N, editors: *Proceedings of the International Symposium on Therapeutic Ultrasound*, Canadian Physiotherapy Association, Winnipeg, 1981.

Reynolds NL: *Reliable ultrasound transmission* (Letter), *Phys Ther* 72(8): 611, 1992.

Roberts M, Rutherford JH, Harris D: The effect of ultrasound on flexor tendon repairs in the rabbit, *Hand* 14: 17, 1982.

Roche C, West J: A controlled trial investigating the effects of ultrasound on venous ulcers referred from general practitioners, *Physiotherapy* 70(12): 475-477, 1984.

Rowe RJ, Gray IM: Ultrasound treatment of plantar warts, *Arch Phys Med Rehabil* 46: 273, 1965.

Shambereer RC, Talbot TL, Tipton HW, et al.: The effect of ultrasonic and thermal treatment of wounds, *Plast Reconstruct Surg* 68(6): 880-890, 1981.

Smith W, Winn F, Farette R: Comparative study using four modalities in shinsplint treatments, *J Orthop Sports Phys Ther* 8: 77, 1986.

Sokoliu A: *Destructive effect of ultrasound on ocular tissues*. In Reid JM, Sikov MR editors: *Interaction of ultrasound and biological tissues*, DHEW Pub (FDA) 73-8008, 1972.

Soren A: Evaluation of ultrasound treatment in musculo-skeletal disorders, *Physiotherapy* 61: 214-217, 1965.

Soren A: Nature and biophysical effects of ultrasound, *J Occup Med* 7: 375, 1965.

Stevenson JH: Functional, mechanical, and biochemical assessment of ultrasound therapy on tendon healing in chicken toe, *Plast Reconstr Surg* 77: 965, 1986.

Stewart HF: Survey of use and performance of ultrasonic therapy equipment in Pinellas County, *Phys Ther* 54: 707, 1974.

Stewart HF, Abzug JL, Harris GF: Considerations in ultrasound therapy and equipment performance, *Phys Ther* 80(4): 424-428, 1980.

Stoller DW, Markholf KL, Zager SA, et al.: The effects of exercise ice and ultrasonography on torsional laxity of the knee joint, *Clin Orthop* 174: 142-150, 1983.

Stratford PW, Cevy DR, Gauldie S, et al.: The evaluation of phonophoresis and friction massage as treatments for extensor carpi radialis tendinitis: a randomized controlled trial, *Physiother Can* 41: 93, 1989.

Stratton SA, Heckmann R, Francis RS: Therapeutic ultrasound: its effect on the integrity of a nonpenetrating wound, *J Orthop Sports Phys Ther* 5: 278, 1984.

Talaat AM, El-Dibany MM, El-Garf A: Physical therapy in the management of myofascial pain dysfunction syndrome, *Am Otol Rhinol Laryngol* 95: 225, 1986.

Taylor E, Humphry R: Survey of physical agent modality use, *Am J Occup Ther* 46(10): 924-931, 1991.

ter Haar G: Basic physics of therapeutic ultrasound, *Physiotherapy* 64(4): 100-103, 1978.

ter Haar G, Dyson M, Oakley EM: The use of ultrasound by physiotherapists in Britain, 1985, *Ultrasound Med Biol* 13: 659, 1987.

ter Haar G, Wyard SJ: Blood cell banding in ultrasonic standing waves: a physical analysis, *Ultrasound Med Biol* 4: 111-123, 1978.

van Levieveld DW: Evaluation of ultrasonics and electrical stimulation in the treatment of sprained ankles: a controlled study, *Ugesrk-Laeger* 141(16): 1077-1080, 1979.

Warren CG, Koblanski IN, Sigelmann RA: Ultrasound coupling media: their relative transmissivity, *Arch Phys Med Rehabil* 57: 218, 1976.

Warren CG, Lehmann JF, Koblanski N: Heat and stretch procedures: an evaluation using rat tail tendon, *Arch Phys Med Rehabil* 57: 122, 1976.

Wells PN: *Biomedical ultrasonics,* London, 1977, Academic Press.

Wells PN, Frampton V, Bowsher D, editors: *Pain: management and control in physiotherapy,* London, 1988, Heinemann.

Williams AR, McHale I, Bowditch M: Effects of MHz ultrasound on electrical pain threshold perception in humans, *Ultrasound Med Biol* 13: 249, 1987.

Williamson JB, George TK, Simpson DC, et al.: Ultrasound in the treatment of ankle sprains, *Injury* 17: 176-178, 1986.

Wilson AG, Jamieson S, Saunders R: The physical behaviour of ultrasound, *NZ J Physiother* 12(1): 30-31, 1984.

Wood RW, Loomis AL: The physical and biological effects of high frequency waves of great intensity, *Philosoph Mag* 4: 417, 1927.

Wright ET, Haase KH: Keloid and ultrasound, *Arch Phys Med Rehabil* 52: 280, 1971.

Wyper DJ, McNiven DR, Donnelly TJ: Therapeutic ultrasound and muscle blood flow, *Physiotherapy* 64: 321, 1978.

Zankei HT: Effects of physical agents on motor conduction velocity of the ulnar nerve, *Arch Phys Med Rehabil* 47: 787-792, 1966.

Traction as a Specialized Modality

13

Daniel N. Hooker

OBJECTIVES

After completion of this chapter, the student will be able to do the following:

- Discuss the effect and therapeutic value of traction on bone, muscle, ligaments, joint structures, nerve, blood vessels, and intervertebral disk.

- Describe the parameters of traction.

- Discuss the effect that changing a parameter might have on treatment results.

- Outline the set-up procedure for mechanical, positional, and manual traction to both the lumbar and the cervical spine.

In the care of the athletic population, **traction** has not traditionally been one of the more frequently used treatments. The age, vigor, and condition of the athletic population, along with the expense of the equipment, time-consuming set-up, and lack of data supporting traction's effectiveness, all led to the low use of and interest in traction by the sports therapist. New clinical and home use equipment have raised the interest and acceptance of the athletic population in the use of traction for both preventive and therapeutic treatment programs. Some of the concepts of traction discussed in this chapter are generalizable to the treatment of the extremities, but the discussion has been aimed specifically at cervical and lumbar spinal traction.

Traction has been used since ancient times in the treatment of painful spinal conditions, but the literature on traction and its clinical effectiveness is limited.* Most of the clinical studies go into great depth about the pathology being treated and give only a cursory description of the traction set-up, making duplication of the traction method difficult. Traction can be defined as a drawing tension applied to a body segment.[4]

---

* References 6, 8, 12, 22, 27, 33, 39.

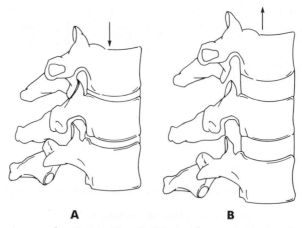

Fig. 13-1. A, Spine in normal resting position. **B,** Spine under traction load with overall increase in length and overall increased separation between vertebrae.

EFFECTS ON SPINAL MOVEMENT

Traction encourages movement of the spine both overall and between each individual spinal segment.[2] Changes in overall spinal length and the amount of separation or space between each vertebra have been shown in studies of both the lumbar and the cervical spine* (Figure 13-1, *A* and *B*).

The amount of movement varies according to the position of the spine, the amount of force, and the length of time the force is applied. Separations of 1 to 2 mm per intervertebral space have been reported. This change is very transient, and the spine quickly returns to the previous intervertebral space relationships when traction is released and the erect posture is assumed.[10,17,21,27] Decreases in pain, paresthesia, or tingling while traction is applied may be caused by the physical separation of the vertebral segments and the resultant decrease in pressure on sensitive structures. If these changes occur while the patient is being treated with traction, the prognosis for the patient is good and traction should be continued as part of the treatment plan.[2,5,26] Any lasting therapeutic changes must be assumed to occur from adjustments or adaptations of the structures around the vertebrae in response to the traction.

EFFECTS ON BONE

Bone changes, according to **Wolff's law,** usually occur in response to compressive or distractive loads. Traction would place a distractive load on each of the vertebrae affected by the traction load. Although bone tissue adapts relatively quickly, bony changes do not occur fast enough to cause the symptomatic changes that occur with traction application. An intermittent traction with a rhythmic on and off load cycle not only provides distraction load but also promotes movement. The major effect of

* References 1, 6, 21, 26, 27, 32, 33.

traction on the bone may come from the increase in spinal movement that reverses any immobilization-related bone weakness by increasing or maintaining bone density.

EFFECTS ON LIGAMENTS

The ligamentous structures of the spinal column will be stretched by traction. Structural changes of the ligaments occur relatively slowly in response to mechanical stresses because ligaments have **viscoelastic properties** that allow them to resist shear forces and to return to their original form after deforming load is removed.[2,5,25]

With rapid loading, the ligaments become stiffer or resistant to changes in length and will be able to absorb a high load or force before failure occurs. With this type of loading, overstress could produce a significant injury.[5] The Wild West and the cervical traction of hanged horse thieves gives us a great example of this type of loading. The sudden drop of body weight as the horse rides out and leaves the thief suspended by a rope around his neck places a rapid load on the ligaments and bones of the cervical spine. This overstress produces no adaptive change as it overwhelms the ligamentous and bony structures, causing a fracture dislocation of the upper cervical spine with spinal cord compression and resulting in the death of the thief.

Slow loading rates will allow the ligament to lengthen as it absorbs the force of the load. Overstress can still produce injury, but it will not be as severe as in the high loading rates. The amount of **ligament deformation** accompanying a low rate of loading will be higher than in rapid loading situations. Loading should be slow and comfortable.[5] The ligament deformation will allow the spinal vertebrae to move apart.

In ligaments shortened or contracted by an injury or a long-term postural problem, traction is important in restoring normal length. The traction force provides the stress that encourages the ligament to make adaptive changes in length and strength. The traction force in this instance would have to be heavy enough to stimulate adaptive changes but not heavy enough to overwhelm the ligament. In acute severely sprained ligaments, a traction force may overwhelm the ligament and have a negative effect on the healing process. Traction treatment should be a part of an overall treatment program that includes strengthening and flexibility exercises.[2]

When ligaments are stretched, they put pressure on or move other structures within the ligamentous structure (**proprioceptive nervous system**) and external to the ligament structure (**disk material, synovial fringes,** vascular structures, and nerve roots). This pressure or movement can significantly reduce pain if pressure on a sensitive structure (nerve, vascular) is reduced. Activation of the proprioceptive nervous system will also relieve pain by providing a gating effect similar to a transcutaneous electrical nerve stimulation (TENS) treatment.[2,8]

EFFECTS ON THE DISK

The mechanical tension created by the traction has a good effect on **disk protrusions** and disk-related pain. Normally the disk helps to dissipate compressive forces while the spine is in an erect posture (Figure 13-2, A).

In the normal disk, internal pressure increases, but the nucleus pulposus (fluidlike center of the fibrocartilaginous vertebral disk) does not move with changes

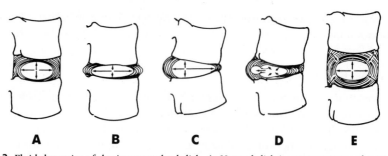

Fig. 13-2. Fluid dynamics of the intervertebral disk. **A,** Normal disk in noncompressed position; internal pressure, indicated by arrows, is exerted relatively equally in all directions. The internal annular fibers contain the nuclear materials. **B,** Sitting or standing with compression of an injured disk causes the nucleus to become flatter. Pressure in this instance still remains relatively equal in all directions. **C,** In an injured disk, movement in the weight-bearing position causes a horizontal shift in the nuclear material. If this was forward bending, the bulge to the left would take place at the posterior annular fibers while the anterior annular fibers would be slackened and narrow. **D,** Weakness of the annular wall would allow the nuclear material to create a herniation and possibly put pressure on sensitive structures in the area. **E,** When placed under traction, the intervertebral space expands, lowering the disk pressure. The taut annulus creates a centripetally directed force. Both these factors encourage the nuclear material to move and decrease the herniation and its effects.

in the weight-bearing forces as the spine moves from flexion to extension.[27] When an injury occurs to the disk structures and the disk loses its normal fullness, the vertebrae can move closer together. The annular fibers bulge just as an underinflated car tire bulges when compared with a normally inflated one[27] (Figure 13-2, *B*).

If the disk is damaged and movement occurs in a weight-bearing position, the disk nucleus will shift according to fluid-dynamic principles. Pressure on one side squeezes the nucleus in the opposite direction (Figure 13-2, *C*). If tears develop in the annular fibers, the nucleus will tend to take the path of least resistance and move in this direction (Figure 13-2, *D*).

Traction that increases the separation of the vertebral bodies decreases the central pressure in the disk space and encourages the **disk nucleus** to return to a central position. The mechanical tension of the **annulus fibrosus** and ligaments surrounding the disk also tends to force the nuclear material and cartilage fragments toward the center.*

Movement of these materials relieves pain and symptoms if they are compressing nervous or vascular structures. Decreasing the compressive forces also allows for better fluid interchange within the disk and spinal canal.[2,8] The reduction in **disk herniation** is unstable and tends to return when compressive forces return[21,22] (Figure 13-2, *D* and *E*).

The positive effect of traction in this instance may be destroyed by allowing the patient to sit after treatment. Minimizing compressive forces after treatment may be equally as important to the treatment's success as the traction.[2] The sitting posture

---

* References 2, 8, 12, 17, 22, 25, 27.

increases the disk pressure, causing the nucleus to follow the path of least resistance and the disk herniation to return.

EFFECTS ON ARTICULAR FACET JOINTS

The articular joints of the spine **(facet joints)** can be affected by traction, primarily through increased separation of the joint surfaces. **Meniscoid structures,** synovial fringes, or osteochondral fragments (calcified bone chips) impinged between joint surfaces are released and a dramatic reduction in symptoms is noticed when joint surfaces are separated. Increased joint separation decompresses the articular cartilage, allowing the synovial fluid exchange to nourish the cartilage. The separation may also decrease the rate of degenerative changes from osteoarthritis. Increased proprioceptive discharge from the facet joint structures provides some decrease in pain perception.[2,5,10,22]

EFFECTS ON THE MUSCULAR SYSTEM

The vertebral muscles can be effectively stretched by traction, provided that the positions of the spine during traction are selected to optimize the stretch of particular muscle groups. The initial stretch should come from body positioning, and the addition of traction will then provide some additional stretch. EMG recordings of the spinal erector muscles during traction showed some decrease in EMG activity in most patients, indicating a muscular relaxation.[11,24] This effect can be enhanced by palpating the erector muscles and focusing the athlete's attention on relaxing them. The muscular stretch would lengthen tight muscle structures or create relaxation of contraction, allowing better muscular blood flow, and also activate muscle proprioceptors, providing even more of a gating influence on the pain. All these properties lead to a decrease in muscular irritation.*

EFFECTS ON THE NERVES

The nerve is the structure to which traction's effects are most often directed. Pressure on nerves or roots from bulging disk material, irritated facet joints, bony spurs, or narrowed foramen size causes the neurologic malfunctioning often associated with spinal pain. Tingling is usually the first clinical sign indicating that there is pressure on a nerve structure. If the pressure is not relieved or if damage of the nerve as a result of trauma or **anoxia** has resulted in inflammation, the tingling may not respond to traction.†

Unrelieved pressure on a nerve will cause slowing and eventual loss of impulse conduction. The signs of motor weakness, numbness, and loss of reflex become progressively more apparent and are indicative of nerve degeneration. Pain, tenderness, and muscular spasm are also associated with continued pressure on the nerve.

Anything that decreases the pressure on the nerve increases the blood's

---

* References 2, 10, 11, 13, 20, 23.
† References 10, 12, 26, 27, 32, 34.

circulation to the nerve, decreasing edema and allowing the nerve to return to normal functioning. Some degenerative changes are reversible, depending on the amount of degeneration and the amount of **fibrosis** that occurs during the repair process.[2,10,32,34]

EFFECTS ON THE ENTIRE BODY PART

The previous discussion outlined the effect of traction on the major systems involved in spine-related pain and dysfunction. The complexity and interrelationships among these systems make determining specific causes of pain and dysfunction very difficult. Traction is not specific to one system but has an effect on each system, and collectively the effect can be very good. Traction can affect the pathologic process in any of the systems, and then all the structures involved can begin to normalize. Traction should not stand alone as a treatment but should be considered as part of an overall treatment plan, and each component of any spine-related dysfunction should be treated with other appropriate modalities.*

CLINICAL APPLICATION

The discussion of specific traction set-ups is organized according to lumbar and cervical traction. Each of these areas will contain discussions of postural, manual, and machine-assisted traction. The traction set-ups mentioned in this chapter should be used as starting points in a treatment plan. The parameters of time, position, and traction force should be adapted to the patient, rather than forcing the patient to adapt to a predetermined traction set-up.

The treatment plan should include the clinical criteria for judging the success and continued use of traction. Positive changes should occur within 5 to 8 treatment days if traction is going to be successful; for example, if an athlete has a positive straight leg raise sign (i.e., pain in the back with a passive straight leg raise). This is a measurable clinical criterion that can be used to judge the treatment's success. If the straight leg raise test is positive at 20 degrees of hip flexion before and after traction and after successive treatments the straight leg raise test is positive at increasing degrees of hip flexion, then the treatment can be considered successful.

Lumbar Traction

Spinal **nerve root impingement,** with causes ranging from disk herniation or prolapse to **spondylolisthesis,** is the leading diagnosis for which traction is prescribed. Traction has also been used to treat joint hypomobility, arthritic conditions of the facet joints, mechanically produced muscle spasm, and joint pain.†

LUMBAR POSITIONAL TRACTION. Normal spinal mechanics allow movements to occur that narrow or enlarge the intervertebral foramina. If the patient is placed in the backlying position with hips and knees flexed, the lumbar spine bends forward and the spinous processes separate. This movement increases the size of the intervertebral foramen bilaterally (Figure 13-3). The flexed postures used to treat low-back pain are examples of this positional traction.

---

* References 1, 2, 5, 8, 20, 26, 27, 28, 32.
† References 2, 11, 12, 26, 27, 34, 36, 39.

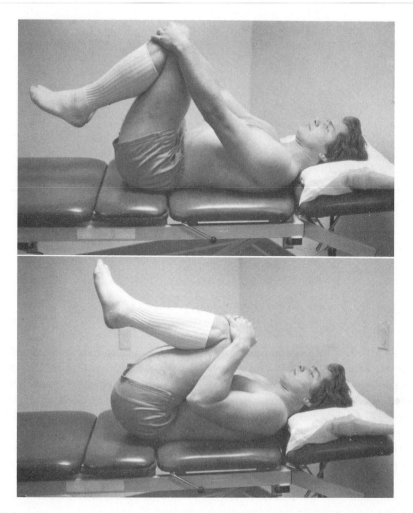

Fig. 13-3. Positional traction; knees to chest posture can be used to increase the size of the lumbar intervertebral foramen bilaterally.

The greatest **unilateral foramen opening** occurs by positioning the patient sidelying with a pillow or blanket roll between the iliac crest and the lower border of the rib cage. The side on which increased foramen opening is desired should be superior. The roll should be close to the level of the spine where the traction separation is desired. The spine side bends around the roll (Figure 13-4). The patient's hips and knees are then flexed until the lumbar spine is in a forward-bent position (Figure 13-5, *A*). This accentuates the opening of a foramen. Maximal opening can be achieved by adding trunk rotation toward the side of the superior shoulder[27,32,33,34] (Figure 13-5, *B*).

Positional traction is normally used when the patient is on a very restricted activity program because of low-back pain. The positions are used on a trial-and-error basis to determine maximum comfort and to attempt to relieve pressure on nerve roots.

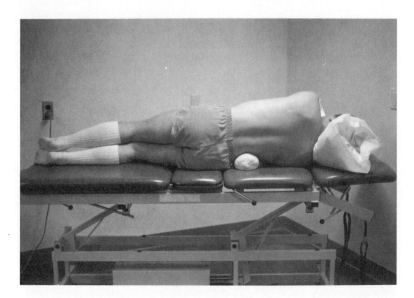

Fig. 13-4. Positional traction; patient positioned sidelying with a blanket roll between iliac crest and rib cage. This increases the intervertebral foramen size of the left side of the lumbar spine.

The results of the patient evaluation should be used to determine whether the painful side should be up or down when using the sidelying positional traction technique. Protective scoliosis is the most obvious sign that will help determine patient position. If the patient leans away from the painful side, the painful side should be up (Figure 13-6, *A*); if the patient leans toward the painful side, the painful side should be down (Figure 13-6, *B*).

The location of the pressure from the disk herniation was previously believed to cause these signs. Further research suggests that hand dominance may be more of a factor than herniation location in producing this scoliosis. However, the athlete may be more compliant with the treatment regimen if simple mechanical explanations, such as pushing the herniation back into place, are used.[29]

Patients with these symptoms may also be good candidates for unilateral traction* (see Figure 13-13). Facet irritation may cause similar scoliotic curves; in most instances the scoliosis is convex toward the painful side.

INVERSION TRACTION. Inversion traction, another positional traction, is being used for prevention and treatment of back problems. Specialized equipment or simply hanging upside down from a chinning bar will place a person in the inverted position. The spinal column is lengthened because of the stretch provided by the weight of the trunk. The force of the trunk in this position is usually calculated to be approximately 40% of body weight (Figure 13-7).

When the person is comfortable and able to relax, the length of the spinal column will increase. These length changes will coincide with decreases in spinal muscle activity.†

---

* References 2, 5, 25, 27, 31, 32.
† References 1, 2, 6, 7, 16, 18, 19, 24.

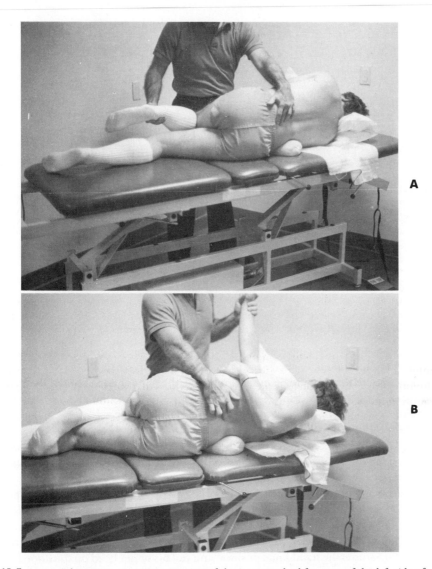

Fig. 13-5. Positional traction; maximum opening of the intervertebral foramen of the left side of the patient's lumbar spine is achieved by flexing the upper hip and knee and rotating the patient's shoulders so he is looking over the left shoulder (left rotation).

No research-supported protocols exist for this method of traction, although a slow progression of time in the inverted position seems to be best. One study suggests the electromyographic activity decreases after 70 seconds in the inverted position. If the patient is comfortable completely inverted, 70 seconds may be used as a minimum treatment time. The inverted position may be repeated 2 or 3 times at a treatment session, with a 2- to 3-minute rest between bouts. Longer treatment times may also enhance results. Maximum treatment times range from 10 to 30 minutes. Set-up procedures are equipment-dependent, and the manufacturer's protocols should be

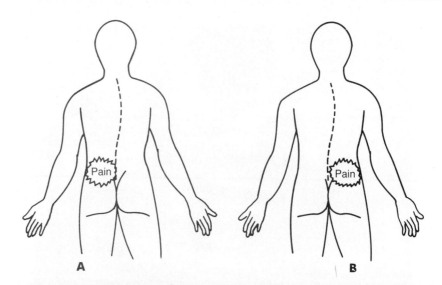

Fig. 13-6. A, Patient leaning away from the painful side. The patient's left side should be placed up while sidelying over a blanket roll to open up the upper foramen or the nerve roots away from the lateral herniation or both. **B,** Patient leaning toward the painful side. The patient's left side should be placed up while sidelying over a blanket roll to pull the nerve roots away from a medial herniation.

followed and modified as necessary to meet the patient's needs.[1,2,3,9,24]

Blood pressure should be monitored while the patient is in the inverted position. If a rise of 20 mm Hg above the resting diastolic pressure is found, the therapist should stop the treatment for that session.[2,3,24]

Contraindications include hypertensive (140/90) individuals and anyone with heart disease or glaucoma. Patients with sinus problems, diabetes, thyroid conditions, asthma, migraine headaches, detached retinas, or hiatal hernias should consult their physicians before treatment is initiated.

Recent lower limb surgery or musculoskeletal problems may require modification of the inversion apparatus. In addition, meals or snacks should not be eaten during the hour before treatment to keep the patient comfortable.

One method of testing the patient's tolerance to the inverted position is to have the patient assume the hand-knee position and put his or her head on the floor, holding that position for 60 seconds. Any vertigo, dizziness, or nausea may indicate that this patient is a poor candidate for inversion and that the treatment progression should be very slow* (Figure 13-8).

MANUAL LUMBAR TRACTION. Manual lumbar traction is used for lumbar spine problems to test the patient's tolerance to traction, to arrive at the most comfortable treatment set-up, to make the traction as specific to one vertebral level as possible, and to provide the specificity needed for a traction mobilization of the spine. If the athlete's back pain is diminished by having the sports therapist flex the athlete's hips and knees to 90 degrees each and apply enough pressure under the calves to lift their buttocks

---

* References 1, 2, 3, 6, 7, 9, 16, 18, 19, 24.

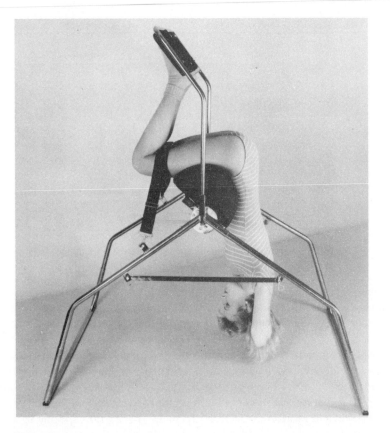

Fig. 13-7. Inversion traction apparatus.
(Courtesy Lossing Orthopaedic, Minneapolis, MN 55404.)

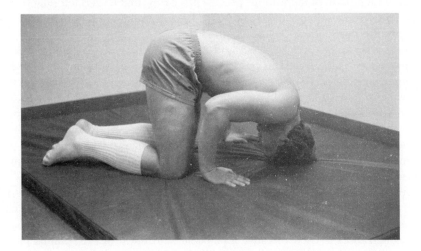

Fig. 13-8. Inversion tolerance test position. Any vertigo, dizziness, or nausea may indicate that this patient is a poor candidate for inversion treatment.

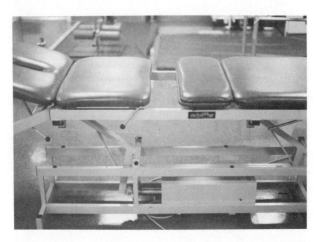

Fig. 13-9. Split table with movable section to decrease frictional forces.

off the table, then the athlete is a good candidate for spine 90-90 degree traction. The disadvantage is that maintaining the large forces necessary for separation of the lumbar vertebrae for a period of time is difficult and energy consuming for the sports therapist.[2,31,32]

Having a split table will eliminate most of the friction between the patient's body segments and the treatment table and is essential for effective delivery of manual lumbar traction[2,5,21,32,34] (Figure 13-9). The sports therapist's effort does not cause separation of the vertebral segments unless the frictional forces are overcome first.

LEVEL-SPECIFIC MANUAL TRACTION. To make the traction specific to a vertebral level, the patient is positioned sidelying on the split table. For traction specific to L3-4, L4-5, and L5-S1 levels, the patient's upper leg is used as a lever and the lumbar spine is flexed until motion of the spinous process just below that level is felt (Figure 13-10). The patient's trunk is then rotated toward the upper shoulder until the spinous process just above the desired level is felt (Figure 13-11).

If lumbar levels T12, L1, L1-2, and L2-3 are to be given specific traction, the patient is again positioned sidelying. These levels require positioning in reverse order from the lower levels. First the trunk is rotated (see Figure 13-11), then the lumbar spine is flexed[2,5] (see Figure 13-10).

In both instances the rotation and flexion tighten and lock joint structures in which these motions have taken place, leaving the desired segment with more movement available than the upper or lower levels. When traction is applied, greater movement of the desired level occurs while movement at other levels is minimized because of the joint locking created by the preliminary positioning.

The split table is then released, and the sports therapist palpates the spinous processes of the selected intervertebral level, places his or her chest against the anterosuperior iliac spine of the patient's upper hip, and leans toward the patient's feet. Enough force is used to cause a palpable separation of the spinous processes (Figure 13-12). Intermittent movement is most easily accomplished, while sustained traction becomes physically more difficult.[2,5]

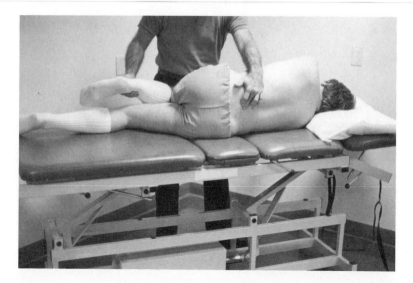

Fig. 13-10. Positioning the patient for maximum effect at a specific level. The lumbar spine is flexed, using the patient's upper leg as a lever. The sports therapist palpates the interspinous area between two spinous processes. The upper spinous process is the one at which maximum effect is desired. When the lumbar spine flexes and the sports therapist feels the motion of the lower spinous process with the palpating hand, the foot is placed against the opposite leg so that further flexion is not allowed.

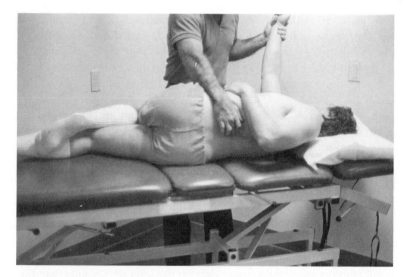

Fig. 13-11. Positioning the patient for maximum effect at a specific level. The patient's trunk is rotated by the sports therapist until motion of the upper spinous process is felt by the sports therapist. Trunk rotation should be passively produced by the sports therapist, positioning the patient's upper arm with hand on the rib cage, and pulling on the patient's lower arm, creating trunk rotation toward the upper arm. In this case it is rotation to the left.

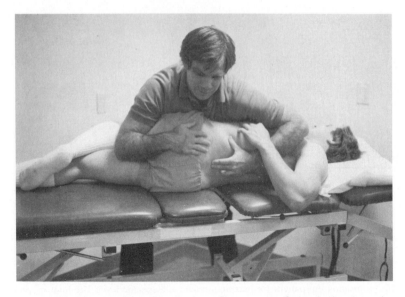

Fig. 13-12. Manual lumbar traction with maximum effect at a specific level. The sports therapist has positioned the patient for maximum effect and is palpating the interspinous area between the two spinous processes where maximum traction effect is desired. The sports therapist then places his or her chest against the anterior superior iliac spine and the patient's upper hip. The split table is released and the sports therapist leans toward the patient's feet, using enough force to cause a palpable separation of the spinous processes at the desired level.

UNILATERAL LEG PULL MANUAL TRACTION. Unilateral leg pull manual traction has been used to treat hip joint problems or difficult lateral shift corrections. A thoracic countertraction harness is used to secure the patient to the table. The sports therapist grasps the patient's ankle and brings the patient's hip into 30-degree flexion, 30-degree abduction, and full external rotation. A steady pull is applied until a noticeable distraction is felt[5] (Figure 13-13).

In suspected sacroiliac joint problems, a similar set-up can be used. A banana strap is placed through the groin on the side to be stretched. This strap will secure the patient in position. The sports therapist grasps the patient's ankle, brings his or her hip into 30-degree flexion and 15-degree abduction, and then applies a sustained or intermittent pull to create a mobilizing effect on the sacroiliac joint[5] (Figure 13-14).

As a preliminary to mechanical traction, manual traction is helpful in determining what degree of lumbar flexion, extension, or sidebending is most comfortable and will also give an indication of the treatment's success. The most comfortable position is usually the best therapeutic position.[5,31,33]

Patient comfort may have more impact on the traction's results than the angle of pull, the force used, the mode, or the duration of the treatment. The inability of the patient to relax in any traction set-up will affect the traction's ability to cause a separation of the vertebrae. The lack of vertebral separation would minimize some of the traction's therapeutic benefits.[5,31,33]

MECHANICAL LUMBAR TRACTION. When using mechanical lumbar traction, the

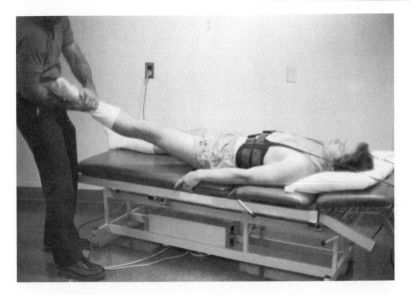

Fig. 13-13. Unilateral leg pull traction. With the patient secured to the table with a thoracic countertraction harness, the sports therapist brings the patient's hip into 30-degree flexion, 30-degree abduction, and maximum external rotation. A steady pull is then applied.

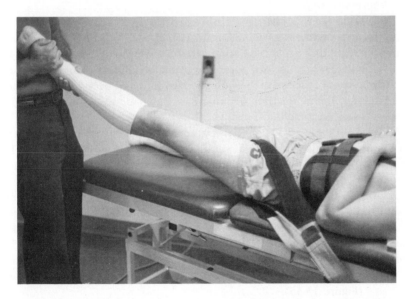

Fig. 13-14. Unilateral leg pull traction for sacroiliac joint problems. A strap is placed through the groin and secured to the table. The sports therapist brings the patient's hip into 30-degree flexion and 15-degree abduction, and then applies a traction force to the leg.

sports therapist will have to select and adjust the following parameters of the traction equipment and patient position:

    1. Body position: prone, supine, hip position, bilateral or unilateral direction of pull

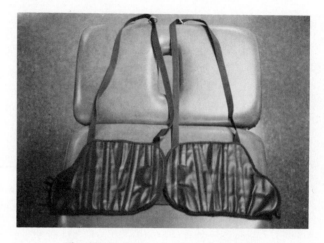

Fig. 13-15. Vinyl-backed traction harness.

2. Force used
3. Intermittent traction: traction time and rest time
4. Sustained traction
5. Duration of treatment
6. Progressive steps
7. Regressive steps

The research on mechanical lumbar traction gives us a strong protocol for using traction to decrease disk protrusion and nerve root symptoms. The protocols for use in other pathologies are not supported by research, but clinical empiricism and inference from some of the research give a good working protocol. The sports therapist will need to match the traction treatment to the patient's symptoms and make adjustments based on the clinical results.[5,12,25,31]

PATIENT SET-UP AND EQUIPMENT. A split table or other mechanism to eliminate friction between body segments and the table surface is a prerequisite to effective lumbar traction. Otherwise, most of the force applied would be spent overcoming the coefficient of friction* (see Figure 13-9).

A nonslip traction harness is needed to transfer the traction force comfortably to the patient and to stabilize the trunk while the lumbar spine is placed under traction. A harness lined with a vinyl material is best because it adheres to the patient's skin and does not slip like the cotton-lined harness. Clothing between the harness and the skin will also promote slipping. The vinyl-sided harness does not have to be as constricting as the cotton-backed harness to prevent slippage, thus increasing the patient's comfort[5,32,34] (Figure 13-15).

The harness can be applied when the patient is standing next to the traction table before treatment. The pelvic harness is applied so that the contact pads and upper belt are at or just above the level of the iliac crest (Figure 13-16).

Shirts should never be tucked under the pelvic harness because some of the

---

* References 1, 2, 5, 15, 21, 32, 34.

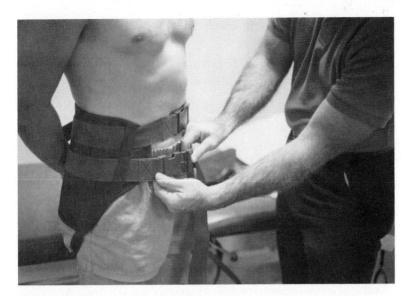

Fig. 13-16. Pelvic harness for mechanical lumbar traction. The contact pads are applied so that the upper belt is at or just above the level of the iliac crest.

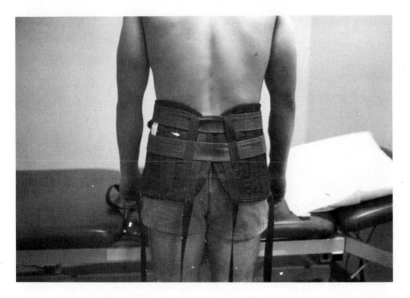

Fig. 13-17. The traction straps from the pelvic harness should bracket the patient's buttocks if a lumbar flexion pull is desired. If a straight pull is desired, the pelvic harness should be adjusted so that the straps bracket the patient's lateral hip area.

tractive force would be dissipated pulling on the shirt material. The contact pads should be adjusted so that the harness loops will provide a posteriorly directed pull, encouraging lumbar flexion (Figure 13-17). The harness firmly adheres to the patient's hips.[5,32,34]

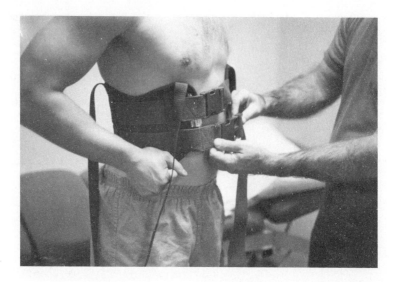

Fig. 13-18. Thoracic countertraction harness. Rib pads are positioned over the lower rib cage.

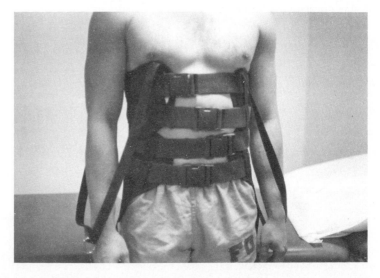

Fig. 13-19. Applying the pelvic and thoracic harnesses may be easier if done while the patient is standing.

The rib belt is then applied in a similar manner with the rib pads positioned over the lower rib cage in a comfortable manner. The rib belt is then snugged up and the patient is positioned on the table[5,32,34] (Figure 13-18).

The standing application of the traction harness is easier and more effective if the patient is placed in prone position for treatment[5,32,34] (Figure 13-19). The traction harness can also be applied by laying it out on the traction table and having the patient lie down on top of it. The pads are then adjusted and the belts tightened with the patient lying down.

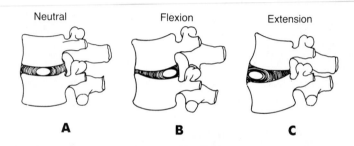

Neutral   Flexion   Extension

A   B   C

Fig. 13-20. **A,** Neutral lumbar spine position allows for the largest intervertebral foramen opening before traction is applied. **B,** Flexion, while it may tend to increase the posterior opening, puts pressure on the disk nucleus to move posterior. Other soft tissue may also close the foramen opening. **C,** Extension beyond neutral tends to close the foramen down as the bony arches come closer together.

BODY POSITION. Body position has reportedly affected traction results, but this has been empirically derived rather than research supported. The sports therapist needs a good understanding of the mechanics of the lumbar spine to make decisions about position that will best affect a patient's symptoms.*

Generally, the neutral spinal position allows for the largest intervertebral foramen opening, and it is usually the position of choice whether the patient is prone or supine. Extension beyond neutral lumbar spine causes the bony elements of the foramen to create a narrower opening. Lumbar spinal flexion beyond neutral causes the ligamentum flavum and other soft tissues to constrict the foramen's opening[31,33] (Figure 13-20, *A* to *C*).

Saunders[32,34] recommends the prone position with a normal to slightly flattened lumbar lordosis (an abnormal anterior curve) as the position of choice in disk protrusions. The amount of lordosis may be controlled by using pillows under the abdomen. The prone position also allows the easy application of other modalities to the painful area and an easier assessment of the amount of spinous process separations[5,32,34] (Figure 13-21).

In traction applied to a patient in the supine position, hip position was found to affect vertebral separation. As hip flexion increased from 0 to 90 degrees, traction produced a greater posterior intervertebral space separation[30] (Figure 13-22).

Unilateral pelvic traction has also been recommended when a stronger force is desired on one side of the spine. Patients with protective scoliosis, unilateral joint dysfunction, or unilateral lumbar muscle spasm with scoliosis may do quite well with this approach. Only one side of the pelvic harness is hooked to the traction device to accomplish this technique[32] (Figure 13-23).

In patients with protective scoliosis, when the patient leans away from the painful side, the traction should be applied on the painful side. When the patient leans toward the painful side, the traction should be applied on the nonpainful side (see Figure 13-6).

In patients with scoliosis caused by muscle spasm, the traction force should be applied from the side with the muscle spasm (Figure 13-24). In unilateral facet joint dysfunction, the traction should be applied from the side of most complaint.[33]

---

* References 2, 5, 22, 27, 32, 34.

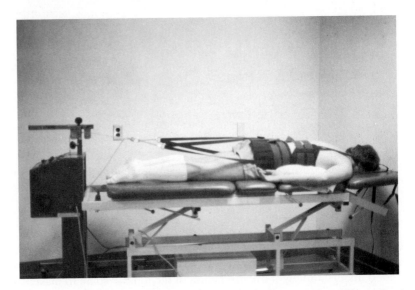

Fig. 13-21. Mechanical lumbar traction; patient in the prone position with a pillow under the abdomen to help control lumbar spine extension.

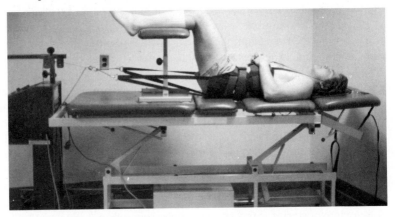

Fig. 13-22. Mechanical lumbar traction; patient in the supine position with hips flexed to approximately 90 degrees.

Overall, patient positioning for traction should be varied according to a patient's needs and comfort. Experimentation with positioning is encouraged so that the traction's effect on the patient will be maximized. Patient comfort is far more important than relative position in making patient position decisions. If the patient cannot relax, the traction will not be successful in causing vertebral separation.[5,32,34]

TRACTION FORCE. Several researchers have indicated that no lumbar vertebral separation will occur with traction forces less than one quarter of the patient's body weight. The traction force necessary to cause effective vertebral separation will range between 65 and 200 pounds.* This force does not have to be used on the first

---

* References 1, 2, 21, 22, 32, 34.

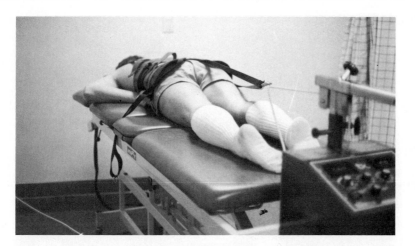

Fig. 13-23. Mechanical lumbar traction with a unilateral pull; only one of the pelvic straps is hooked to the traction device.

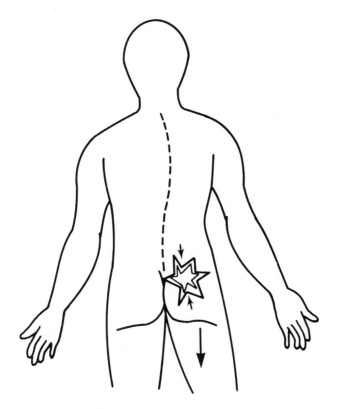

Fig. 13-24. In a patient with scoliosis caused by muscle spasm *(right)*, the unilateral traction force should be applied using only the right pelvic strap.

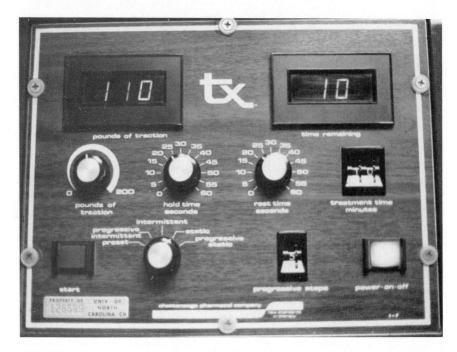

Fig. 13-25. Traction device set for traction with 100 pounds of static traction for 10 minutes with 6 progressive steps.

treatment, and progressive steps both during and between treatments are often necessary to comfortably reach these therapeutic loads. A force equal to half the patient's body weight is a good guideline to use in selecting a force high enough to cause vertebral separation. These high weight levels pose no danger, since cadaver research indicates a force of 440 pounds or greater is necessary to cause damage to the lumbar spine components[21,22] (Figure 13-25).

Caution must be used when using traction of the lumbar spine because there is a tendency for the nucleus pulposus gel to imbibe fluid from the vertebral body, thus increasing pressure within the disk. This happens in a very short period of time. When pressure is released and weight is applied to the disk, this excess fluid increases pressure on the annulus and exacerbates the patient's symptoms. Therefore it is recommended that during an initial treatment with lumbar traction a maximum of 30 pounds be used to determine whether traction will have a negative effect on the symptoms.[10]

The research has been aimed at forces necessary to cause vertebral separation. Traction certainly has effects that are not associated with vertebral separation, and if these effects are desired, less force may be necessary to get them.

INTERMITTENT VERSUS SUSTAINED. Good results have been reported with both intermittent and sustained traction. In most cases of lumbar disk problems, sustained traction seems to be the treatment of choice. Partial reduction in disk protrusions was observed in 4 minutes of sustained traction.[21,22,26,32,34] Good results were also reported using intermittent traction in the treatment of ruptured intervertebral disk.[12]

Separation of the posterior intervertebral space was noted with a 10-second-hold intermittent traction.[30] Posterior intervertebral separations using 100 pounds of force were similar when intermittent and sustained traction modes were compared.[22] The electromyographic activity of the sacrospinalis musculature showed similar patterns when sustained and intermittent traction were compared.[11]

Sustained traction is favored in treating intervertebral disk herniation because it allows more time with the disk uncompressed to cause the disk nuclear material to move centripetally and reduce the disk herniation's pressure on nerve structures. When used for this purpose, sustained traction may be superior to intermittent traction.[5,32,34]

In deciding on sustained versus intermittent traction, the sports therapist should follow the guidelines for treating diagnosed disk herniations with sustained traction, while most other traction-appropriate diagnoses may be treated with intermittent traction. Intermittent traction, in any case, is usually more comfortable when using higher forces, and increased comfort will be one of the primary considerations because there is no conclusive evidence supporting the choice of one method over the other.*

The timing of the traction and rest phases of intermittent traction has not been researched. Short (less than 10 seconds) traction phases will cause only minimal interspace separation but will activate joint and muscle receptors and create facet joint movements.[5,8] Longer (more than 10 seconds) traction phases will tend to stretch the ligamentous and muscular tissues long enough to overcome their resistance to movement and create a longer lasting mechanical separation. When using high traction forces, the comfort of the patient may dictate the adjustment of the traction time. Longer total treatment time will also be tolerated with intermittent traction.[5,8,10,22,32]

Rest phase times should be relatively short but should also be comfort oriented. The rest time should be adjusted to allow the patient to recover and feel relaxed before the next traction cycle. The sports therapist should monitor the traction patient frequently to adjust traction and rest time to maintain the patient in a relaxed, comfortable state.

DURATION OF TREATMENT. The total treatment times of sustained traction and intermittent traction are only partially research-based. With sustained traction, Mathews[21] found reduction in disk protrusion after 4 minutes with further reduction at 20 minutes. Complete reduction in protrusions was seen at 38 minutes. Other researchers found no difference in separation of the cervical spine when times of 7, 30, and 60 seconds were compared.[8,21,22]

When dealing with suspected disk protrusions, the total treatment time should be relatively short. As the disk space widens, the pressure inside the disk decreases and the disk nucleus will move centripetally. The projected time for pressure within a disk to equalize is 8 to 10 minutes. At this point the nuclear material is no longer moving centripetally. With longer time in this position, osmotic forces will equalize the pressure within the disk with that of the surrounding tissue. When the pressure equalization occurs, the traction effect on the protrusion is lost. The intradiskal pressure may increase when the traction is released if the traction stays on too long. This increased pressure would result in increased symptoms. This situation has not been reported

---

* References 1, 2, 5, 12, 22, 30, 32, 34.

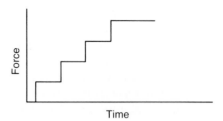

Fig. 13-26. Progressive steps for lumbar traction of X pounds. Four steps are used: the first is ¼ X pounds, the second ²⁄₄ X, etc. Each lasts for an equal time.

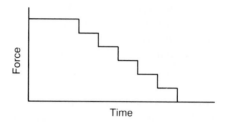

Fig. 13-27. Regressive steps for lumbar traction of X pounds. Six equal regressive steps are used: the first drops the traction force from X to ⁵⁄₆ X, the second to ⁴⁄₆ X, etc. Each lasts for an equal time.

when treatment times are kept at 10 minutes or less.[32,34] If this reaction does occur, shorter treatment times or long-hold (60 seconds traction, 10 to 20 seconds rest) intermittent traction may be necessary to control the symptoms.

Some sources advocate traction times of up to 30 minutes.[5,21,22] The contradiction in philosophy may be because of pathology or the individual anatomy of each patient. An adverse reaction to traction (i.e., a dramatic increase in symptoms when the traction is released) is something the sports therapist should avoid.

Total treatment time for sustained traction when treating disk-related symptoms should start at less than 10 minutes. If the treatment is successful in reducing symptoms, the time should be left at 10 minutes or less. If the treatment is partially successful or unsuccessful in relieving symptoms, the sports therapist may increase the time gradually over several treatments to 30 minutes.

PROGRESSIVE AND REGRESSIVE STEPS. Some traction equipment is built with progressive and regressive modes. The machine will progressively increase the traction force in a preselected number of steps. A gradual increase in pressure lets patients accommodate slowly to the traction and helps them stay relaxed. A gradual progression of force also allows the sports therapist to release the split table after the slack in the system has been taken up by several progressions[2,5,28] (Figure 13-26).

Regressive steps do just the opposite and allow the patient to come down gradually from the high loads. Again, patient comfort is the primary consideration because no research supports any protocol[2,5,28] (Figure 13-27).

Some equipment has the capability to be programmed for progressive and regressive steps and also to have minimum traction forces allowing a sustained force

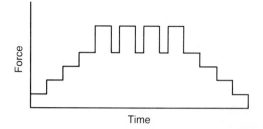

Fig. 13-28. Progressive and regressive steps with a minimum sustained traction force.

with intermittent peaks[2,5,28] (Figure 13-28). To achieve these traction set-ups with a machine that is not programmable, manual operation and timing will be necessary.

Throughout the discussion on lumbar traction, patient comfort comes up again and again in regard to the parameters of the treatment set-up. One of the primary keys to successful traction treatment is patient relaxation. The use of appropriate modalities before and during the traction treatment will add to the total effectiveness of the treatment plan. Bracing or appropriate exercise after traction may also enhance the results and prolong the benefits gained. Better technology and more research will help refine traction and provide better results from this type of treatment.

Cervical Traction

The objectives for using traction in the cervical region do not vary much from the objectives for using traction in the lumbar region. Reasonable objectives for cervical traction include stretch of the muscles and joint structures of the vertebral column, enlargement of the intervertebral spaces and foramina, centripetally directed forces on the disk and soft tissue around the disk, mobilization of vertebral joints, increases and changes in joint proprioception, relief of compressive effects of normal posture, and improvement in arterial venous and lymphatic flow.* In athletics, diagnoses and symptoms requiring traction are found infrequently.[25] These diagnoses are usually found in older populations. The literature does provide a relatively clear protocol to use in trying to achieve vertebral separation using a mechanical traction apparatus.

The patient should be supine or long-sitting with the neck flexed between 20 and 30 degrees (Figure 13-29). A sitting posture can be used but is clinically more cumbersome and not supported by the research as an optimal cervical traction position.[35]

A traction force above 20 pounds, applied intermittently for a minimum of 7 seconds traction time and with adequate rest time for recovery, is recommended. This traction should be continued over 20 to 25 minutes. Higher forces up to 50 pounds may produce increased separation, but the other parameters should remain the same. The average separation at the posterior vertebral area is 1 to 1.5 mm per space, while the anterior vertebral area separates approximately 0.4 mm per space. Greater separations are expected in the younger population than in the older population. Within 20 to 25 minutes from the time traction is stopped and normal sitting or standing postures are resumed, the vertebral separation returns to its previous heights.

---

* References 5, 10, 22, 31, 36, 37, 38.

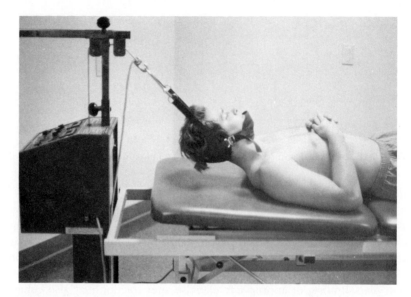

Fig. 13-29. Mechanical cervical traction; patient in the supine position with traction harness placed so that maximum pull is exerted on the occiput and the patient is in a position of approximately 20 to 30 degrees of neck flexion.

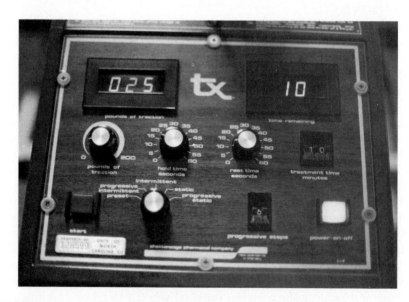

Fig. 13-30. Control panel of traction machine with parameters adjusted for intermittent cervical traction.

The upper cervical segments do not separate as easily as lower cervical segments.[8,10,22] This traction force can be applied either manually or mechanically.

    MECHANICAL TRACTION PROTOCOL. The traction harness must be arranged comfortably so that the majority of pull is placed on the occiput rather than the chin (see Figure 13-29). Some cervical traction harnesses do not have a chinpiece. These

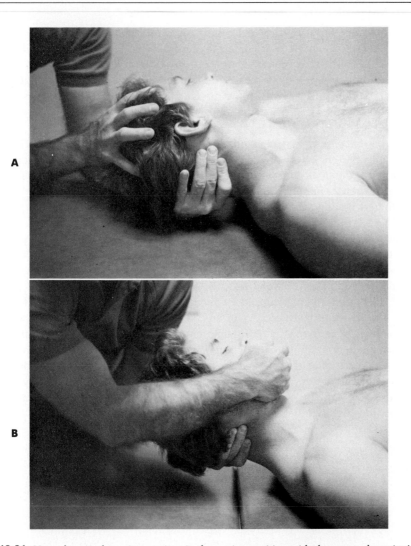

Fig. 13-31. Manual cervical traction; patient in the supine position with the sports therapists's fingertips and thenar eminence contacting the mastoid process of the patient's skull.

harnesses may have an advantage, provided that the traction force is effectively transferred to the structures of the cervical spine.[8,10]

For diagnoses or symptoms that require stretching the posterior neck and ligamentous structures, the following parameters should be used:

1. The neck-trunk angle should be positioned at less than 30 degrees. Various rotations and sidebendings can also be used.
2. Force should be 20 pounds or more applied intermittently with a 20-second traction time.
3. Treatment duration should be 10 minutes or longer.
4. The addition of pain-reducing and heating modalities will add to the benefits gained by the traction[1,2,5,10,22] (Figure 13-30).

MANUAL CERVICAL TRACTION. In most cases in athletics (sprains and strains), simple manual traction used to produce a rhythmic longitudinal movement will be very successful in helping decrease pain, muscle spasm, stiffness, and inflammation and also in reducing joint compressive forces. Manual traction is much more adaptable than mechanical traction, and changes in the direction, force, duration of the traction, and patient position can be made instantaneously as the sports therapist senses relaxation or resistance.[1,2,5,8,22]

The patient's head and neck are supported by the sports therapist. The hand should cradle the neck and provide adequate grip for the effective transfer of the traction force to the mastoid processes. One hand should be placed under the patient's neck with the thenar eminence (base of the thumb) in contact with one mastoid process and the fingers cradling the neck reaching across toward the other mastoid process[2] (Figure 13-31, A).

The sports therapist then provides a gentle (less than 20 pounds) pull in a cephalic direction. Intervertebral separation is not desired because of the damage to the ligaments or capsule it could cause. A head halter or similar harness may also be used to deliver the force (Figure 13-31, B).

The force should be intermittent, with the traction time between 3 and 10 seconds. The rest time may be very brief, but the tractive force should be released almost completely. The total treatment time should be between 3 and 10 minutes.[1,2,5,8]

When pain is limiting or affecting movement, a bout of traction should be followed by a reassessment of the painful motion to determine increases or decreases in pain or motion. Successive bouts of traction can be used as long as the symptoms are improving. When the symptoms stabilize or are worse upon reassessment, the traction should be discontinued.[5]

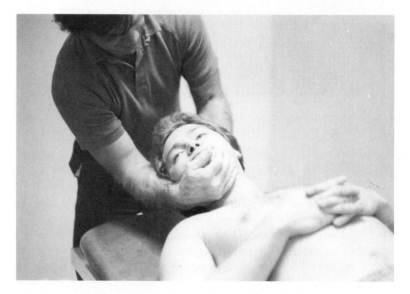

Fig. 13-32. Manual cervical traction; patient is positioned with neck in flexion and with some neck rotation to the right. Laterally flexed positions may also be used.

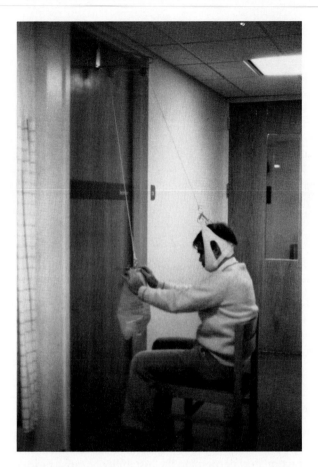

Fig. 13-33. Cervical traction using a wall-mounted unit.

A variety of patient head and neck positions can be used in cervical traction. Different head and neck positions will place some vertebral structures under more tension than others. Good knowledge of cervical kinesiology and biomechanics and good knowledge and skill in joint mobilization are required before the sports therapist should experiment with extensive position changes[2,5,8] (Figure 13-32).

At the completion of the traction treatment in cases of strain or sprain, protection of the neck with a soft collar is often desirable to prevent extremes of motion, minimize compressive forces, and encourage muscle relaxation. Instructions in sleeping positions and regular support postures are also important in caring for athletes with cervical problems.[2,5]

WALL MOUNTED TRACTION. A mechanical traction device can be very costly and is beyond the budgetary limitations of many institutions. Thus knowledge of manual traction techniques will be necessary. A third option is a wall-mounted traction device that can provide cervical traction. These units are relatively inexpensive and can be effective if used appropriately. Weight can be applied via weight plates, sand bags, or water bags. The patient should be placed in a comfortable position (sitting, prone) with

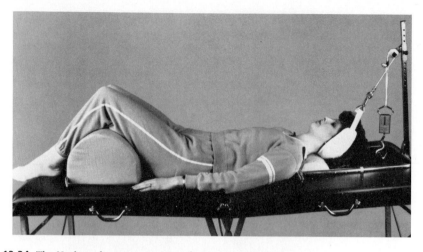

Fig. 13-34. The Necktrac home-use traction device.
(Courtesy Lossing Orthopedic 777 Harding St. NE Minneapolis, MN 55418)

10 to 20 pounds of traction applied for 20 to 25 minutes. Static traction is most easily used, although intermittent traction may also be used, if desired, by simply lifting the weight and releasing tension periodically (Figure 13-33).

The Necktrac is another example of a fairly inexpensive home-use traction device (Figure 13-34).

CONTRAINDICATIONS

Traction, except as a light mobilization, is contraindicated in acute sprains (first 3 to 5 days) or in any conditions in which movement is undesirable. In cases of vertebral joint instability, traction may perpetuate the instability or cause further strain. Certainly the serious problems associated with tumors, bone diseases, osteoporosis, and infections in bones or joints are also contraindications.

SUMMARY

1. Traction has been used to treat a variety of cervical and lumbar spine problems. The effect of traction on each system involved in the complex anatomic make-up of the spine needs to be considered when selecting traction as a part of a therapeutic treatment plan.

2. The traction protocol should be set up to manage a particular problem rather than applied in the same manner regardless of the patient or pathology. Traction is a flexible modality with an infinite number of variations available. This flexibility should allow sports therapists to adjust their protocols to match the patient's symptoms and diagnosis.

3. Traction is capable of producing a separation of vertebral bodies; a centripetal force on the soft tissues surrounding the vertebrae; a mobilization of vertebral joints; a change in proprioceptive discharge of the spinal complex; a stretch of connective tissue; a stretch of muscle tissue; an improvement in arterial, venous, and lymphatic flow; and a lessening of the compressive effects of

posture. Any of these effects can change the symptoms of the patient under treatment and help to normalize the patient's lumbar or cervical spine.

GLOSSARY

annulus fibrosus The interlacing cross-fibers of fibroelastic tissue that are attached to adjacent vertebral bodies that contain the nucleus pulposus.

anoxia Reduction of oxygen in body tissues below physiologic levels.

disk herniation The protrusion of the nucleus pulposus through a defect in the annulus fibrosus.

disk material Cartilaginous material from vertebral body surfaces, disk nucleus, or annulus fibrosus.

disk nucleus The protein polysaccharide gel that is contained between the cartilaginous end plates of the vertebrae and the annulus fibrosus.

disk protrusion The abnormal projection of the disk nucleus through some or all of the annular rings.

facet joints Articular joints of the spine.

fibrosis The formation of fibrous tissue in the injury repair process.

ligament deformation Lengthening distortion of ligament caused by traction loading.

meniscoid structures A cartilage tip found on the synovial fringes of some facet joints.

nerve root impingement Abnormal encroachment of some body tissue into the space occupied by the nerve root.

proprioceptive nervous system System of nerves that provides information on joint movement, pressure, and muscle tension.

spondylolisthesis Forward displacement of one vertebra over another.

synovial fringes Folds of synovial tissue that move in and out of the joint space.

traction Drawing tension applied to a body segment.

unilateral foramen opening Enlargement of the foramen on one side of a vertebral segment.

viscoelastic properties The property of a material to show sensitivity to rate of loading.

Wolff's law Bone remodels itself and provides increased strength along the lines of the mechanical forces placed on it.

REFERENCES

1 Bridger RS: Effect of lumbar traction on stature, *Spine* 15: 522-524, 1990.

2 Burkhardt S: *Course notes, cervical and lumbar traction seminar,* Morgantown, W Va, 1983.

3 Cooperman J, Scheid D: Guidelines for the use of inversion, *Clin Manage* 4(1): 6, 1984.

4 *Dorland's illustrated medical dictionary,* ed 24, Philadelphia, 1965, WB Saunders.

5 Erhard R: *Course notes, cervical and lumbar traction seminar,* Morgantown, W Va, 1983.

6 Gianakopoulos G: Inversion devices: their role in producing lumbar distraction, *Arch Phys Med Rehabil* 68: 100-102, 1985.

7 Goldman RM: The effects of oscillating inversion on systemic blood pressure, pulse, intraocular pressure and central retinal arterial pressure, *Phys Sportsmed* 13(3): 93-96, 1985.

8 Grieve GP: Neck traction, *Physiotherapy* 6: 260-265, 1982.

9 Gudenhoven RC: Gravitational lumbar traction, *Arch Phys Med Rehabil* 59: 510-512, 1978.

10 Harris PR: Cervical traction: review of the literature and treatment guidelines, *Phys Ther* 57: 910-914, 1977.

11 Hood CJ: Comparison of EMG activity in normal lumbar sacrospinalis musculature during continuous and intermittent pelvic traction, *J Orthop Sports Phys Ther* 2: 137-141, 1981.

12 Hood LD, Chrisman D: Intermittent pelvic traction in the treatment of the ruptured intervertebral disk, *Phys Ther* 48: 2 1-30, 1968.

13 Jette DU: Effect of intermittent, supine cervical traction on the myoelectric activity of the upper trapezius muscle in subjects with neck pain, *Phys Ther* 65: 1173-1176, 1985.

14 Klatz RM: Effects of gravity inversion on hypertensive subjects, *Phys Sportsmed* 13(3): 85-89, 1985.

15 KeKosz, UN: Cervical and lumbopelvic traction, *Postgrad Med J* 80(8): 187-194, 1986.

16 Kent BE: Anatomy of the trunk, I, *Phys Ther* 54: 722-744, 1974.

17 Kent BE: Anatomy of the trunk, II, *Phys Ther* 54: 850-859, 1974.

18 LaBan MM: Intermittent traction: a progenetor of lumbar radicular pain, *Arch Phys Med Rehabil* 73: 295-296, 1992.

19 LeMarr JD: Cardiorepiratory responses to inversion, *Phys Sportsmed* 11(11): 51-57, 1983.

20 Letchuman R, Deusinger RH: Comparison of sacrospinalis myoelectric activity and pain levels in patients undergoing static and intermittent lumbar traction, *Spine* 18: 1261-1265, 1993.

21 Mathews JA: Dynamic discography: a study of lumbar traction, *Ann Phys Med* 9: 275-279, 1968.

22 Mathews JA: The effects of spinal traction, *Physiotherapy* 58: 64-66, 1972.

23 Murphy MJ: Effects of cervical traction on muscle activity, *JOSPT* 13: 220-225, 1991.

24 Nosse LJ: Inverted spinal traction, *Arch Phys Med Rehabil* 59: 367-370, 1978.

25 O'Donoghue DH: *Treatment of injuries to athletes,* ed 3, Philadelphia, 1978, WB Saunders.

26 Onel D: Computed tomographic investigation of the effects of traction on lumbar disc herniations, *Spine* 14: 82-90, 1989.

27 Paris S: *Course notes: basic course in spinal mobilization,* Atlanta, Ga, 1977.

28 Petulla LR: Clinical observations with respect to progressive/regressive traction, *JOSPT* 7: 261-263, 1986.

29 Porter RW, Miller CG: Back pain and trunk list, *Spine* 11: 596-600, 1986.

30 Reilly J: Pelvic femoral position on vertebral separation produced by lumbar traction, *Phys Ther* 59: 282-286, 1979.

31 Roaf R: A study of the mechanics of spinal injuries, *J Bone Joint Surg* 42[B]: 810-819, 1960.

32 Saunders HD: Lumbar traction, *J Orthop Sports Phys Ther* 1: 36-45, 1979.

33 Saunders HD: Unilateral lumbar traction, *Phys Ther* 61: 221-225, 1981.

34 Saunders HD: Use of spinal traction in the treatment of neck and back conditions, *Clin Orthop* 179: 31-38, 1983.

35 Sood NA: Prone cervical traction, *Clin Manage Phys Ther* 7(6): 37, 1987.

36 Stoddard A: Traction for cervical nerve root irritation, *Physiotherapy* 40: 48-49, 1954.

37 Varma SK: The role of traction in cervical spondylosis, *Physiotherapy* 59: 248-249, 1973.

38 Walker GL: Goodley polyaxial cervical traction: a new approach to a traditional treatment, *Phys Ther* 66: 1255-1259, 1986.

39 Weinert AM, Rizzo TD: Non-operative management of multilevel lumbar disk herniations in an adolescent athlete, *Mayo Clin Proc* 67: 137-141, 1992.

Intermittent Compression Devices

14

Daniel N. Hooker

OBJECTIVES

After completion of this chapter, the student will be able to do the following:

- Discuss the effects of external compression on the accumulation and the reabsorption of edema after an athletic injury.

- Outline the set-up procedure for intermittent external compression.

- Describe the effects that changing a parameter might have on edema reduction.

- Know when intermittent compression devices may best be used.

Edema accumulation after athletic trauma is one of the clinical signs toward which considerable attention is directed in first aid and therapeutic rehabilitation programs. **Edema** is defined as the presence of abnormal amounts of fluid in the extracellular tissue spaces of the body. Intermittent compression is one of the clinical modalities that is used to help reduce the accumulation of edema.

There are two distinct kinds of tissue swelling that are usually associated with athletic injuries. **Joint swelling,** marked by the presence of blood and joint fluid accumulated within the joint capsule, is one kind. This type of swelling occurs immediately after joint injury. Joint swelling is usually contained by the joint capsule and will appear and feel like a water balloon. If pressure is placed on the swelling, the fluid moves but immediately returns when the pressure is released.

Lymphedema is the other variety of swelling encountered in athletic injuries. This type of swelling in the subcutaneous tissues results from an excessive accumulation of **lymph** and usually occurs over several hours after the injury. Intermittent compression can be used with both varieties, but it is usually more successful with **pitting edema.** The lymphatic system is the primary body system that deals with these injury induced changes.

THE LYMPHATIC SYSTEM
Purposes of the Lymphatic System

The lymphatic system has four major purposes:

1. The fluid in the interstitial spaces is continuously circulating. As plasma and

plasma proteins escape from the small blood vessels, they are picked up by the lymphatic system and returned to the blood circulation.

2. The lymphatic system acts as a safety valve for fluid overload and helps keep edema from forming. As the interstitial fluid increases, the interstitial fluid pressure increases, which causes an increase in the local lymph flow. The local lymphatic system can be overwhelmed by sudden local increases in the interstitial fluid, resulting in pitting edema.[24]

3. The homeostasis of the extracellular environment is maintained by the lymphatic system. The lymphatic system removes excess protein molecules and waste from the interstitial fluid. The large protein molecules and fluids that cannot reenter the circulatory vessels gain entry back into the blood circulation through the terminal lymphatics.

4. The lymphatic system also cleanses the interstitial fluid and provides a blockade to the spread of infection or malignant cells in the lymph nodes. The function of the lymph nodes is not clearly understood and is highly variable.[13]

Structure of the Lymphatic System

The lymphatic system is a closed vascular system of **endothelial cell** lined tubes that parallel the arterial and nervous systems. The lymphatic capillaries are made of single layered endothelial cells with **fibrils** radiating from the junctions of the endothelial cells (Figure 14-1). These fibrils support the lymphatic capillaries and anchor them to the surrounding connective tissue. The capillary is surrounded by the interstitial fluid and tissues. These lymphatic capillaries are called the terminal lymphatics, and they provide the entry way into the lymphatic system for the excess interstitial fluid and plasma proteins.

These lymphatic capillaries join together in a network of lymphatic vessels that eventually lead to larger collecting vessels in the extremities. The collecting vessels connect with the thoracic duct or the right lymphatic duct, which join the venous

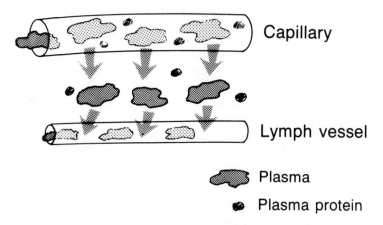

Fig. 14-1. Plasma proteins outside the capillaries attract fluid to the intercellular space, leading to an abnormal "wet state" in the intercellular spaces. Plasma is absorbed back into the lymphatic vessel and moves away from the injured area.

system in the left and right cervical area. As the lymph flows centrally up the system, it moves through one or more lymph nodes. These nodes remove the foreign substances and are the primary area of lymphocytic activity.[13]

Peripheral Lymphatic Structure and Function

Deep and superficial lymphatic collecting systems are found in the extremities. The terminal lymphatics in the skin and subcutaneous tissue drain into the superficial branches. Lymph channels in the fascial and bony layers drain into the deep branches.

In the superficial branches, the dermis is packed with two types of lymphatic channels. The channels closer to the surface have no valves, while those lying under the dermis and in the subcutaneous tissue do have valves. The valves are located approximately a centimeter apart and are similar in construction to the valves in veins. These structures prevent the back flow of lymph when pressure is applied. As with the blood vessels, the lymph system is concentrated on the medial side of the limbs.[13]

As the lymphatic system changes from the entry channels to the collecting channels, the lymphatic vessel changes to look similar to venous tissue. These vessels have smooth muscle and appear to have innervation from the sympathetic nervous system.

As the fluid or tissues move in the interstitial spaces, they push or pull on the fibrils supporting the terminal lymphatics (Figure 14-2). This activity forces the endothelial cells to gap apart at their junctions, creating an opening in the terminal lymphatics for the entry of interstitial fluid, cellular waste, large protein molecules, plasma proteins, extracellular particles, and cells into the lymphatic channels. These junctions are constantly being pushed and pulled open and are then allowed to close, depending on the local activity. Once the interstitial fluid and proteins enter these channels, they become lymph. Terminal lymphatics in inflamed areas are dilated, and an increased number of gaps in the capillary are present (see Figure 14-2).[9,13,16,31,32]

If no tissue activity or interstitial volume increase takes place, these endothelial junctions remain closed. The interstitial fluid, however, can still enter the terminal

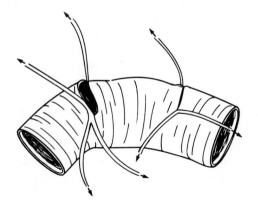

Fig. 14-2. Lymphatic capillary with pore open to allow movement of plasma protein out of the intercellular space. As the intercellular fluid accumulates, the fibrils radiating from the seams in the lymphatic capillary pull the seam open to create a pore large enough for plasma proteins to enter.

lymphatics by moving across the endothelial cell or by being transported across in a vesicle or cell organelle. This permeability is similar to the small blood vessels or capillaries (see Figure 14-1).

Muscle activity, active and passive movements, elevated positions, respiration, and blood vessel pulsation all aid in the movement of lymph by compressing the lymphatic vessels. This allows gravity to pull the lymph down the channels. The valves help by maintaining a unidirectional flow of lymph in response to pressure. The collecting lymph channels all have smooth muscle in their walls. These muscles can provide contractible activity that promotes lymph flow. These muscles have a natural firing frequency that stimulates a rhythmic pumping action. There are also studies that indicate increased lymph flow during heating of animal limbs.*

INJURY EDEMA

After a closed injury, changes in and around the injury site occur that affect the accumulation of extracellular fluid and proteins in the local interstitial spaces. The direct effects of the injury include cell death, bleeding, the release of chemical mediators to initiate and guide the healing process, and changes in local tissue electric currents. The first stage of the healing process is inflammation, which is characterized by local redness, heat, swelling, and pain. In addition, loss of function frequently occurs.

These changes are brought about by changes in the local circulation. Local edema is formed by the plasma, plasma proteins, and cell debris from the damaged cells all moving into the interstitial spaces. This sudden volume change is compounded by the intact local circulatory responses to the chemical mediators of the inflammatory process. The hormones released by the injured cells stimulate the small anterioles, capillaries, and venules to vasodialate, enlarging the size of the vascular pool. This causes the local blood flow to slow down, and the pressure within the blood vessels increases. The endothelial cells in the blood vessel walls then separate or become more loosely bound to their neighboring cell. The permeability of the vessel increases, allowing more plasma, plasma proteins, and leukocytes to escape into the local area. The increase in the plasma proteins in the interstitial spaces causes the osmotic pressure to push more plasma into the area, forming an inflammatory exudate. This exudate forms too quickly for the lymphatic system to maintain the local equilibrium, and pitting edema is formed (Figure 14-3). This small increase in the plasma protein in the intercellular spaces causes an increase in the intercellular fluid volume by several hundred percent.†

This fluid in the form of a gel is trapped by both collagen fibers and proteoglycan molecules. The gel prevents the free flow of fluid as seen in the joint fluid example. Clinically, this state is recognized as pitting edema. After finger pressure on the swollen part is released, a slight pit is left at the finger's previous location. Fluid is squeezed out of the intercellular space, and time is needed for the fluid to move slowly back into that space (see Figure 14-3).

---

* References 1-8, 10, 11, 15, 26-34.
† References 1, 2, 3, 6, 12, 17, 32, 33.

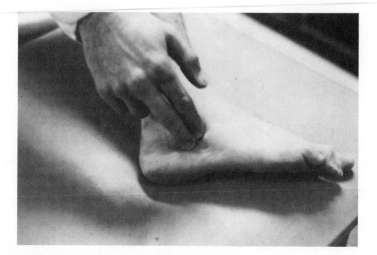

Fig. 14-3. Ankle with pitting edema. Finger pressure squeezes fluid out of the intercellular space; an indentation is left when the pressure is removed.

As the intercellular fluid volume increases, the lymph begins to flow. If the edema causes an overdistention of the lymph capillaries, the entry pores become ineffective, and lymphedema results. Constriction of lymph capillaries or larger lymphatic vessels from increased pressure will also discourage lymph flow and cause intercellular fluid to increase.*

Using computerized tomography cross sectional images, Airaksinen reported a 23% increase in the subcutaneous tissue, thickened skin, and muscular atrophy in patients after lower leg fracture and casting. He reported an 8% edema decrease in the subcutaneous compartment after intermittent compression. The mean area of the subfascial compartment remained the same, but the density of the muscle tissue increased after treatment. This study indicates that injury edema will follow the path of least resistance and that tissues that have the least natural pressure exerted on them will demonstrate the greatest accumulation of extra fluid. The skin and subcutaneous tissue appear to be the major site for pitting edema; the deep muscle and connective tissue have enough pressure to inhibit major accumulations in the deeper tissues.[3]

Clinical measurement of edema is reasonably accurate and correlates very well with both CT scan and volumetric measures. The standard clinical circumferential measurement of limb and joint is adequate to determine the treatment effects.[3,4]

Edema compounds the extent of an injury by causing the secondary hypoxic cellular death in the tissues surrounding the injured area. The edema increases the distance nutrients and oxygen must travel to nourish the remaining cells. This in turn adds to the injury debris in the damaged area and causes further edema to accumulate, perpetuating this cycle.[9]

Other ill effects of edema include the physical separation of torn tissue ends, pain, and restricted joint range of motion. Recovery times become more prolonged. If the edema persists, further problems with extremity function can occur, including

---

* References 1, 2, 3, 6, 12, 17, 32, 33.

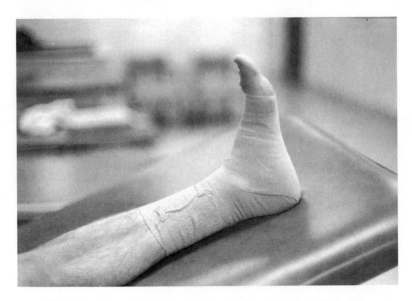

Fig. 14-4. Ankle with elastic wrap compression in an elevated position.

infection, muscle atrophy, joint contractures, interstitial fibrosis, and reflex sympathetic dystrophy.[6,9,11]

TREATMENT OF EDEMA

Good first aid can minimize edema (Figure 14-4). The use of ice, compression, electricity, elevation, and early gentle motion retards the accumulation of fluid and keeps the lymphatic system operating at an optimum level. Any treatment that encourages lymph flow will decrease plasma protein content in the intercellular spaces and therefore decrease edema in that part.[20] The standard methods of treatment in most sports therapy settings include elevation, compression, and muscular contraction.

The force of gravity can be used to augment normal lymph flow. The swollen part can be elevated so that gravity does not resist the lymph flow but encourages its movement. Elevation of the injured swollen part above heart level is all that is necessary. The higher the elevation, the greater the effect on the lymph flow.[22,25]

In an uninjured population, placing their legs in an elevated position significantly decreased ankle volume after 20 minutes, while the dependent position significantly increased ankle volumes. These findings could be expected to be the same in injured subjects. The dependent position may markedly increase volume, while the elevated position may not decrease volumes as well because of the tissue injury. In studies using postacute ankle sprain edema, elevation alone provided a significant reduction in ankle volume after treatment.[4,19,22,25]

Rhythmic internal compression provided by muscle contraction will also squeeze the lymph through the lymph vessels, improving its flow back to the vascular system. This muscle contraction can be accomplished through isometric or active exercise or through electrically induced muscle contraction. Several authors also advocate the use of noncontractible electric current for edema control and reduction. (See Chapter 5 for a discussion of electrical therapy for edema control.) When elevation is combined with muscle contraction, lymph flow is increased.[5,10]

External pressure can also be used to increase lymph flow. Massage, elastic compression, and intermittent pressure devices are the external pressure devices most used. This external compression not only moves the lymph along but also may spread the intercellular edema over a larger area, enabling more lymph capillaries to become involved in removing the plasma proteins and water. External pressure from horseshoe, pads, and elastic wraps also helps minimize the accumulation or reaccumulation of edema in the injured area.[7,31,32,33]

Gardner has proposed that weight-bearing activities activate a powerful venous pump. The pump consists of the venae comitantes of the lateral plantar artery. It is emptied immediately upon weight bearing and flattening of the plantar arch. Because this emptying occurs so rapidly, he believes that this process is mediated by the release of an **endothelial-derived relaxing factor** (EDRF) and is not related to muscular activity of the limb. The EDRF is liberated by sudden pressure changes, and it diffuses locally. Its major action is to relax the smooth muscle and stimulate blood flow rates in the veins.[14]

This phenomena may explain the rapid decrease in edema that occurs when athletes switch from a nonweight-bearing gait to a weight-bearing gait. Using this venous pump on lower leg edema is a reason early weight bearing would be included in a variety of injury treatment protocols.

Using an intermittent compression device to decrease postacute injury edema has recently been shown to have a good effect. The addition of cryotherapy to the intermittent compression has shown the best results in the reduction of postacute injury edema.*

CLINICAL PARAMETERS

There are three parameters available for adjustment when using most intermittent pressure devices: inflation pressure, on-off time sequence, and total treatment time (Figure 14-5). There are also intermittent pressure devices with multiple compartments that inflate distal to proximal with gradual reduced pressure in each compartment. These devices try to mimic the massage strokes used in edema removal.[15,16,19,29] Reduction in postacute injury edema does not require this graded sequential action, nor is postinjury edema reduction significantly enhanced by these devices.[19,29] All intermittent compression devices seem to have similar influences on edema.

Little research has been done comparing adjustments of these parameters with volumetric results. Empiricism and clinical trials have been used to design the established protocols. Pressure settings have been loosely correlated with blood pressure and patient comfort to arrive at the therapeutic pressure. A pressure approximating the patient's diastolic blood pressure has been used in most treatment protocols. The arterial capillary pressures are approximately 30 mm Hg, and any pressure that exceeds this should encourage reabsorption of the edema and movement

---

* References 1, 2, 3, 4, 15, 16, 19, 21, 26, 27, 34.

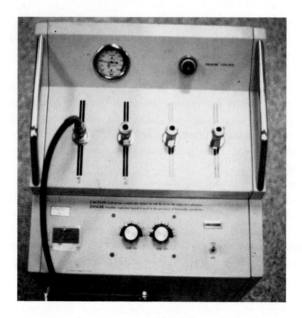

Fig. 14-5. Pressure gauge and pressure control knob for an intermittent compression unit.

of the lymph. Maximum pressure should correspond to the systolic blood pressure. Higher pressure would shut off arterial blood flow and create a potentially uncomfortable tissue response as a result of low blood flow.*

More may not necessarily be better. Enough pressure is needed to squeeze the lymphatic vessels and force the lymph to move. This should be accomplished with relatively low pressures between 30 and 40 mm Hg. The other mechanism in operation is the force of the hydrostatic pressure. Pressure in the range of 40 to 50 mm Hg should suffice to raise the interstitial fluid pressure higher than the blood vessel pressures. [11,17,18]

On- and off-time sequences are even more variable, with some protocols calling for a sequence of 30 seconds on, 30 seconds off; 1 minute on, 2 minutes off; while others reverse this to 2 minutes on, 1 minute off. Others use a 4 minutes on to 1 minute off ratio. If lymphatic massage is the primary vehicle used in this therapy, shorter on-off time sequences may have an advantage. The hydrostatic pressure vehicle would require the longer on times. These time periods are not research-based, and the sports therapist is left to his or her own empirical judgment as to the optimum time sequence for each patient. Patient comfort should be a primary deciding factor here. Total treatment times have some basis in research, but again this is convenience or empirically based in many instances. Most of the protocols for primary lymphedema call for long 3- to 4-hour treatments. This time frame has been effective for many patients.†

Researchers have shown a marked increase in lymph flow on initiation of massage; this flow decreases over a 10-minute period and stops when the massage is

---

* References 1, 2, 3, 9, 11, 17, 18.
† References 1, 2, 3, 4, 10, 11, 15, 16, 18, 19, 21, 22, 23, 26, 27, 29, 34.

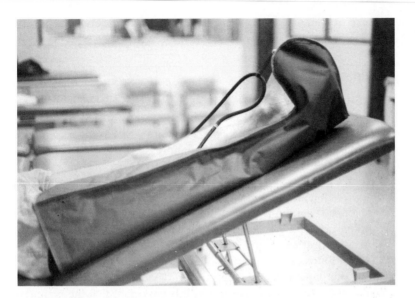

Fig. 14-6. Uninflated compression appliance applied to patient's leg in an elevated position.

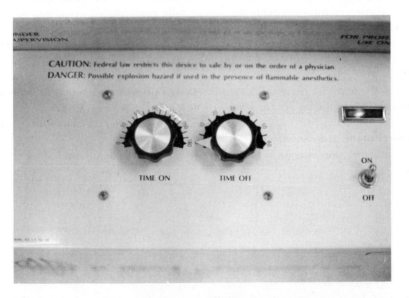

Fig. 14-7. Time setting control knobs for on and off cycles of an intermittent compression unit. This illustrates the setting at the beginning of the treatment when the appliance is uninflated. The off time knob is increased when the proper inflation pressure is reached.

discontinued.[28,34] Clinical studies show significant gains in limb volume reduction after 30 minutes of compression.* In the athletic situation, a 10- to 30-minute treatment seems adequate unless the edema is overwhelming in volume or is resistant to the

---

* References 1, 2, 3, 4, 10, 19, 21, 26, 27, 34.

treatment. More treatment times per day may also be advantageous in controlling and reducing edema from athletic injuries.

PATIENT SET-UP AND INSTRUCTIONS

Patient set-up using an intermittent compression device is relatively simple. The patient should have the appropriate-sized compression appliance fitted on the extremity in an elevated position (Figure 14-6). The compression sleeves come as either half-leg, full-leg, full-arm, or half-arm. The deflated compression sleeve is connected to the compression unit via a rubber hose and connecting valve.

Once the machine has been turned on, three parameters may be adjusted: on/off time, inflation pressure, and treatment time. The on time should be adjusted between 30 and 120 seconds (Figure 14-7). The off time is left at 0 until the sleeve is inflated and the treatment pressure is reached and then may be adjusted between 0 and 120 seconds. When the unit cycles off, the patient should be instructed to move the extremity. A 30-seconds-on, 30-seconds-off setting seems to be both effective and comfortable for the patient. Some compression devices will slowly reach the target pressure, while others respond more rapidly. It is important that the on and off times take the machine's characteristics into account.

When using electrical stimulation in combination with compression, always adjust the current intensity with the sleeve fully pressurized, since this may affect electrode contact and current density (Figure 14-8).

The treatment should last between 20 and 30 minutes. Patients do not seem to comfortably tolerate treatments lasting longer than 30 minutes. On completion of the treatment, the extremity should be measured to see if the desired results have been achieved. The part should be wrapped with elastic compression wraps to help maintain

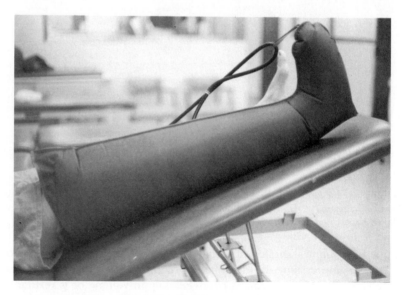

Fig. 14-8. Inflated pressure sleeve.

the reduction. If the edema is not reduced, another treatment may be needed after a short recovery time. If not contraindicated, weight bearing should be encouraged to stimulate the venous pump.

COLD AND COMPRESSION COMBINATION

Some manufacturers have coupled intermittent pressure with a coolant (either water or Freon). These devices have the advantage of cooling the injured part as well as compressing it. The Jobst Cryotemp is a controlled cold/compression unit that has a temperature adjustment ranging between 10° and 25° C. Cooling is accomplished by circulating cold water through the sleeve.

The combination of cold and compression has been shown to be clinically effective in treating some edema conditions.* A study comparing a technique using an intermittent compression unit, cold, and elevation with one using an elastic wrap,

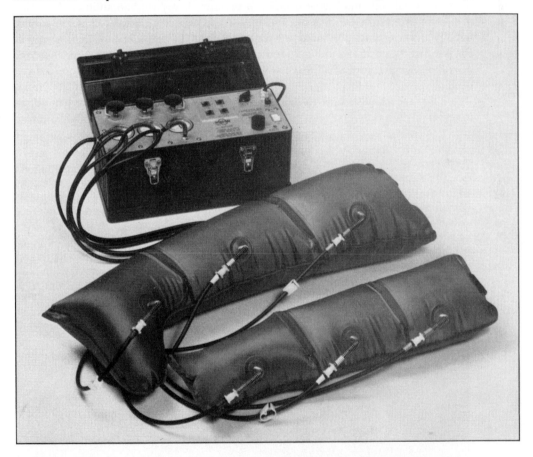

Fig. 14-9. The Wright Linear Pump is a programmable gradient pressure sequential compression system.

---

* References 4, 10, 17, 19, 21, 26, 27.

cold, and elevation showed that the use of the cold-compression device was more effective in edema reduction.[4]

LINEAR COMPRESSION PUMPS

Intermittent compression pumps have incorporated sequentially inflated multiple compartment designs for some time.[16,17,29] Recently these designs have also included a programmable gradient design, for example, the Wright Linear Pump (Figure 14-9). This was designed to incorporate the massage effect of a distal to proximal pressure with a gradual decrease in the pressure gradient.[16]

The highest pressure is in the distal sleeve and, according to the manufacturer's recommendation, is determined by the mean value of systolic to diastolic pressure at the outset of a specifically determined 48-hour protocol whose purpose is to determine the effectiveness of the device in individual cases.[16] The middle cell is set 20 mm lower than the distal cell, and the proximal cell pressure is reduced an additional 20 mm.

The length of each pressure cycle is 120 seconds. The distal cell is pressurized initially and continues pressurization for 90 seconds. Twenty seconds later the middle cell is inflated, and after another 20 seconds the proximal cell inflates. A final 30-second period allows pressure in all three cells to return to 0, after which the cycle repeats itself.

Only a few studies have shown the efficacy of using decreasing pressure in a distal to proximal direction relative to previously existing compression sleeves.[15,16] In a study

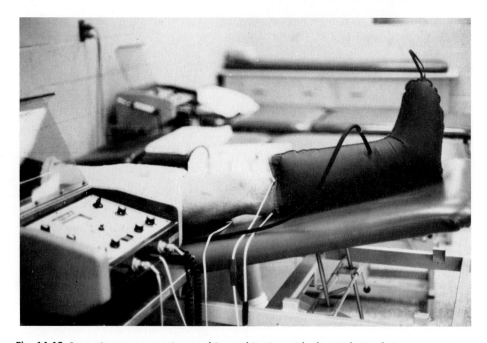

Fig. 14-10. Intermittent compression used in combination with electrical stimulating currents to reduce edema.

comparing linear compression and cold and compression, Lemley found both effective in reducing edema but no significant difference between the devices.[19]

Intermittent compression may also be used in conjunction with a low-frequency pulsed or surging electrical stimulating current set-up to produce muscle pumping contractions. The combination of these two modalities should facilitate resorption of injury byproducts by the lymphatic system (Figure 14-10).[10]

SUMMARY

1. Edema after injury or surgery can be effectively managed using a compression pump program.
2. This treatment, along with external elastic supports, elevation, weight bearing, and exercise, will help reverse the edema and prevent its reaccumulation.
3. Treatment parameters are better understood from clinic empiricism than from research studies. Although the physiologic principles of edema accumulation and reduction should be used to establish minimum and maximum values, specific manipulations of on-off times, pressure, and total treatment time should use patient comfort as the primary guide.

GLOSSARY

edema The presence of abnormal amounts of fluid in the extracellular tissue spaces of the body.
endothelial cell Cells that line the cavities of vessels.
endothelial-derived relaxing factor Relaxes smooth muscle and stimulates blood flow rates in veins.
fibrils Connective tissue fibers supporting the lymphatic capillaries.
joint swelling Accumulation of blood and joint fluid within the joint capsule.

lymph A transparent slightly yellow liquid found in the lymphatic vessels.
lymphedema Swelling of subcutaneous tissues as a result of accumulation of excessive lymph fluid.
pitting edema A type of swelling that leaves a pitlike depression when the skin is compressed.

REFERENCES

1 Airaksinen O: Treatment of post-traumatic edema in lower legs using intermittent pneumatic compression, *Scand J Rehabil Med* 20: 25-28, 1988.
2 Airaksinen O: Changes in post-traumatic ankle joint mobility, pain and edema following intermittent pneumatic compression therapy, *Arch Phys Med Rehabil* 70: 341-344, 1989.
3 Airaksinen O: Intermittent pneumatic compression therapy in post-traumatic lower limb edema: computed tomography and clinical measurements, *Arch Phys Med Rehabil* 72: 667-670, 1991.
4 Brewer K: *The effects of intermittent compression and cold on reducing edema in post-acute ankle sprains.* Unpublished master's thesis, Chapel Hill, NC, 1990, University of North Carolina Press.
5 Brown S: Ankle edema and galvanic muscle stimulation, *Phys Sports Med* 9: 137, 1981.
6 Carriere B: Edema: its development and treatment using lymph drainage massage, *Clin Manage Phys Ther* 8(5): 19-21, 1988.

7 Duffley H, Knight K: Ankle compression variability using elastic wrap, elastic wrap with a horseshoe, edema II boot and air stirrup brace, *Ath Train* 24: 320-323, 1989.
8 Elkins EC, Herrick JF, Grindley JH: Effect of various procedures on the flow of lymph, *Arch Phys Med Rehabil* 34: 31-39, 1953.
9 Evans P: The healing process at the cellular level: a review, *Physiotherapy* 66: 256-259, 1980.
10 Flicker M: *An analysis of cold intermittent compression with simultaneous treatment of electrical stimulation in the reduction of post acute ankle lymphaedema.* Unpublished master's thesis, Chapel Hill, NC, May 1993, University of North Carolina Press.
11 Foldi E, Foldi M, Weissleder H: Conservative treatment of lymphoedema of the limbs, *Angiology* 36: 171-180, 1985.
12 Gardner A: Reduction of post-traumatic swelling and compartment pressure by impulse compression of the foot, *J Bone Joint Surg* 72[B]: 810-815, 1990.
13 Gnepp D: *Lymphatics.* In Staub NC, Taylor AE, editors: *Edema,* New York, 1984, Raven Press.

14 Hurley JV: *Inflammation*. In Staub NC, Taylor AE, editors: *Edema*, New York, 1984, Raven Press.

15 Kim-Sing C, Basco V: Postmastectomy lymphedema treated with the Wright Linear Pump, *Can J Surg* 30(5): 368-370, 1987.

16 Klein M, Alexander M, Wright J, et al.: Treatment of lower extremity lymphedema with the Wright Linear Pump: a statistical analysis of a clinical trial, *Arch Phys Med Rehabil* 69: 202-206, 1988.

17 Kobi P, Denegar C: Traumatic edema and the lymphatic system, *Ath Train* 18: 339-341, 1983.

18 Kruse R, Kruse A, Britton RC: Physical therapy for the patient with peripheral edema: procedures for management, *Phys Ther* 80: 29-33, 1960.

19 Lemley T: *A comparison of two intermittent compression devices on pitting ankle edema*. Unpublished master's thesis, Chapel Hill, NC, 1991, University of North Carolina Press.

20 Liu N, Olszewski W: The influence of local hyperthermia on lymphedema and lymphedematous skin of the human leg, *Lymphology* 26: 28-37, 1993.

21 Quillen WS, Rouiller L: Initial management of acute ankle sprains with rapid pulsed pneumatic compression and cold, *J Orthop Sports Phys Ther* 4: 39-43, 1982.

22 Rucinski TJ, Hooker D, Prentice W: The effects of intermittent compression on edema in post-acute ankle sprains, *JOSPT* 14 (2): 65-69, 1991.

23 Sanderson R, Fletcher W: Conservative management of primary lymphedema, *Northwest Med* 64: 584-588, 1965.

24 Seki K: Lymph flow in human leg, *Lymphology* 12: 2-3, 1979.

25 Sims D: Effects of positioning on ankle edema, *JOSPT* 8: 30-33, 1986.

26 Sloan J, Giddings P, Hain R: Effects of cold and compression on edema, *Phys Sports Med* 16(8): 116-120, 1988.

27 Starkey J: Treatment of ankle sprains by simultaneous use of intermittent compression and ice packs, *Am J Sports Med* 4: 142-144, 1976.

28 Stillwell G: Further studies on the treatment of lymphedema, *Arch Phys Med Rehabil* 38: 435-441, 1957.

29 Wakim KG: Influence of centripetal rhythmic compression on localized edema of an extremity, *Arch Phys Med Rehabil* 36: 98-103, 1955.

30 Wilkerson J: Contrast baths and pressure treatment for ankle sprains, *Phys Sports Med* 7: 143, 1979.

31 Wilkerson J: Treatment of ankle sprains with external compression and early mobilization, *Phys Sports Med* 13(6): 83-90, 1985.

32 Wilkerson J: External compression for controlling traumatic edema, *Phys Sports Med* 13(6): 97-106, 1985.

33 Wilkerson J: Treatment of the inversion ankle sprain through synchronous application of local compression and cold, *Ath Train* 26: 220-237, 1991.

34 Winsor T, Selle W: The effect of venous compression on the circulation of the extremities, *Arch Phys Med Rehabil* 34: 559-565, 1953.

Massage

15

Clairbeth Lehn and William E. Prentice

OBJECTIVES

After completion of this chapter, the student will be able to do the following:

- Discuss the physiologic effects of massage, differentiating between reflexive and mechanical effects.

- Be aware of specific treatment guidelines and considerations when administering massage.

- Discuss the various strokes involved with classic Hoffa massage.

- Describe connective tissue massage.

- Discuss how acupressure massage is most effectively used, and identify the relationship between acupuncture and trigger points.

- Explain how myofascial release can be used to restore normal functional movement patterns.

- Discuss special message techniques, including Rolfing and Tragering.

The earliest available medical records seem to indicate that massage has played an important role in the treatment of sick and injured people.[20] A natural reaction when a part of the body hurts is to rub the injured area with a hand.

In early writings pertaining to medical treatments, little difference is shown between massage as we know it and general body exercise. Although there are very detailed descriptions of techniques, it is difficult to determine exactly what is meant because the terminology is unfamiliar. Language changes with time.

In Europe during the Middle Ages the influence of the Church of Rome and its religious teachings discouraged the use of massage as a healing practice. This brought the art to a halt until enlightened individuals strove to bring medical knowledge into the forefront and scholars in the medical fields started to again delve into how and why the body functions as it does.

The word massage is derived from two sources. One is the Arabic verb *mass,* to touch, and the other is the Greek word *massein,* to knead. However, history shows that this was not an art exclusive to the Greeks and Arabs. Massage was also known and practiced by the Egyptians, Romans, Japanese, Persians, and Chinese.

In Sweden in the early part of the nineteenth century, Peter H. Ling (1776 to 1839), the acknowledged founder of curative gymnastics, used massage as a branch of gymnastics. He appears to be the founder of modern day massage techniques, with some incorporation of French massage techniques into his system.[9]

Massage techniques, are based on the research and teachings of Albert Hoffa (1859 to 1907), James B. Mennell (1880 to 1957), and Gertrude Beard (1887 to 1971), have changed dramatically in the past 50 years. Medical practitioners of the twentieth century have added a scientific basis to massage, along with additional techniques and terms. In modern preventative and rehabilitative therapy, massage is a widely used therapeutic modality that seems to be gaining renewed interest within the sports-medicine community.[25]

PHYSIOLOGIC EFFECTS

Massage is a mechanical stimulation of the tissues by means of rhythmically applied pressure and stretching.[46] Over the years, many claims have been made relative to the therapeutic benefits of massage in the athletic population. Few claims are based on well controlled and designed studies.[4] Athletes have used massage to increase flexibility, coordination, and pain threshold[22]; to decrease neuromuscular excitability[35,40]; to stimulate circulation, thus improving energy transport to the muscle[27]; to facilitate healing and restore joint mobility[22]; and to remove lactic acid, thus alleviating muscle cramps.[26] There is little conclusive evidence of the efficacy of massage as an ergogenic aid in the athletic population.[19]

How these effects may be accomplished is determined by the specific approaches and applications used with massage techniques. Generally the effects of massage may be either reflexive or mechanical.[8] The effect of massage on the nervous system will differ greatly according to the method used, pressure exerted, and the duration of applications. Through the reflex mechanism, sedation is induced. Slow, gentle, rhythmical, and superficial effleurage may relieve tension and soothe, rendering the muscles more relaxed. This indicates a local effect on sensory and motor nerves and some central nervous system response. The mechanical approach seeks to make histologic changes in myofascial structures through direct force applied superficially.[8]

Reflexive Effects

The first approach in massage therapy involves a reflexive mechanism. The reflexive approach attempts to exert its effects through the skin and superficial connective tissues. Mobilization of soft tissue stimulates sensory receptors in the skin and superficial fascia.[8] If hands are passed lightly over the skin, a series of responses occurs as a result of the sensory stimulus of cutaneous receptors. This reflex mechanism is believed to be an autonomic nervous system phenomenon.[3] The reflex stimulus can occur alone (i.e., unaccompanied by the mechanical mechanism). Mennell[34] calls this the reflex effect. In itself, it is not an effect but the cause of an effect, causing sedation, relieving tension, and increasing blood flow.

EFFECTS ON PAIN. The effect of massage on pain is probably regulated by both the gate control theory and through the release of endogenous opiads (see Chapter 3). In gate control, cutaneous stimulation of large-diameter afferent nerve fibers effectively blocks transmission of pain information carried in small diameter nerve fibers. Stimulation of painful areas in the skin or myofascia can facilitate the release of β-endorphins and enkephalin, which essentially affect the transmission of pain-associated information in descending spinal tracts.

EFFECTS ON CIRCULATION. According to Pemberton,[36] the effect of massage on the circulation of the blood takes place through a reflex influence on blood vessels from a sympathetic division in the nervous system. Pemberton believes that vessels in the muscular system are emptied during massage not only by being squeezed but also by this reflex action. Effleurage produces an almost instantaneous reaction through transient dilation of lymphatics and small capillaries. Heavier pressure brings about a more lasting dilation. If capillary dilation occurs, blood volume and blood flow will increase producing an increase in temperature in the area being massaged.[14]

Massage increases lymphatic flow.[16] In the lymphatic system, movement of fluid depends on forces outside of the system. Such factors as gravity, muscle contraction, movement, and massage can affect the flow of lymph. Increased lymphatic flow will assist in the removal of edema.[7] When administering massage to an edematous part, elevation will also help to increase lymph flow.

EFFECTS ON METABOLISM. Massage does not alter general metabolism appreciably.[36] There is no change in acid-base equilibrium of blood. Massage does not appear to have any significant effects on the cardiovascular system.[5] Massage metabolically augments a chemical balance. The increased circulation means increased dispersion of waste products and an increase of fresh blood and oxygen. The mechanical movements assist in the removal and hasten the resynthesis of lactic acid.

Mechanical Effects

The second approach to massage is mechanical in nature. Techniques that stretch a muscle, elongate fascia, or mobilize soft tissue adhesions or restrictions are all mechanical. The mechanical effects are always accompanied by some reflex effects. As the mechanical stimulus becomes more effective, the reflex stimulus becomes less effective. Mechanical techniques should be performed after reflexive techniques. This is not to imply that mechanical techniques are more aggressive forms of massage. However, mechanical techniques are most often directed at deeper tissues, such as adhesions or restrictions in muscle, tendons, and fascia.

EFFECTS ON MUSCLE. The basic goal of massage on muscle tissue is to "maintain the muscle in the best possible state of nutrition, flexibility, and vitality so that after recovery from trauma or disease the muscle can function at its maximum."[46] Muscle massage is done either for mechanical stretching of the intramuscular connective tissue or to relieve pain and discomfort associated with myofascial trigger points. Massage has been shown to increase blood flow to skeletal muscle[13,47] and thus to increase venous return. It has retarded muscle atrophy after injury.[41] Massage has also increased the range of motion in hamstring muscles because of the combined decrease in neuromuscular excitability and stretching of muscle and scar tissue.[11] Massage does not increase muscle strength or bulk, nor does it increase muscle tone.

EFFECTS ON SKIN. Effects of massage on the skin include an increase in skin temperature, possibly as a result of direct mechanical effects, and indirect vasomotor action. Increased sweating and decreased skin resistance to galvanic current also result from massage.

If skin becomes adherent to underlying tissues and scar tissue is formed, friction massage can often be used to mechanically loosen the adhesions and to soften the scar. Massage toughens yet softens the skin. It acts directly on the surface of the skin to remove dead cells that result from prolonged casting (6 to 8 weeks). Massage can stretch and break down fibrous scar tissue. Massage can also break down adhesions between skin and subcutaneous tissue and stretch contracted or adhered tissue.

PSYCHOLOGIC EFFECTS

Psychologic effects of massage can be as beneficial to some patients as the physiologic effects. The "hands on" effect helps patients feel that someone is helping them. A general sedative effect can be most beneficial for the patient. Massage has lowered psychoemotional and somatic arousal, such as tension and anxiety.[29] The sports therapist's approach should inspire a feeling of confidence in the patient, and the patient should respond with a feeling of well being from being helped.

MASSAGE TREATMENT CONSIDERATIONS AND GUIDELINES

The sports therapist must have knowledge of basic anatomy and of the specific area being treated. The physiology of the area to be treated and the total function of the patient must be considered. There should be an understanding of the existing pathology so that the process by which repair occurs is known. The sports therapist needs a thorough knowledge of massage principles and skillful techniques, as well as manual dexterity, coordination, and concentration in the use of massage techniques. The sports therapist also needs to exhibit such traits as patience, a sense of caring, and courteousness both in speech and manner.

Perhaps the most important tools in massage therapy are the clinician's hands. They must be clean, warm, dry, and soft. The nails must be short and smooth. Hands must be washed before and after treatment for sanitary reasons. If the sports therapist's hands are cold, they should be placed in warm water for a short period. Rubbing them together briskly also helps to warm them.

Positioning is also important for the clinician. Correct positioning will allow relaxation, prevent fatigue, and permit free movement of arms, hands, and the body. Good posture will also help prevent fatigue and backache. The weight should rest evenly on both feet with the body in good postural alignment. When massaging a large area, the weight should shift from one foot to the other. You must be able to fit your hands to the contour of the area being treated. A good position is required to allow the correct application of pressure and rhythmic strokes during the procedure (Figure 15-1).

These points are important to consider when administering massage:
1. Pressure regulation should be determined by the type and amount of tissue present. It must also be governed by the patient's condition and which tissues

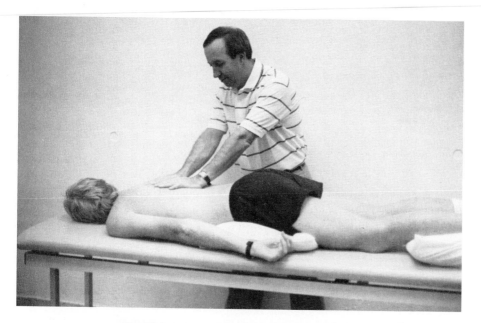

Fig. 15-1. Position of sports therapist for stroking.

are to be affected. The pressure must be delivered from the body, through the soft parts of the hands, and adjusted to contours of the patient's body parts.

2. Rhythm must be steady and even. The time for each stroke and between successive strokes should be equal.

3. Duration depends on the pathology, size of the area being treated, speed of motion, age, size, and condition of the patient. One also should observe the response of the patient to determine duration of the procedure. Massage of the back or the neck area might take 15 to 30 minutes. Massage of a large joint (such as a hip or shoulder) may require less than 10 minutes.

4. If swelling is present in an extremity, treatment should begin with the proximal part. This helps facilitate the lymphatic flow proximally. The subsequent effects of distal massage in removing fluid or edema will be more efficient, since the proximal resistance to lymphatic flow will be reduced. This technique has been referred to as the "uncorking effect."

5. Massage should never be painful, except possibly for friction massage, nor should it be given with such force that it causes ecchymosis (discoloration of the skin resulting from contusion).

6. In general, forces should be applied in the direction of the muscle fibers (Figure 15-2).

7. During a session, the sports therapist should begin and end with effleurage. The maneuvers should increase progressively to the greatest energy possible and end by decreasing energy maneuvers.

8. The sports therapist must consider the position in which massage can best be given and be sure the patient is warm comfortable, and relaxed.

9. The body part may be elevated if necessary and possible (Figure 15-3).

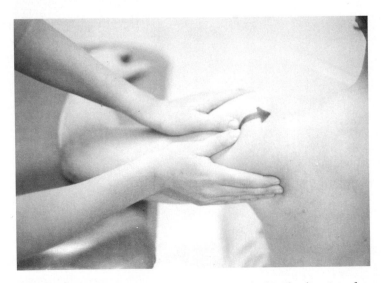

Fig. 15-2. In the application of massage, forces should be applied in the direction of muscle fibers.

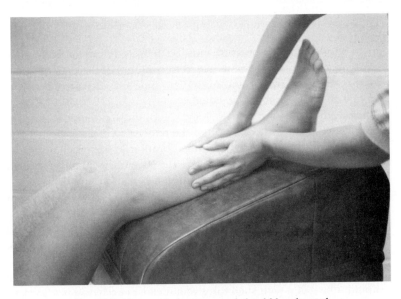

Fig. 15-3. The part being massaged should be elevated.

10. The sports therapist should be in a position in which the whole body, as well as hands and arms, can be relaxed and the procedure accomplished without strain (see Figure 15-1).
11. Sufficient lubricant should be used so that the therapist's hands will move smoothly along the skin surface (except in friction). Guard against using too much lubricant.
12. Massage should begin with superficial stroking; this stroke is used to spread the lubricant over the part being treated.

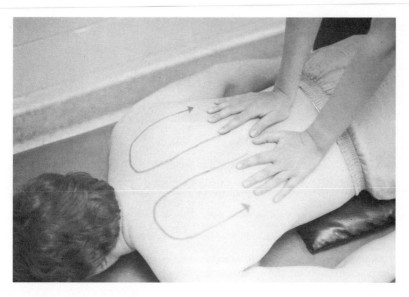

Fig. 15-4. Massage pressure should be in line of venous flow followed by a return stroke without pressure.

13. Each stroke should start at the joint or just below the joint (unless massage over joints is contraindicated) and finish above the joint so that strokes will overlap.

14. The pressure should be in line with venous flow followed by a return stroke without pressure. The pressure should be in the centripetal direction (Figure 15-4).

15. Care should be used over body areas. Hands should be relaxed and pressure adjusted to fit the contour of the area being treated.

16. Bony prominences and painful joints should be avoided if possible.

17. All strokes should be rhythmic. The pressure strokes should end with a swing off, in a small half circle, so that the rhythm will not be broken by an abrupt reversal.

Equipment

TABLE. A firm table, easily accessible from both sides, is most desirable. The height of the table should be reasonably comfortable for the sports therapist; leaning over or reaching up to perform the required movements should not be necessary. An adjustable table is almost a must in this situation. To facilitate cleaning and disinfecting, a washable plastic surface is much preferred. There should be a storage area close by for linens and lubricant. If the table is not padded, a mattress or foam pad should be used for the patient's comfort.

LINENS AND PILLOWS. The patient should be draped with a sheet so that only that part to be massaged is uncovered (Figure 15-5). Towels should be handy for removing the lubricant. A cotton sheet between the plastic surface of the table and the patient is required to absorb perspiration and to facilitate patient comfort. The surface of the plastic material is generally too cool for comfort. Pillows should be available to support the patient.

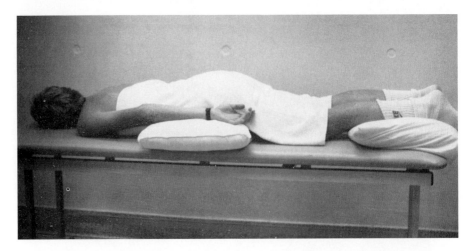

Fig. 15-5. Draping of prone patient. Towels are used for removal of lubricants, sheets are used for draping, and pillows are placed under hips and ankles for patient comfort.

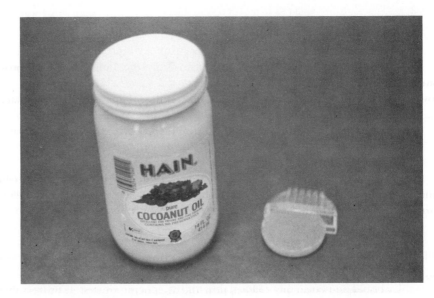

Fig. 15-6. Example of lubricant to be used, beeswax and coconut oil.

LUBRICANT. Some type of lubricant should be used in almost all massage movements to overcome friction and avoid irritation by ensuring smooth contact of hands and skin. If the patient's skin is too oily, it may be desirable to wash the skin first.

The lubricant should be of a type that is absorbed slightly by the skin but does not make it so slippery that the clinician finds it difficult to perform the required strokes. A light oil is recommended for lubrication. One that works well is a combination of one part beeswax to three parts coconut oil. These ingredients should be melted together and allowed to cool (Figure 15-6). It is best to use oil in situations in which (1) the clinician's or patient's skin is too dry, (2) a cast has recently been removed, (3) scar tissue is present, or (4) there is excess hair. Olive oil, mineral oil, cocoa butter, or hydrolanolin may be used. The "warm creams" or analgesic creams are skin irritants and, if used in conjunction with massage, may cause a burn, depending on the patient's skin type. These are also thought to cause blood to come to the surface of the skin, moving away from the muscles, which is the opposite of what we are trying to accomplish through the massage techniques.

Alcohol may be used to remove the lubricant after massage. It is suggested that alcohol be placed in the clinician's hands before application to avoid the dramatic temperature drop that occurs when alcohol is applied directly to the patient's skin.

Sometimes unscented powder should be used if the clinician's hands tend to perspire, or it may be used to prevent skin irritation.

Lubricant should not be used when applying friction movements, since a firm contact between the skin and hands of clinician must take place.

Preparation of the Patient

The patient's position is probably the most important element to ensure a beneficial muscle relaxation from massage. The patient should be in a relaxed, comfortable position. Lying down is most comfortable for the patient and permits gravity to assist in the venous blood flow.

The body part involved in treatment must be adequately supported, and it may be elevated, depending on the pathology. When the patient is treated in the prone position with massage of the neck, shoulders, back, buttocks, or back of the legs, a pillow or roll should be placed under the abdomen. Another pillow should be placed under the ankles so that the knees are slightly flexed (see Figure 15-5). If the patient is in the supine position, small pillows should be placed under the head and knees (Figure 15-7).

Sometimes the prone position will be too painful for a patient to assume for massaging a shoulder, upper back, or neck. The patient may be more comfortable sitting in a chair, facing the table, while leaning forward and supported by pillows on the table. Forearms and hands are on the table for additional support (Figure 15-8). The sports therapist can administer the massage while standing behind the patient.

The body areas not being treated should be covered to keep the patient from being chilled (see Figure 15-5). Clothing should be removed from the part being treated. Towels should cover any clothes near the area being treated to protect them from the lubricant (see Figure 15-5).

SPECIFIC MASSAGE TECHNIQUES
Hoffa Massage

Albert Hoffa's text, published in 1900, provides the basis for the various massage techniques that have developed over the years.[21] Hoffa massage is the classical massage technique, using a variety of superficial strokes including **effleurage, petrissage, tapotement,** and **vibration.** While some clinicians consider this technique to be mechanical, the strokes may be lighter and more superficial, thus making them more

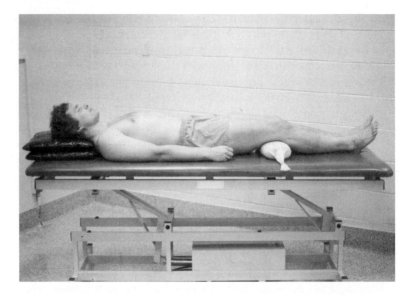

Fig. 15-7. Patient supine with pillow under head and knees.

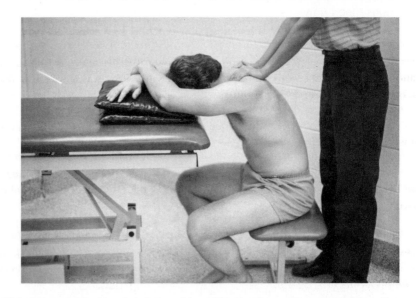

Fig. 15-8. Patient resting in a chair facing table and leaning forward is supported by pillows on the table with forearms and hands on the table for support. Sports therapist stands behind the patient.

reflexive in nature. This technique opens the door for more mechanical techniques directed toward underlying tissues.

EFFLEURAGE. This massage maneuver glides over the skin lightly without attempting to move the deep muscle masses. The main physiologic effect occurs when stroking is begun at the peripheral areas and moves toward the heart. The return flow of the venous and lymphatic systems is probably helped by this process. Circulation to

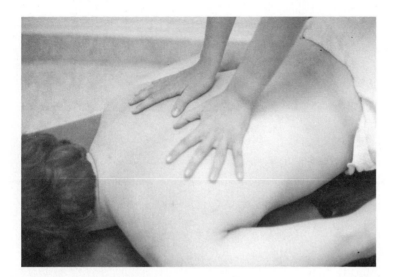

Fig. 15-9. The stroke is performed with the heel of the hand, fingers slightly bent and thumbs spread.

the skin surface is also increased by stroking; the success is traced to the increased rate of metabolic exchange in the peripheral areas.

The primary purpose of effleurage is to accustom the patient to the physical contact of the clinician. Initially effleurage serves to evenly distribute the lubricant. It also allows sensitive fingers to search for areas of muscle spasm or soreness and to locate trigger points and pressure points that can help determine the procedures to be used during the massage.

At the start of the massage, the stroke should be performed with a light pressure coming from the flat of the hand, with fingers slightly bent and thumbs spread (Figure 15-9). Once the unidirectional flow is established, going either centripetally or centrifugally, it should be continued throughout the treatment. The stroke should move toward the heart, and contact should be maintained with the patient at all times to enhance relaxation (Figure 15-10).

Deep stroking massage is also a form of effleurage, except it is given with more pressure to produce a mechanical as well as a reflexing effect (Figure 15-11).

Every massage begins and ends with effleurage. Stroking should also be used between other techniques. Stroking relaxes, decreases the defensive tension against harder massage techniques, and has a generally soothing effect.

PETRISSAGE. Petrissage consists of kneading manipulations that press and roll the muscles under the fingers or hands. There is no gliding over the skin except between progressions from one area to another. The muscles are gently squeezed, lifted, and relaxed. The hands may remain stationary or may travel slowly along the length of the muscle or limb. Petrissage increases venous and lymphatic return and presses metabolic waste products out of affected areas through intensive, vigorous action. This form of massage can also break up adhesions between the skin and underlying tissue, loosen adherent fibrous tissue, and increase skin elasticity.

Petrissage can be described as a kneading technique. It involves repeated

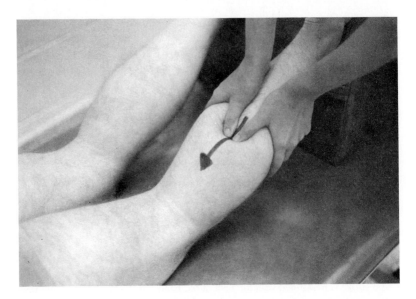

Fig. 15-10. The kneading stroke is directed toward the heart, and contact should be maintained with the patient.

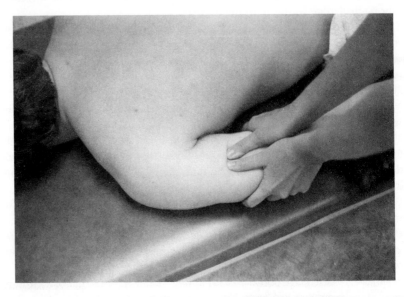

Fig. 15-11. Deep stroking massage.

grasping, application of pressure, releasing in a lifting or rolling motion, then moving an adjacent area (Figure 15-12). Smaller muscles may be kneaded with one hand (Figure 15-13). Larger muscles, such as the hamstrings or muscle groups, will require the use of both hands (Figure 15-14). When kneading, the hands should move from the distal to the proximal point of the muscle insertion, grasping parallel or perpendicular to the muscle fibers (see Figure 15-10).

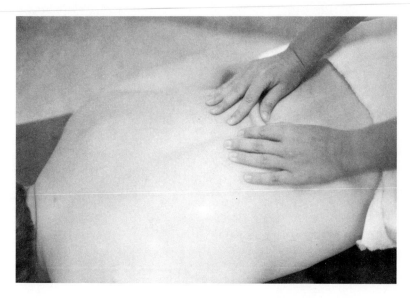

Fig. 15-12. Petrissage application on the back.

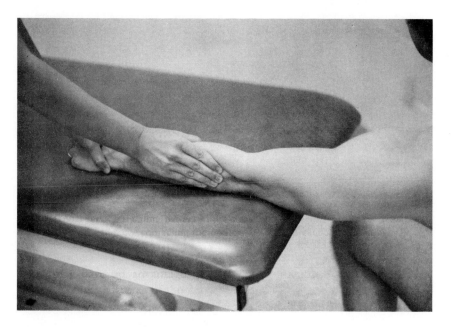

Fig. 15-13. Petrissage kneading with one hand.

TAPOTEMENT OR PERCUSSION. Percussion movements are a series of brisk blows, administered with relaxed hands and following each other in rapid alternating movements. This technique has a penetrating effect that is used to stimulate subcutaneous structures. Percussion is often used to increase circulation or to achieve

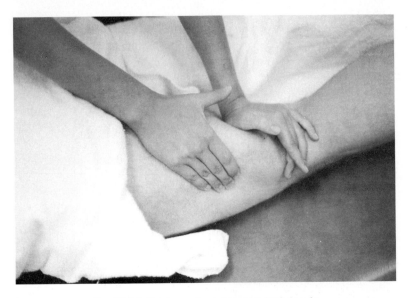

Fig. 15-14. Petrissage kneading with both hands.

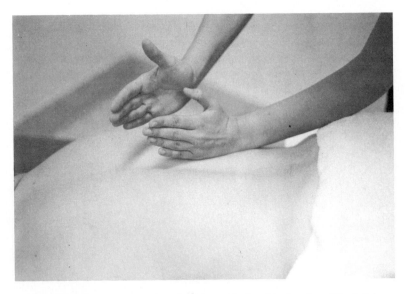

Fig. 15-15. Percussion stroke of striking with the ulnar border of the hand.

a more active blood flow. It stimulates peripheral nerve endings so that they convey impulses more strongly.

Types of percussion techniques are hacking-alternate striking of patient with the ulnar border of the hand (Figure 15-15); slapping-alternate slapping with fingers (Figure 15-16); beating-half-closed fist using the hypothenar eminence of the hand (Figure 15-17); tapping with the tips of the fingers (Figure 15-18); and clapping or

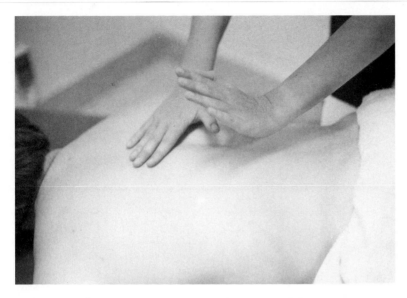

Fig. 15-16. Percussion stroke of slapping with fingers.

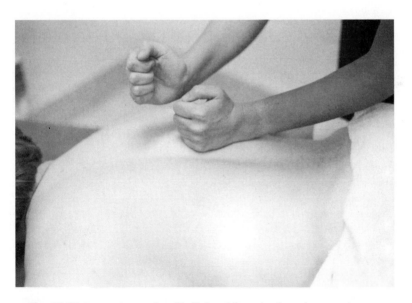

Fig. 15-17. Percussion stroke of half-closed fist using hypothenar eminence.

cupping using fingers, thumb, and palm together to form a concave surface (Figure 15-19). Clapping or cupping is used primarily in postural drainage.

VIBRATION. Vibration technique is a fine tremulous movement made by the hand or fingers placed firmly against a part; this causes the part to vibrate. The hands should remain in contact with the patient and a rhythmical trembling movement will come from the whole forearm through the elbow (Figure 15-20).

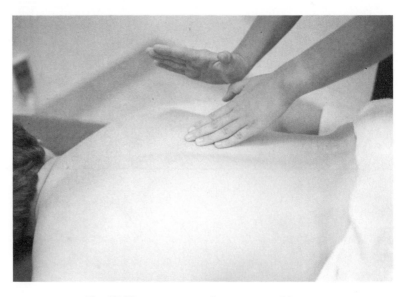

Fig. 15-18. Percussion stroke using tips of fingers.

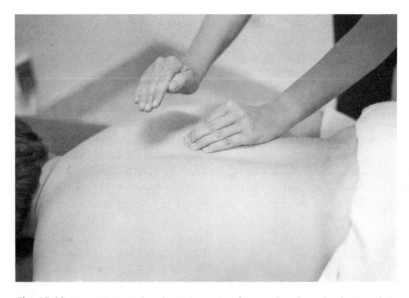

Fig. 15-19. Percussion stroke of cupping using fingers, thumb, and palm together.

ROUTINE. An example of a massage progression or routine would be:
1. Superficial stroking
2. Deep stroking
3. Kneading
4. Optional friction or tapotement
5. Deep stroking
6. Superficial stroking

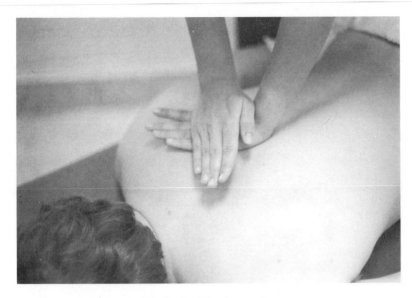

Fig. 15-20. Vibration stroke.

The various individual classic massage techniques alone, however, do not make for a good massage. A proper program, intensity, tempo, and rhythm, as well as the proper starting, climax, and closing of the massage, are all important. The form of the massage depends on the requirements of the patient.

INDICATIONS AND CONTRAINDICATIONS. The areas of treatment that sports therapists will most often see patients for are muscle, tendon, and joint conditions. Adhesions, muscle spasm, myositis, bursitis, fibrositis, tendinitis or tenosynovitis, and postural strain of the back all generally fall into this category.

Areas of concern that indicate that a patient should not be treated with massage include arteriosclerosis, thrombosis or embolism, severe varicose veins, acute phlebitis, cellulitis, synovitis, abscesses, skin injections, and cancers. Acute inflammatory conditions of the skin, soft tissues, or joints are also contraindications.

Friction Massage

James Cyriax and Gillean Russell[12] have used a deep **friction massage** to affect musculoskeletal ligament, tendon, and muscle structures to provide therapeutic movement over a small area. The purposes for friction movements are to loosen adherent fibrous tissue (scar), aid in the absorption of local edema or effusions, and reduce local muscular spasm. Inflammation around joints is softened and more readily broken down so that the formation of adhesions is prevented. Another purpose is to provide deep pressure over trigger points to produce reflex effects. This technique is performed by making small circular movements using the tips of the fingers, the thumb, or the heel of the hand (Figure 15-21). The superficial tissues are moved over the underlying structures by keeping the hand or fingers in firm contact with the skin (Figure 15-22).

Transverse friction massage is a technique for treating chronic tendon inflammations.[12] Inflammation is an important part of the healing process. It must occur

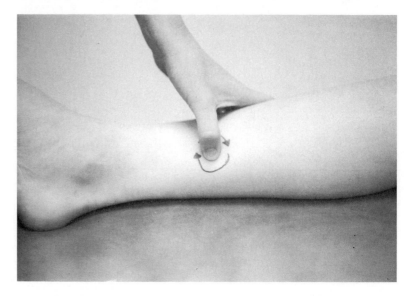

Fig. 15-21. Thumb movement in a circle on an acupressure point.

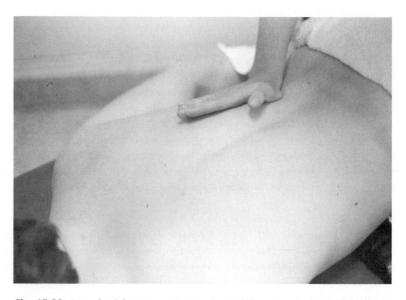

Fig. 15-22. Superficial friction applied to the back by using the heel of the hand.

before the healing process can advance to the fibroblastic stage. In chronic inflammations, however, the inflammatory process "gets stuck" and never really accomplishes what it is supposed to. The purpose of transverse friction massage is to increase the inflammation to a point where the inflammatory process is complete and the injury can progress to the later stages of the healing process. This technique is used

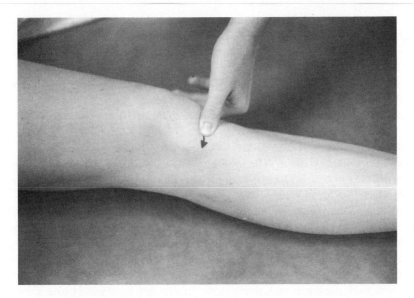

Fig. 15-23. Transverse tendon friction massage on the patellar tendon.

most often in chronic overuse problems, such as lateral or medial humeral epicondylitis, "jumper's knee," and rotator cuff tendinitis.

The technique involves placing the tendon on a slight stretch. Massage is done using the thumb or index finger to exert intense pressure in a direction perpendicular to the direction of the fibers being massaged (Figure 15-23). The massage should last for 7 to 10 minutes and should be done every other day. Since transverse friction massage is a painful technique, ice may be applied to the treatment area before massage for analgesic purposes.

Connective Tissue Massage

Connective tissue massage (Bindegewebsmassage) was developed by Elizabeth Dicke, a German physical therapist who suffered from decreased circulation in her right lower extremity for which amputation was advised. In trying to relieve her lower back pain, she massaged the area with pulling strokes. She found that with the continued stroking there was a relaxation of the muscular tension and a prickling warmth in the area. She continued the technique on herself, and after 3 months, she had no low back pain and she had restored circulation to her right leg.

Connective tissue massage is a stroking technique carried out in the layers of connective tissue on the body surface. This stimulates the nerve endings of the autonomic nervous system. Afferent impulses travel to the spinal cord and the brain, causing a change in reaction susceptibility.[34]

Connective tissue is an organ of metabolism, therefore abnormal tension in one part of the tissue is reflected in other parts. All pathologic changes involve an inflammatory reaction in the affected part. One of the changes caused by inflammatory reaction is accumulation of fluid in the affected area. The area where these changes can most readily be detected is on the body surface. These changes are often seen as flattened areas or depressed bands that may be surrounded by elevated areas. The flat areas are the areas of main response, and the connective tissue is tight, resisting pulling in any direction with movement.

The technique of connective tissue massage is not used as much in the United States as it is in European countries, especially Germany. As more results are seen, especially in the treatment of diseases associated with the pathology of circulation, this technique should become more widely accepted and used in this country.

GENERAL PRINCIPLES OF CONNECTIVE TISSUE MASSAGE

Position of the patient. The patient is usually in the sitting position for a connective tissue massage. Occasionally patients may be treated in a sidelying or prone position when they cannot be treated in a sitting position.

Position of the therapist. The sports therapist should be in a position, seated or standing, that provides good body mechanics, is comfortable, and avoids fatigue.

Application technique. The basic pulling stroke is performed with the tips, or pads, of the middle and ring fingers of either hand. Fingernails must be very short. The stroking technique is characterized by a tangential pull on the skin and subcutaneous tissues away from the fascia with the fingers. This technique should cause a sharp pain in the tissue. The stroke is a pull, not a push of the tissue. No lubricant is used. All treatments are started by the basic strokes from the coccyx to the first lumbar vertebra. Treatments last about 15 to 25 minutes. After 15 treatments, which are carried out two to three times per week, there should be a rest period of at least 4 weeks.

Other considerations. Before any logical plan for treatment can be made, it is important to determine where any alterations in the optimum function of connective tissue have taken place, where the changes started, and if possible the cause of the alteration.

Evaluation is a most important part of an effective connective tissue massage program. The technique of stroking with two fingers of one hand along each side of the vertebral column will give much information about the sensory changes that are caused by alterations in the tension of surface tissues.

INDICATIONS AND CONTRAINDICATIONS. There are numerous arterial and venous disorders that may respond to connective tissue massage. Specific disabilities include: (1) scars on the skin; (2) fractures and arthritis in the bones and joints; (3) lower back pain and torticollis in the muscles; (4) varicose symptoms, thrombophlebitis (subacute), hemorrhoids, and edema in the blood and lymph; (5) Raynaud's disease, intermittent claudication, frostbite, and trophic changes in the circulatory system. Connective tissue massage can also be used for myocardial dysfunctions, respiratory disturbances, intestinal disorders, ulcers, hepatitis, infections of the ovaries and uterus (subacute), amenorrhea, dysmenorrhea, genital infantilism, multiple sclerosis, Parkinson's disease, headaches, migraines, and allergies. Connective tissue massage is recommended to help in the process of revascularization after orthopedic complications, such as fractures, dislocations, and sprains.

Contraindications to connective tissue massage include tuberculosis, tumors, and mental illnesses that result from psychologic dependence.

Connective tissue massage must be learned and performed initially under the direct supervision of someone who has been taught these highly specialized techniques. More detailed information about connective tissue massage can be found in the bibliography.[15,28,42]

Acupressure and Trigger Point Massage

Acupressure is a type of massage based on the ancient Chinese art of acupuncture. Acupuncture, along with herbal medicine, comprises traditional Chinese medicine. Only recently has the amount of research, publication, and interest in acupuncture in Western medical literature increased dramatically.

The Chinese make no distinction between arteries, veins, or nerves when explaining the functions of the body.[30] They concentrate instead on an elaborate system of forces whose interplay is thought to regulate all bodily functions. The traditional, philosophical Chinese explanation has little correlation with the more scientifically oriented Western concepts of medicine, which rely heavily on anatomic and physiologic principles. Consequently, use of acupuncture as a therapeutic technique in Western medical practice has encountered considerable skepticism.

The Chinese believe that an essential life force known as Qi (pronounced che) exists in everyone and controls all aspects of life. Qi is governed by the interplay of two opposing forces, the yang (positive) forces and the yin (negative) forces. Disease and pain result from some imbalance between the two.[31] The yin and yang flow through body passageways or lines called jing by the Chinese and known as meridians in the west. The twelve meridians within the body are named according to the part of the body with which they are associated. The meridians on one side of the body are duplicated by those on the other; however, two additional meridians exist that cannot be paired.[32]

1. Lung (L)
2. Large Intestine (LI)
3. Stomach (ST)
4. Spleen (SP)
5. Heart (H)
6. Small intestine (SI)
7. Urinary bladder (UB)
8. Kidney (K)
9. Pericardium (P)
10. Triple warmet (TW)
11. Gallbladder (GB)
12. Liver (LIV)
13. Governing Vessel (GV)*
14. Conception Vessel (CV)*

Along these meridians lie the acupuncture points that are associated with each particular meridian. These points are named according to the meridian on which they lie. Whenever there is pain or illness, certain points on the surface of the body become tender.[32] When pain is eliminated or the disease is cured, these tender points seem to disappear.[1] According to acupuncture theory, stimulation of specific points through needling can dramatically reduce pain in areas of the body known to be associated with a particular point. Thousands of acupuncture points have been identified by the Chinese. In the Nei Ching,[23] a classical text on Chinese medicine, 365 points that lie on the meridians have been enumerated. Additional acupuncture points have been identified on the auricle as well as the hand.

There is some evidence for the physical existence of these points.[45] The electrical resistance of the skin at certain points corresponding to the acupuncture points is lower than that of the surrounding skin, especially when a disease state is present.

---

* Not paired.

Examining acupuncture points by sectioning indicated increases nerve endings at these points. Russian investigators have reportedly discovered differences in skin temperature at these points. Despite this evidence, there is no definite physical attribute of all acupuncture points, nor is there a thoroughly demonstrated mode of action for the technique. Whatever the explanation, it appears that the locations and effects of stimulating specific acupuncture points for the relief of pain were determined empirically.[33]

In Western medicine, the counterpart of the acupuncture point is the **trigger point.** Trigger points may be found in skeletal muscle and tendons, in myofascia, in ligaments and capsules surrounding joints, in periosteum, and in the skin. Trigger points may activate and become painful due to some trauma to the muscle occurring either from direct trauma or from overuse that results in some inflammatory response.[44] Like acupuncture points, pain is usually referred to areas that follow a specific pattern associated with a particular point. Stimulation of these points has also been demonstrated to result in pain relief.[17]

Acupuncture and trigger points are not necessarily one and the same. However, a study by Melzack, Stillwell and Fox,[33] attempted to develop a correlation coefficient between acupuncture and trigger points on the basis of two criteria: spatial distribution and associated pain patterns. They found a remarkably high correlation coefficient of .84, which suggested that acupuncture and trigger points used for pain relief, although discovered independently, labeled by totally different methods, and derived from such different concepts of medicine, represent a similar phenomenon and may be explained by the same underlying neural mechanisms.[33]

Physiologic explanations of the effectiveness of acupressure massage may be attributed to some interaction of the various mechanisms of pain modulation discussed in Chapter 3.[1] There is considerable evidence that intense, low-frequency stimulation of these points triggers the release of β-endorphin.[37,39,42]

ACUPRESSURE MASSAGE TECHNIQUES. By using acupuncture charts (Figure 15-24) or trigger point charts[44], specific points are selected that are described in the literature as having some relationship to the area of pain. The charts provide the sports therapist with a general idea of where these points are located. Two techniques may be used to specifically locate acupressure and trigger points. Since electrical impedance is reduced at these points, an ohmmeter may be used to locate the points. Perhaps the easiest technique is simply to palpate the area until either a small fibrous nodule or a strip of tense muscle tissue that is tender to the touch is felt.[6,9,10]

Once the point is located, massage is begun using the index or middle fingers, the thumb, or perhaps the elbow. Small circular motions are used on the point. The amount of pressure applied to these acupressure points should be determined by patient tolerance; however, it must be intense and will likely be painful to the patient. Generally, the more pressure the patient can tolerate, the more effective the treatment.

Effective treatment times range from 1 to 5 minutes at a single point per treatment. It may be necessary to massage several points during the treatment to obtain the greatest effects. If this is the case, it is best to work distal points first and then move proximally.

During the massage, the patient will report a dulling or numbing effect and will frequently indicate that the pain diminishes or subsides totally during the massage. The lingering effects of acupressure massage vary tremendously from patient to patient. The

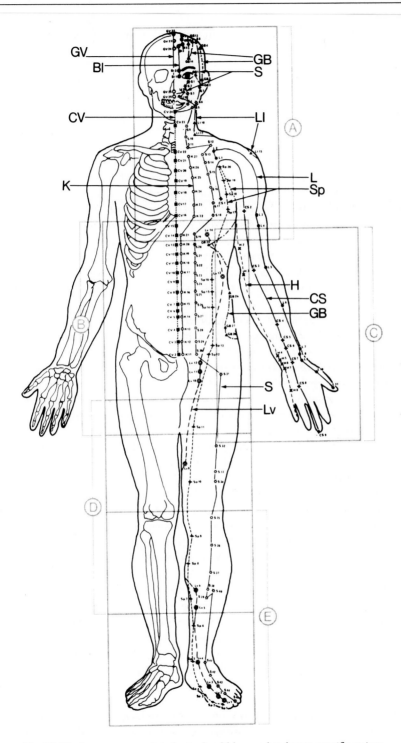

Fig. 15-24. Acupuncture point charts should be used to locate specific points.

effects may last for only a few minutes in some but may persist in others for several hours.

Myofascial Release

Myofascial release refers to a group of techniques used to relieve soft tissue from the abnormal grip of tight fascia.[24] It is essentially a form of stretching that has had significant impact in treating a variety of conditions. In addition to an in-depth understanding of the fascial system, some specialized training is necessary for the sports therapist to understand specific techniques of myofascial release.[2]

Fascia is a type of connective tissue that surrounds muscles, tendons, nerves, bones, and organs. It is essentially continuous from head to toe and is interconnected in various sheaths or planes. Fascia is composed primarily of collagen along with some elastic fibers. During movement the fascia must stretch and move freely. If there is damage to the fascia caused by injury, disease, or inflammation, it will not only affect local adjacent structures but may also affect areas far removed from the injury site. Thus it may be necessary to release tightness in both the area of injury and in distant areas.[24] Fascia tends to soften and release in response to gentle pressure over a relatively long period of time.[24]

Myofascial release has also been referred to as soft tissue mobilization, although technically all forms of massage involve mobilization of soft tissue. Soft tissue mobilization should not be confused with joint mobilization, although the two are closely related. Joint mobilization is used to restore normal joint arthrokinematics, and specific rules exist regarding direction of movement and joint position based on the shape of the articulating surfaces. Myofascial restrictions are considerably more unpredictable and may occur in many different planes and directions. Myofascial treatment is based on localizing the restriction and moving into the direction of the restriction, regardless of whether that follows the arthrokinematics of a nearby joint.[8] Thus myofascial manipulation is considerably more subjective and relies heavily on the clinician's experience.

Myofascial manipulation focuses on large treatment areas, while joint mobilization focuses on a specific joint. Releasing myofascial restrictions over a large treatment area can significantly impact joint mobility.[18] Once a myofascial restriction is located, the massage should be applied directly through the restriction. The progression of the technique is from superficial to deep. Once more superficial restrictions are released, the deep restrictions can be located and released without causing any damage to superficial tissues. Joint mobilization should follow myofascial release and will likely be more effective once soft tissue restrictions are eliminated.

As the extensibility is improved in the myofascia, elongation and stretching of the musculotendinous unit should be incorporated. In addition, strengthening exercises are recommended to enhance neuromuscular reeducation, which helps promote new, more efficient movement patterns. As freedom of movement improves, postural reduction may help to ensure the maintenance of the less restricted movement patterns.

Generally, release is accomplished by using an extremely mild combination of pressure and stretch. Acute cases tend to resolve in just a few treatments. The longer a condition has been present, the longer it will take to resolve. Occasionally dramatic

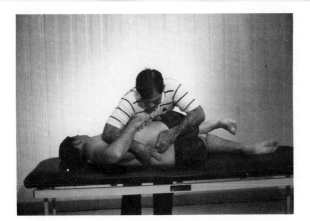

Fig. 15-25. Myofascial release is a mild combination of pressure and stretch used to free soft tissue restrictions.

results will occur immediately after treatment. It is usually recommended that treatment be done at least three times per week.[11]

TREATMENT CONSIDERATIONS

Protecting the hands. The hands are certainly the primary treatment modality in all forms of massage. In myofascial release they are constantly subjected to stress and strain, and consideration must be given to their protection. It is essential to avoid constant hyperextension or hyperflexion of any joints, which may lead to hypermobility. If it is necessary to work in deeper tissues where more force is necessary, the fist or elbow may be substituted for the thumb and fingers.[8]

Use of lubricant. It is necessary to use a small amount of lubricant, particularly if large areas are to be treated using long stroking movements. Enough lubricant should be used to allow for traction while reducing painful friction without allowing the hands to slip on the skin.[8]

Positioning of the patient. As with the other forms of massage, it is critical to appropriately position the athlete such that the effects of the treatment may be maximized. Pillows or towel rolls may aid in establishing effective treatment position even before the hands contact the patient (Figure 15-25). The sports therapist should make certain that good body mechanics and positioning are considered to protect him or her as well as the patient.

Rolfing®

Rolfing, also referred to as *structural integration,* is a system devised by Ida Rolf that is used to correct inefficient structure or to "integrate structure." The goal of this technique is to balance the body within a gravitational field through a technique involving manual soft tissue manipulation.[8] The basic principle of treatment is that if balanced movement is essential at a particular joint yet nearby tissue is restrained, both the tissue and the joint will relocate to a position that accomplishes a more appropriate equilibrium.[38]

Rolfing is a standardized approach that is administered without regard to symptoms or specific pathologies. The technique involves 10-hour sessions, each of which emphasizes some aspect of posture with the massage directed toward the myofascia. The 10 sessions include the following:

1. Respiration
2. Balance under the body (legs and feet)
3. Sagittal plane balance—lateral line from front to back
4. Balance left to right—base of body to midline
5. Pelvic balance—rectus abdominis and psoas
6. Weight transfer from head to feet—sacrum
7. Relationship of head to rest of body—occiput and atlas
8. and 9. Upper half of the body to lower half of the body relationship
10. Balance throughout the system

Once these 10 treatments are completed, advanced sessions may be performed in addition to periodic "tune-up" sessions.

A major aspect of this treatment approach is to integrate the structural with the psychologic. An emotional state may be seen as the projection of structural imbalances. The easiest and most effecient method for changing the physical body is through direct intervention in the body. Changing the structural imbalances can alter the psychologic component.[38]

Trager®

Developed by Milton Trager, **Tragering** combines mechanical soft tissue mobilization and neurophysiologic reeducation.[43] Unlike Rolfing, Tragering has no standardized protocols or procedures. The Trager system uses gentle, passive, rocking oscillations of a body part. This is essentially a mobilization technique emphasizing traction and rotation as a relaxation technique to encourage the patient to relinquish control. This relaxation technique is followed by a series of active movements designed to alter the patient's neurophysiologic control of movement, thus providing a basis for maintaining these changes. This technique does not attempt to make mechanical changes in the soft tissues, but it attempts to establish neuromuscular control so that more normal movement patterns can be routinely performed. Essentially it uses the nervous system to make changes rather than making mechanical changes in the tissues themselves.

SUMMARY

1. Massage, as we know it today, is an improved and more scientific version of the various procedures that go back for thousands of years to the Greeks, Egyptians, and others.
2. Massage is the mechanical stimulation of tissue by means of rhythmically applied pressure and stretching. It allows the sports therapist, as a health-care provider, to assist a patient to overcome pain and to relax through the application of the therapeutic massage techniques.
3. Massage has effects on the circulation, the lymphatic system, the nervous system, the muscles, myofascia, the skin, scar tissue, psychologic responses, relaxation feelings, and pain.

4. Hoffa massage is the classic form of massage and uses strokes including effleurage, petrissage, percussion or tapotement, and vibration.

5. Friction massage is used to increase the inflammatory response, particularly in cases of chronic tendinitis or tenosynovitis.

6. Massage of acupuncture and trigger points is used to reduce pain and irritation in anatomic areas known to be associated with specific points.

7. Connective tissue massage is a reflex zone massage. It is a relatively new form of treatment in this country and has its best effects on circulatory pathologies.

8. Myofascial release is a massage technique used to relieve soft tissue from the abnormal grip of tight fascia.

9. Rolfing is a system devised to correct inefficient structure by balancing the body within a gravitational field through a technique involving manual soft tissue manipulation.

10. Trager attempts to establish neuromuscular control so that more normal movement patterns can be routinely performed.

GLOSSARY

acupressure The technique of using finger pressure over acupuncture points to decrease pain.

Bindegewebsmassage Reflex zone massage; uses a pulling stroke across connective tissue to effect change.

effleurage To stroke; any stroke that glides over the skin without attempting to move the deep muscle masses. The hand is molded to the part, stroking with more or less constant pressure, usually upward. Any degree of pressure may be applied, varying from the lightest possible touch to very deep pressure.

friction massage A technique that affects fibrositic adhesions in tendon, muscle, or ligament. It is performed by small circular movements that penetrate into the depth of a muscle, not by moving the finger on the skin, but by moving the tissues under the skin.

massage The act of rubbing, kneading, or stroking the superficial parts of the body with the hand or with an instrument for the purpose of modifying nutrition, restoring power of movement, or breaking up adhesions.

myofascial release A group of techniques used to relieve soft tissue from the abnormal grip of tight fascia.

petrissage Massage technique that is a kneading manipulation. Consists of repeatedly grasping and releasing the tissue with one or both hands or parts thereof in a lifting, rolling, or pressing movement. The outside characteristic of this movement as contrasted to stroking movements is that the pressure is applied intermittently.

Rolfing A system devised to correct inefficient structure by balancing the body within a gravitational field through a technique involving manual soft tissue manipulation.

tapotement A percussion massage; any series of brisk blows following each other in a rapid alternating fashion: hacking, cupping, slapping, beating, tapping, and pinchment. It is used when stimulation is the objective.

Trager A technique that attempts to establish neuromuscular control so that more normal movement patterns can be routinely performed.

trigger point A spot of exquisite tenderness within a band of muscle.

vibration A shaking massage technique; a fine tremulous movement made by the hand or fingers placed firmly against a part that will cause the part to vibrate. Often used for a soothing effect; may be stimulating when more energy is applied.

REFERENCES

1 Baldry PE: *Acupuncture, trigger points and musculoskeletal pain,* London, 1993, Churchill Livingstone.

2 Barnes J: Five years of myofascial release, *Phys Ther* 6(37): 12-14, 1987.

3 Barr J, Taslitz N: Influence of back massage on autonomic functions, *Phys Ther* 50: 1679-1691, 1970.

4 Birukov AA: Training massage during contemporary sports loads, *Soviet Sports Review* 22: 42-44, 1987.

5 Boone T, Cooper R, Thompson W: A physiologic evaluation of the sports massage, *Ath Train* 26(1): 51-54, 1991.

6 Brickey R, Yao J: *Acupuncture and transcutaneous electrical stimulation techniques,* course manual in acutherapy post graduate seminars, Raleigh, NC, 1978.

7 Cafarelli E: Vibratory massage and short-term recovery from muscular fatigue, *Inter J Sports Med* 11: 474, 1990.

8 Cantu RI, Grodin AJ: *Myofascial manipulation: theory and*

clinical applications, Gaithersburg, Md, 1992, Aspen Publications.

9 Castel J: *Pain management with acupuncture and transcutaneous electrical nerve stimulation techniques and photo stimulation* (Laser), course manual, 1982.

10 Cheng R, Pomerantz B: Electroacupuncture analgesia could be mediated by at least two pain relieving mechanisms: endorphin and non-endorphin systems, *Life Sci* 25: 1957-1962, 1979.

11 Crosman LJ, Chateauvert SR, Weisberg J: The effects of massage to the hamstring muscle group on range of motion, *J Orthop Sport Phys Ther* 6: 168, 1984.

12 Cyriax J, Russell G: *Textbook of orthopedic medicine*, vol II., ed 10, Baltimore, 1980, Williams & Wilkins.

13 Dubrovsky VI: Changes in muscle and venous blood flow after massage, *Soviet Sports Review* 18: 134-135, 1983.

14 Ebel A, Wisham LH: Effect of massage on muscle temperature and radiosodium clearance, *Arch Phys Med Rehabil* 33: 399-405, 1952.

15 Ebner M: *Connective tissue manipulations*, Malibar, Fla, 1985, RE Krieger.

16 Elkins EC: Effects of various procedures on flow of lymph, *Arch Phys Med Rehabil* 34: 31-39, 1953.

17 Fox E, Melzack R: Transcutaneous electrical stimulation and acupuncture: comparison of treatment for low back pain, *Pain* 2: 357-373, 1976.

18 Gordon P: *Myofascial reorganization*, Brookline, Mass, 1988, The Gordon Group.

19 Harmer PA: The effect of pre-performance massage on stride frequency in sprinters, *Ath Train* 26(1): 55-59, 1991.

20 Head H: Die *sensibilitatorungen der haut bei viszeral erkran kungen*, Berlin, 1898.

21 Hoffa AJ: *Technik der massage*, ed 14, Stuttgart, Germany, 1900, Ferdinand Enke.

22 Hungerford MH, Bornstein R: Sports massage, *Sports Med Guide* 4: 4-6, 1985.

23 *Hwang Ti Nei Ching (translation)*, Berkeley, 1973, University of California Press.

24 Juett T: Myofascial release: an introduction for the patient, *Phys Ther* 7(41): 7-8, 1988.

25 King RK: *Performance massage*, Champaign, Ill, 1993, Human Kinetics.

26 Kopysov VS: Use of vibrational massage in regulating the pre-competition condition of weight lifters, *Soviet Sports Review* 14: 82-84, 1979.

27 Kuprian W: *Massage*. In Kuprian W, editor: *Physical therapy for sports*, Philadelphia, 1981, WB Saunders.

28 Licht S: *Massage, manipulation and traction*, New Haven, 1960, Elizabeth Licht.

29 Longworth JC: Psychophysiological effects of slow stroke back massage in normotensive females, *Adv Nurs Science* 10: 44-61, 1982.

30 Man P, Chen C: Acupuncture anesthesia: a new theory and clinical study, *Curr Ther Res* 14: 390-394, 1972.

31 Manaka Y: On certain electrical phenomena for the interpretation of Chi in Chinese literature, *Am J Chin Med* 3: 71-74, 1975.

32 Mann F: *Acupuncture: the ancient Chinese art of healing and how it works scientifically*, New York, 1973, Random House.

33 Melzack R, Stillwell D, Fox E: Trigger points and acupuncture points for pain: correlations and implications, *Pain* 3: 3-23, 1977.

34 Mennell JB: *Physical treatment*, ed 5, Philadelphia, 1968, Blakiston.

35 Morelli M, Seaborne PT, Sullivan SJ: Changes in H-reflex amplitude during massage of triceps surae in healthy subjects, *J Orthop Sports Phys Ther* 12(2): 55-59, 1990.

36 Pemberton R: *The physiologic influence of massage*. In Mock HE, Pemberton R, Coulter JS, editors: *Principles and practices of physical therapy*, vol I, Hagerstown, Md, 1939, WF Prior.

37 Prentice W: The use of electroacutherapy in the treatment of inversion ankle sprains, *J Nat Athl Train Assoc* 17(1): 15-21, 1982.

38 Rolf IP: *Rolfing: the integration of human structures*, Rochester, Vt, 1977, Healing Arts Press.

39 Sjolund B, Eriksson M: Electroacupuncture and endogenous morphines, *Lancet* 2: 1085, 1976.

40 Sullivan SJ: Effects of massage on alpha motorneuron excitability, *Phys Ther* 71: 555, 1991.

41 Suskind MI, Hajek N, Hinds H: Effects of massage on denervated muscle, *Arch Phys Med Rehabil* 27: 133-135, 1946.

42 Tappan F: *Healing massage techniques: holistic, classic, and emerging methods*, East Norwalk, Conn, 1988, Appleton & Lange.

43 Trager M: Trager psychophysical integration and mentastics, *Trager Journal*, 5: 10, 1982.

44 Travell JG, Simons DG: *Myofascial pain and dysfunction: the trigger point manual*, Baltimore, 1983, Williams & Wilkins.

45 Wei L: Scientific advances in Chinese medicine *Am J Chin Med* 7: 53-75, 1979.

46 Wood E, Becker P: *Beard's massage*, Philadelphia, 1981, WB Saunders.

47 Wyper DJ, McNiven D: Effects of some physiotherapeutic agents on skeletal muscle blood flow, *Phys Ther* 62: 83-85, 1976.

SUGGESTED READINGS

Bean B, Henderson H, Martinsen M: Massage: how to do it and what it can do for you, *Scholastic Coach* 52(5): 10-11, 1982.

Beard G: A history of massage technique, *Phys Ther* 32: 613-624, 1952.

Beard G, Wood EC: *Massage: principles and techniques*, Philadelphia, 1964, WB Saunders.

Breakey BM: An overlooked therapy you can use ad lib, *RN* 45: 7, 1982.

Chamberlain G: Cyriax's friction massage: a review, *J Orthop Sports Phys Ther* 4(1): 16-22, 1982.

Cyriax J: *Textbook of orthopedic medicine*, vol I, ed 8, New York, 1982, Macmillan Publishing.

Day JA, Mason PR, Chesrow SE: Effect of massage on serum level of β-endorphin and β-lipotrophin in healthy adults, *Phys Ther* 67: 926-930, 1987.

Ebner M: Connective tissue massage, *Physiotherapy* 64: 208-210, 1978.

Ernst E, Matra A, Magyarosy I: Massages cause changes in blood fluidity, *Physiotherapy* 73: 43-45, 1987.

Hall D: A practical guide to the art of massage, *Runner's World,* 14(10): 5-59, 1979.

Hollis M: *Massage for therapists,* Oxford, England, 1987, Blackwell Scientific Publications.

Hovind H, Neilson SL: Effect of massage on blood flow in skeletal muscle, *Scand J Rehabil Med* 6: 74-77, 1974.

Kewley M: What you should know about massage, *International Swimmer* September: 29-30, 1982.

Martin D: Massage, *Jogger* 10(5): 8-15, 1978.

McKeechie AA: Anxiety states: a preliminary report on the value of connective tissue massage, *J Psychosomatic Res* 27(2): 125-129, 1983.

Meagher J, Boughton P: *Sportsmassage,* New York, 1980, Doubleday.

Morelli M, Seaborne PT, Sullivan SJ: H-reflex modulation during massage of triceps surae in healthy subjects, *Arch Phys Med Rehabil* 72: 915, 1991.

Phaigh R, Perry P: *Athletic massage,* New York, 1984, Simon & Schuster.

Rogoff J: *Manipulation, traction and massage,* ed 2, Baltimore, 1980, Williams & Wilkins.

Ryan J: The neglected art of massage, *Phys Sports Med* 18(12): 25, 1980.

Stamford B: Massage for athletes, *Phys Sports Med* 13(10): 178, 1985.

Tappan F: *Healing massage techniques: a study of eastern and western methods,* Reston, Va., 1978, Reston.

Wakim KG, Martin GM, Terrier JC: The effects of massage in normal and paralyzed extremities, *Arch Phys Med Rehabil* 30: 135-144, 1949.

Wiktorrson-Moeller M, Oberg B, Ekstrand J: Effects of warming up, massage and stretching on range of motion and muscle strength in the lower extremity, *Am J Sports Med* 11: 249-251, 1983.

Locations of the Motor Points

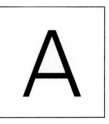

The illustrations in this appendix show the locations of the motor points located on the extremities and the torso. (Courtesy Mettler Electronics Corporation, 1333 S. Claudina Street, Anaheim, CA 92805.)

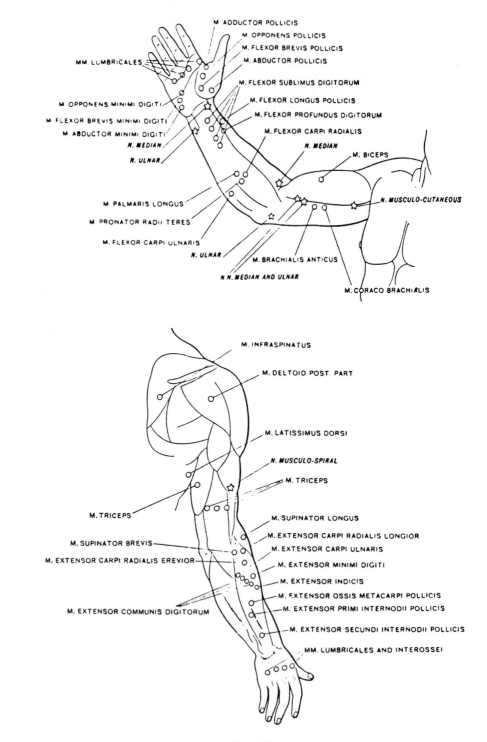

Fig. A-1.

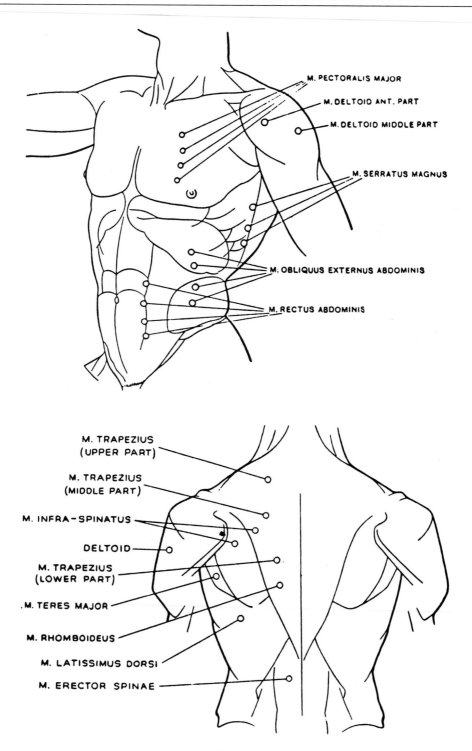

M. PECTORALIS MAJOR

M. DELTOID ANT. PART

M. DELTOID MIDDLE PART

M. SERRATUS MAGNUS

M. OBLIQUUS EXTERNUS ABDOMINIS

M. RECTUS ABDOMINIS

M. TRAPEZIUS
(UPPER PART)

M. TRAPEZIUS
(MIDDLE PART)

M. INFRA-SPINATUS

DELTOID

M. TRAPEZIUS
(LOWER PART)

.M. TERES MAJOR

M. RHOMBOIDEUS

M. LATISSIMUS DORSI

M. ERECTOR SPINAE

Fig. A-2.

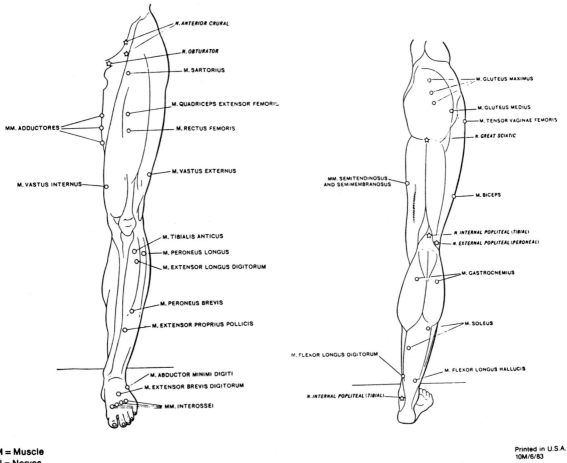

M = Muscle
N = Nerves

Printed in U.S.A.
10M/6/83

Fig. A-3.

List of Therapeutic Modality Equipment Manufacturers and Distributors

B

ELECTROTHERAPY
Electrodes

AdvanTeq Development Corp
12509 Crenshaw Blvd
Hawthorne, CA 90250
800/234-7846

AliMed Inc
297 High St
Dedham, MA 02026
617/329-2900

American Imex
16520 Aston St
Irvine, CA 92714
800/521-8286
714/553-8885

Anodyne Inc
7300 France Ave S, Ste 403
Edina, MN 55435
800/736-8367
612/831-6130

Austin Medical Equipment Inc
5947 S Oak Park Ave
Chicago, IL 60638
800/382-0300

BioMedical Life Systems Inc
1120 Sycamore Ave, Ste F
Vista, CA 92085
800/726-8367
619/727-5600

Chattanooga Group Inc
4717 Adams Rd
PO Box 489
Hixson, TN 37343
800/592-7329
615/870-2281

Comfort Technologies Inc
PO Box 7
Pittstown, NJ 08867
800/321-STIM
908/735-0344

CONMED Corp
310 Broad St
Utica, NY 13501
315/797-8375

Davicon Inc
79 Second Ave
Burlington, MA 01803
800/DAVICON
617/229-2800

AR Davis Co Inc
PO Box 219
Irvington, AL 36544
800/872-5804
205/957-3214
FAX: 205/957-2031

Dynatronics
470 W Lawndale Dr
Bldg D
Salt Lake City, UT 84115
801/485-4739

DynaWave Corp
2520 Kaneville Ct
Geneva, IL 60134
708/232-4945
FAX: 708/232-7042

The Electrode Store
PO Box 188
Enumclaw, WA 98022
800/537-1093
206/735-9259
FAX: 206/735-9343

Electro-Med Health Industries
11601 Biscayne Blvd, Ste 200A
Miami, FL 33181
305/892-2866
FAX: 305/892-2980

Electronic Waveform Lab Inc
15683 Chemical Ln
Huntington Beach, CA 92649
800/874-9283

ELMED Inc
60 W Fay Ave
Addison, IL 60101
312/543-2792

Empi Inc
1275 Grey Fox Rd
St Paul, MN 55112
800/328-2536
612/636-6600

Excel Tech Ltd
1200-11 Aerowood Dr
Mississauga, Ontario, Canada
L4W 2S7
800/387-7516

Henley International, A Division of Maxxim Medical
104 Industrial Blvd
Sugar Land, TX 77478
800/477-7342
FAX: 713/240-2577

IOMED Inc
1290 W 2320 S
Salt Lake City, UT 84119
800/621-3347
801/975-1191

Life-Tech Inc
10920 Kinghurst
Houston, TX 77099
713/495-9411

William B McBeth Co
PO Box 267
Telford, PA 18969
800/346-2171
215/723-0824

MECI Electrotherapeutics
810-B NW Main St
PO Box 1149
Lee's Summit, MO 64063
800/527-0748

Medical Devices Inc
833 Third St SW
St Paul, MN 55112
800/328-0875

Medical Science Products Inc
PO Box 381
Canal Fulton, OH 44614
800/456-1971

Mettler Electronics Corp
1333 S Claudina St
Anaheim, CA 92805
800/854-9305
714/533-2221
FAX: 714/635-7539

Monad Corp
908 E Holt Ave
Pomona, CA 91767
800/34MONAD
800/233MENS (in CA)

Nemectron Medical Inc
28069 Diaz Rd, Unit A
Temecula, CA 92590
800/428-4010

Physical Health Devices Inc
417 Corporate Sq
1500 W Cypress Creek Rd
Ft Lauderdale, FL 33309
305/351-0303
FAX: 305/351-0598

JA Preston Corp
PO Box 89
Jackson, MI 49204
800/631-7277
517/787-1600
See ad on page 45.

Promatek Medical Systems Inc
1851 Black Rd
Joliet, IL 60435
800/327-3422
815/725-6766

PTI
PO Box 19005
Topeka, KS 66619-0005
800/255-3554

Rich-Mar Corp
PO Box 879
Inola, OK 74036
800/762-4665
918/543-2222
See ad on page 140.

Self Regulation Systems Inc (SRS)
14770 NE 95th St
Redmond, WA 98052
800/345-5642
206/882-1101
FAX: 206/882-1935

Sentry Medical Products Inc
17171 Murphy Ave
Irvine, CA 92714
800/854-6004 (outside CA)
714/250-0233

Sparta Surgical Corp
26602 Corporate Ave
Hayward, CA 94545
510/887-7717

Staodyn Inc
1225 Florida Ave
PO Box 1379
Longmont, CO 80502-1379
800/525-2114
303/772-3631

TC Medical Inc
6565 City W Pkwy
Minneapolis, MN 55344-3248
800/826-3342
FAX: 612/829-8284

Thera-Kinetics Inc
1300 Rte 73
Mount Laurel, NJ 08054
800/234-0900

3M Health Care/Electrotherapy Products
3M Ctr, Bldg 275-4W-02
St Paul, MN 55144-1000
800/228-3957

TMD, A Division of Staodyn Inc
3625 Queen Palm Dr
PO Box 30244
Tampa, FL 33630-3244
800/343-0488

Uni-Patch Inc
1313 Grant Blvd W
PO Box 271
Wabasha, MN 55981
800/328-9454
612/565-2601

Verimed Inc
1401 E Broward Blvd
Ste 200
Ft Lauderdale, FL 33301
800/999-9797
305/768-9990

Electrotherapy Equipment

AdvanTeq Development Corp
12509 Crenshaw Blvd
Hawthorne, CA 90250
800/234-7846

American Imex
16520 Aston St
Irvine, CA 92714
800/521-8286
714/553-8885

Anodyne Inc
7300 France Ave S, Ste 403
Edina, MN 55435
800/736-8367
612/831-6130

Austin Medical Equipment Inc
5947 S Oak Park Ave
Chicago, IL 60638
800/382-0300

BioMedical Life Systems Inc
1120 Sycamore Ave, Ste F
Vista, CA 92085
800/726-8367
619/727-5600

Chattanooga Group Inc
4717 Adams Rd
PO Box 489
Hixson, TN 37343
800/592-7329
615/870-2281

Comfort Technologies Inc
PO Box 7
Pittstown, NJ 08867
800/321-STIM
908/735-0344

Davicon Inc
79 Second Ave
Burlington, MA 01803
800/DAVICON
617/229-2800

Dynatronics
470 W Lawndale Dr
Bldg D
Salt Lake City, UT 84115
801/485-4739

DynaWave Corp
2520 Kaneville Ct
Geneva, IL 60134
708/232-4945
FAX: 708/232-7042

Electro-Med Health Industries
11601 Biscayne Blvd
Ste 200A
Miami, FL 33181
305/892-2866
FAX: 305/892-2980

Electro Medical Inc
18433 Amistad
Fountain Valley, CA 92708
800/422-8726
714/964-6776
FAX: 714/968-0712

Electronic Waveform Lab Inc
15683 Chemical Ln
Huntington Beach, CA 92649
800/874-9283

ELMED Inc
60 W Fay Ave
Addison, IL 60101
312/543-2792

Empi Inc
1275 Grey Fox Rd
St Paul, MN 55112
800/328-2536
612/636-6600

Ergometrics Inc
3753 Varsity Dr
Ann Arbor, MI 48014
800/447-3009
313/971-7111

Excel Tech Ltd
1200-11 Aerowood Dr
Mississauga, Ontario, Canada
L4W 2S7
800/387-7516

GNR Health Systems Inc
1203 SW 12th St
Bldg H
Ocala, FL 32674
800/523-0912

Ideal Medical Products Inc
County Rd 623
Rte 1, PO Box 56
Broseley, MO 63932
800/321-5490
314/686-0003

IOMED Inc
1290 W 2320 S
Salt Lake City, UT 84119
800/621-3347
801/975-1191

I-REP Inc
29885 Second St, #G
Lake Elsinore, CA 92532
800/828-0852

Med Labs Inc
28 Vereda Cordillera
Goleta, CA 93117
805/968-2486

Mettler Electronics Corp
1333 S Claudina St
Anaheim, CA 92805
800/854-9305
714/533-2221
FAX: 714/635-7539

Microcurrent Research Inc
10443 N Cave Creek Rd
Ste 211
Phoenix, AZ 85020
800/872-6789
FAX: 602/943-6409

Monad Corp
908 E Holt Ave
Pomona, CA 91767
800/34MONAD
800/233MENS (in CA)

David Nelson, PT
1602 35th Ave
Vero Beach, FL 32960
407/562-5316

Nemectron Medical Inc
28069 Diaz Rd, Unit A
Temecula, CA 92590
800/428-4010

JA Preston Corp
PO Box 89
Jackson, MI 49204
800/631-7277
517/787-1600

Promatek Medical Systems Inc
1851 Black Rd
Joliet, IL 60435
800/327-3422
815/725-6766

PTI
PO Box 19005
Topeka, KS 66619-0005
800/255-3554

Rich-Mar Corp
PO Box 879
Inola, OK 74036
800/762-4665
918/543-2222

Rothhammer International
PO Box 5579
Santa Maria, CA 93456
800/235-2156

Thera-Kinetics Inc
1300 Rte 73
Mount Laurel, NJ 08054
800/234-0900

TMD, A Division of Staodyn Inc
3625 Queen Palm Dr
PO Box 30244
Tampa, FL 33630-3244
800/343-0488

Verimed Inc
1401 E Broward Blvd
Ste 200
Ft Lauderdale, FL 33301
800/999-9797
305/768-9990

Galvanic Stimulators

Anodyne Inc
7300 France Ave S, Ste 403
Edina, MN 55435
800/736-8367
612/831-6130

BioMedical Life Systems Inc
1120 Sycamore Ave, Ste F
Vista, CA 92085
800/726-8367
619/727-5600

Comfort Technologies Inc
PO Box 7
Pittstown, NJ 08867
800/321-STIM
908/735-0344

DynaWave Corp
2520 Kaneville Ct
Geneva, IL 60134
708/232-4945
FAX: 708/232-7042

Electro-Med Health Industries
11601 Biscayne Blvd, Ste 200A
Miami, FL 33181
305/892-2866
FAX: 305/892-2980

ELMED Inc
60 W Fay Ave
Addison, IL 60101
312/543-2792

Excel Tech Ltd
1200-11 Aerowood Dr
Mississauga, Ontario, Canada
L4W 2S7
800/387-7516

William B McBeth Co
PO Box 267
Telford, PA 18969
800/346-2171
215/723-0824

MECI Electrotherapeutics
810-B NW Main St
PO Box 1149
Lee's Summit, MO 64063
800/527-0748

Medical Devices Inc
833 Third St SW
St Paul, MN 55112
800/328-0875

Med Labs Inc
28 Vereda Cordillera
Goleta, CA 93117
805/968-2486

Mettler Electronics Corp
1333 S Claudina St
Anaheim, CA 92805
800/854-9305
714/533-2221
FAX: 714/635-7539

Physio Therapeutix Inc
3500 N Causeway Blvd
Ste 160
Metairie, LA 70002
800/274-9746

Rich-Mar Corp
PO Box 879
Inola, OK 74036
800/762-4665
918/543-2222

Staodyn Inc
1225 Florida Ave
PO Box 1379
Longmont, CO 80502-1379
800/525-2114
303/772-3631

Thera-Kinetics Inc
1300 Rte 73
Mount Laurel, NJ 08054
800/234-0900

TMD, A Division of Staodyn Inc
3625 Queen Palm Dr
PO Box 30244
Tampa, FL 33630-3244
800/343-0488

Gels/Sprays

AdvanTeq Development Corp
12509 Crenshaw Blvd
Hawthorne, CA 90250
800/234-7846

AliMed Inc
297 High St
Dedham, MA 02026
617/329-2900

AloeTran Products Inc
PO Box 337
Farmerville, LA 71241
800/328-8367
318/368-7266

American Imex
16520 Aston St
Irvine, CA 92714
800/521-8286
714/553-8885

CONMED Corp
310 Broad St
Utica, NY 13501
315/979-8375

AR Davis Co Inc
PO Box 219
Irvington, AL 36544
800/872-5804
205/957-3214
FAX: 205/957-2031

Dynatronics
470 W Lawndale Dr
Bldg D
Salt Lake City, UT 84115
801/485-4739

The Electrode Store
PO Box 188
Enumclaw, WA 98022
800/537-1093
206/735-9259
FAX: 206/735-9343

Electro-Med Health Industries
11601 Biscayne Blvd, Ste 200A
Miami, FL 33181
305/892-2866
FAX: 305/892-2980

Electronic Waveform Lab Inc
15683 Chemical Ln
Huntington Beach, CA 92649
800/874-9283

ELMED Inc
60 W Fay Ave
Addison, IL 60101
312/543-2792

Excel Tech Ltd
1200-11 Aerowood Dr
Mississauga, Ontario, Canada
L4W 2S7
800/387-7516

Ideal Medical Products Inc
County Rd 623
Rte 1, PO Box 56
Broseley, MO 63932
800/321-5490
314/686-0003

William B McBeth Co
PO Box 267
Telford, PA 18969
800/346-2171
215/723-0824

Medical Devices Inc
833 Third St SW
St Paul, MN 55112
800/328-0875

Medical Science Products Inc
PO Box 381
Canal Fulton, OH 44614
800/456-1971

Parker Laboratories Inc
307 Washington St
Orange, NJ 07050
201/676-5000
FAX: 201/676-0784

Pharmaceutical Innovations Inc
897 Frelinghuysen Ave
Newark, NJ 07114
201/242-2900
FAX: 201/242-0578

Rich-Mar Corp
PO Box 879
Inola, OK 74036
800/762-4665
918/543-2222
See ad on page 140.

Self Regulation Systems Inc (SRS)
14770 NE 95th St
Redmond, WA 98052
800/345-5642
206/882-1101
FAX: 206/882-1935

TC Medical Inc
6565 City West Pkwy
Minneapolis, MN 55344
800/826-3342
FAX: 612/829-8284

Thera-Kinetics Inc
1300 Rte 73
Mount Laurel, NJ 08054
800/234-0900

Uni-Patch Inc
1313 Grant Blvd W
PO Box 271
Wabasha, MN 55981
800/328-9454
612/565-2601

Interferential Therapy

AdvanTeq Development Corp
12509 Crenshaw Blvd
Hawthorne, CA 90250
800/234-7846

American Imex
16520 Aston St
Irvine CA 92714
800/521-8286
714/553-8885

Anodyne Inc
7300 France Ave S, Ste 403
Edina, MN 55435
800/736-8367
612/831-6130

Austin Medical Equipment Inc
5947 S Oak Park Ave
Chicago, IL 60638
800/382-0300

BioMedical Life Systems Inc
1120 Sycamore Ave, Ste F
Vista, CA 92085
800/726-8367
619/727-5600

Chattanooga Group Inc
4717 Adams Rd
PO Box 489
Hixson, TN 37343
800/592-7329
615/870-2281

Comfort Technologies Inc
PO Box 7
Pittstown, NJ 08867
800/321-STIM
908/735-0344

Dynatronics
470 W Lawndale Dr
Bldg D
Salt Lake City, UT 84115
801/485-4739

ELMED Inc
60 W Fay Ave
Addison, IL 60101
312/543-2792

Excel Tech Ltd
1200-11 Aerowood Dr
Mississauga, Ontario, Canada
L4W 2S7
800/387-7516

Ideal Medical Products Inc
County Rd 623
Rte 1, PO Box 56
Broseley, MO 63932
800/321-5490
314/686-0003

I-REP Inc
29885 Second St, #G
Lake Elsinore, CA 92532
800/828-0852

William B McBeth Co
PO Box 267
Telford, PA 18969
800/346-2171
215/723-0824

Medical Devices Inc
833 Third St SW
St Paul, MN 55112
800/328-0875

Mettler Electronics Corp
1333 S Claudina St
Anaheim, CA 92805
800/854-9305
714/533-2221
FAX: 714/635-7539

Microcurrent Research Inc
10443 N Cave Creek Rd
Ste 211
Phoenix, AZ 85020
800/872-6789
FAX: 602/943-6409

Monad Corp
908 E Holt Ave
Pomona, CA 91767
800/34MONAD
800/233MENS (in CA)

Nemectron Medical Inc
28069 Diaz Rd, Unit A
Temecula, CA 92590
800/428-4010

Promatek Medical Systems Inc
1851 Black Rd
Joliet, IL 60435
800/327-3422
815/725-6766

PTI
PO Box 19005
Topeka, KS 66619-0005
800/255-3554

Rich-Mar Corp
PO Box 879
Inola, OK 74036
800/762-4665
918/543-2222

Iontophoretic Systems

Anodyne Inc
7300 France Ave S, Ste 403
Edina, MN 55435
800/736-8367
612/831-6130

ELMED Inc
60 W Fay Ave
Addison, IL 60101
312/543-2792

Empi Inc
1275 Grey Fox Rd
St Paul, MN 55112
800/328-2536
612/636-6600

General Medical Co
1935 Armacost Ave
Los Angeles, CA 90025-5296
310/820-5881

General Medical Manufacturing Co
8741 Landmark Rd
Richmond, VA 23228
804/264-7500

**Henley International, A
Division of Maxxim Medical**
104 Industrial Blvd
Sugar Land, TX 77478
800/477-7342
FAX: 713/240-2577

IOMED Inc
1290 W 2320 S
Salt Lake City, UT 84119
800/621-3347
801/975-1191

Life-Tech Inc
10920 Kinghurst
Houston, TX 77099
713/495-9411

William B McBeth Co
PO Box 267
Telford, PA 18969
800/346-2171
215/723-0824

Medical Science Products Inc
PO Box 381
Canal Fulton, OH 44614
800/456-1971

Monad Corp
908 E Holt Ave
Pomona, CA 91767
800/34MONAD
800/233MENS (in CA)

Muscle Stimulators

AdvanTeq Development Corp
12509 Crenshaw Blvd
Hawthorne, CA 90250
800/234-7846

American Imex
16520 Aston St
Irvine, CA 92714
800/521-8286
714/553-8885

Anodyne Inc
7300 France Ave S, Ste 403
Edina, MN 55435
800/736-8367
612/831-6130

Austin Medical Equipment Inc
5947 S Oak Park Ave
Chicago, IL 60638
800/382-0300

Ballert International Inc
3645 Woodhead Dr
Northbrook, IL 60062-1816
800/345-3456
FAX: 312/480-1088

BioMedical Life Systems Inc
1120 Sycamore Ave, Ste F
Vista, CA 92085
800/726-8367
619/727-5600

Chattanooga Group Inc
4717 Adams Rd
PO Box 489
Hixson, TN 37343
800/592-7329
615/870-2281

Comfort Technologies Inc
PO Box 7
Pittstown, NJ 08867
800/321-STIM
908/735-0344

Complete Medical Products Inc
2052 N Decatur Rd
Decatur, GA 30033
800/525-4119

Dynatronics
470 W Lawndale Dr
Bldg D
Salt Lake City, UT 84115
801/485-4739

DynaWave Corp
2520 Kaneville Ct
Geneva, IL 60134
708/232-4945
FAX: 708/232-7042

Electro-Med Health Industries
11601 Biscayne Blvd, Ste 200A
Miami, FL 33181
305/892-2866
FAX: 305/892-2980

Electro Medical Inc
18433 Amistad
Fountain Valley, CA 92708
800/422-8726
714/964-6776
FAX: 714/968-0712

Electronic Waveform Lab Inc
15683 Chemical Ln
Huntington Beach, CA 92649
800/874-9283

ELMED Inc
60 W Fay Ave
Addison, IL 60101
312/543-2792

Empi Inc
1275 Grey Fox Rd
St Paul, MN 55112
800/328-2536
612/636-6600

Excel Tech Ltd
1200-11 Aerowood Dr
Mississauga, Ontario, Canada
L4W 2S7
800/387-7516

General Physiotherapy Inc
13222 Lakefront Dr
St Louis, MO 63045-1504
800/237-1832
314/291-1442

Ideal Medical Products Inc
County Rd 623
Rte 1, PO Box 56
Broseley, MO 63932
800/321-5490
314/686-0003

MECI Electrotherapeutics
810-B NW Main St
PO Box 1149
Lee's Summit, MO 64063
800/527-0748

Med Labs Inc
28 Vereda Cordillera
Goleta, CA 93117
805/968-2486

Mettler Electronics Corp
1333 S Claudina St
Anaheim, CA 92805
800/854-9305
714/533-2221
FAX: 714/635-7539

Nemectron Medical Inc
28069 Diaz Rd, Unit A
Temecula, CA 92590
800/428-4010

JA Preston Corp
PO Box 89
Jackson, MI 49204
800/631-7277
517/787-1600
See ad on page 45.

Promatek Medical Systems Inc
1851 Black Rd
Joliet, IL 60435
800/327-3422
815/725-6766

PTI
PO Box 19005
Topeka, KS 66619-0005
800/255-3554

Rich-Mar Corp
PO Box 879
Inola, OK 74036
800/762-4665
918/543-2222
See ad on page 140.

Sparta Surgical Corp
26602 Corporate Ave
Hayward, CA 94545
510/887-7717

Sportmaster
PO Box 5000
Pittsburgh, PA 15206
412/441-0200

Staodyn Inc
1225 Florida Ave
PO Box 1379
Longmont, CO 80502-1379
800/525-2114
303/772-3631

Sutter Corp
9425 Chesapeake Dr
San Diego, CA 92123
800/854-2216
619/569-8148

TC Medical Inc
6565 City West Pkwy
Minneapolis, MN 55344-3248
800/826-3342
FAX: 612/829-8284

Thera-Kinetics Inc
1300 Rte 73
Mount Laurel, NJ 08054
800/234-0900

TMD, A Division of Staodyn Inc
3625 Queen Palm Dr
PO Box 30244
Tampa, FL 33630-3244
800/343-0488

Neuromuscular Stimulators

AdvanTeq Development Corp
12509 Crenshaw Blvd
Hawthorne, CA 90250
800/234-7846

American Imex
16520 Aston St
Irvine, CA 92714
800/521-8286
714/553-8885

Anodyne Inc
7300 France Ave S, Ste 403
Edina, MN 55435
800/736-8367
612/831-6130

BioMedical Life Systems Inc
1120 Sycamore Ave, Ste F
Vista, CA 92085
800/726-8367
619/727-5600

Chattanooga Group Inc
4717 Adams Rd
PO Box 489
Hixson, TN 37343
800/592-7329
615/870-2281

Comfort Technologies Inc
PO Box 7
Pittstown, NJ 08867
800/321-STIM
908/735-0344

Electro-Med Health Industries
11601 Biscayne Blvd, Ste
200A
Miami, FL 33181
305/892-2866
FAX: 305/892-2980

Electro Medical Inc
18433 Amistad
Fountain Valley, CA 92708
800/422-8726
714/964-6776
FAX: 714/968-0712

Electronic Waveform Lab Inc
15683 Chemical Ln
Huntington Beach, CA 92649
800/874-9283

ELMED Inc
60 W Fay Ave
Addison, IL 60101
312/543-2792

Empi Inc
1275 Grey Fox Rd
St Paul, MN 55112
800/328-2536
612/636-6600

Excel Tech Ltd
1200-11 Aerowood Dr
Mississauga, Ontario, Canada
L4W 2S7
800/387-7516

**Henley International, A
Division of Maxxim Medical**
104 Industrial Blvd
Sugar Land, TX 77478
800/477-7342
FAX: 713/240-2577

Ideal Medical Products Inc
County Rd 623
Rte 1, PO Box 56
Broseley, MO 63932
800/321-5490
314/686-0003

MECI Electrotherapeutics
810-B NW Main St
PO Box 1149
Lee's Summit, MO 64063
800/527-0748

Medical Devices Inc
833 Third St SW
St Paul, MN 55112
800/328-0875

Med Labs Inc
28 Vereda Cordillera
Goleta, CA 93117
805/968-2486

Mettler Electronics Corp
1333 S Claudina St
Anaheim, CA 92805
800/854-9305
714/533-2221
FAX: 714/635-7539

Monad Corp
908 E Holt Ave
Pomona, CA 91767
800/34MONAD
800/233MENS (in CA)

NAPCOR
9852 Crescent Ctr Dr
Ste 801
Rancho Cucamonga, CA 91730
909/989-1641

Nemectron Medical Inc
28069 Diaz Rd, Unit A
Temecula, CA 92590
800/428-4010

Promatek Medical Systems Inc
1851 Black Rd
Joliet, IL 60435
800/327-3422
815/725-6766

PTI
PO Box 19005
Topeka, KS 66619-0005
800/255-3554

Rich-Mar Corp
PO Box 879
Inola, OK 74036
800/762-4665
918/543-2222

Sparta Surgical Corp
26602 Corporate Ave
Hayward, CA 94545
510/887-7717

Sportmaster
PO Box 5000
Pittsburgh, PA 15206
412/441-0200

Staodyn Inc
1225 Florida Ave
PO Box 1379
Longmont, CO 80502-1379
800/525-2114
303/772-3631

Thera-Kinetics Inc
1300 Rte 73
Mount Laurel, NJ 08054
800/234-0900

TMD, A Division of Staodyn Inc
3625 Queen Palm Dr
PO Box 30244
Tampa, FL 33630-3244
800/343-0488

Verimed Inc
1401 E Broward Blvd
Ste 200
Ft Lauderdale, FL 33301
800/999-9797
305/768-9990

TENS Units

AdvanTeq Development Corp
12509 Crenshaw Blvd
Hawthorne, CA 90250
800/234-7846

AGAR USA Inc
1915 Eye St, #500
Washington, DC 20006
202/296-1111

American Imex
16520 Aston St
Irvine, CA 92714
800/521-8286
714/553-8885

Anodyne Inc
7300 France Ave S, Ste 403
Edina, MN 55435
800/736-8367
612/831-6130

Austin Medical Equipment Inc
5947 S Oak Park Ave
Chicago, IL 60638
800/382-0300

BioMedical Life Systems Inc
1120 Sycamore Ave, Ste F
Vista, CA 92085
800/726-8367
619/727-5600

Comfort Technologies Inc
PO Box 7
Pittstown, NJ 08867
800/321-STIM
908/735-0344

AR Davis Co Inc
PO Box 219
Irvington, AL 36544
800/872-5804
205/957-3214
FAX: 205/957-2031

Electro-Med Health Industries
11601 Biscayne Blvd, Ste 200A
Miami, FL 33181
305/892-2866
FAX: 305/892-2980

Electro Medical Inc
18433 Amistad
Fountain Valley, CA 92708
800/422-8726
714/964-6776
FAX: 714/968-0712

Electronic Research Devices Corp
9320 SW Barbur Blvd
Ste 150
Portland, OR 97219
800/547-0366
503/245-7241
FAX: 503/245-4863

ELMED Inc
60 W Fay Ave
Addison, IL 60101
312/543-2792

Empi Inc
1275 Grey Fox Rd
St Paul, MN 55112
800/328-2536
612/636-6600

Excel Tech Ltd
1200-11 Aerowood Dr
Mississauga, Ontario, Canada
L4W 2S7
800/387-7516

Henley International, A
Division of Maxxim Medical
104 Industrial Blvd
Sugar Land, TX 77478
800/477-7342
FAX: 713/240-2577

MECI Electrotherapeutics
810-B NW Main St
PO Box 1149
Lee's Summit, MO 64063
800/527-0748

Medical Devices Inc
833 Third St SW
St Paul, MN 55112
800/328-0875

Medical Science Products Inc
PO Box 381
Canal Fulton, OH 44614
800/456-1971

Monad Corp
908 E Holt Ave
Pomona, CA 91767
800/34MONAD
800/233MENS (in CA)

JA Preston Corp
PO Box 89
Jackson, MI 49204
800/631-7277
517/787-1600

Sparta Surgical Corp
26602 Corporate Ave
Hayward, CA 94545
510/887-7717

Sportmaster
PO Box 5000
Pittsburgh, PA 15206
412/441-0200

Staodyn Inc
1225 Florida Ave
PO Box 1379
Longmont, CO 80502
800/525-2114
303/772-3631

TC Medical Inc
6565 City West Pkwy
Minneapolis, MN 55344-3248
800/826-3342
FAX: 612/829-8284

Thera-Kinetics Inc
1300 Rte 73
Mount Laurel, NJ 08054
800/234-0900

3M Health Care/ Electrotherapy Products
3M Ctr, Bldg 275-4W-02
St Paul, MN 55144-1000
800/228-3957

TMD, A Division of Staodyn Inc
3625 Queen Palm Dr
PO Box 30244
Tampa, FL 33630-3244
800/343-0488

Uni-Patch Inc
1313 Grant Blvd W
PO Box 271
Wabasha, MN 55981
800/328-9454
612/565-2601

Biofeedback Instrumentation

Anodyne Inc
7300 France Ave S, Ste 403
Edina, MN 55435
800/736-8367
612/831-6130

BioMedical Life Systems Inc
1120 Sycamore Ave, Ste F
Vista, CA 92085
800/726-8367
619/727-5600

Davicon Inc
79 Second Ave
Burlington, MA 01803
800/DAVICON
617/229-2800

Ergometrics Inc
3753 Varsity Dr
Ann Arbor, MI 48014
800/447-3009
313/971-7111

Innovative Systems for Rehabilitation (ISR)
1711 W County Rd B
Ste 208 N
St Paul, MN 55113
612/636-8212

Lafayette Instrument Co
3700 Sagamore Pkwy N
PO Box 5729
Lafayette, IN 47903
800/428-7545
317/423-1505

William B McBeth Co
PO Box 267
Telford, PA 18969
800/346-2171
215/723-0824

NeuroCom International Inc
9570 SE Lawnfield Rd
Clackamas, OR 97015
800/767-6744
503/653-2144
FAX: 503/653-1992

Physical Health Devices Inc
417 Corporate Sq
1500 W Cypress Creek Rd
Ft Lauderdale, FL 33309
305/351-0303
FAX: 305/351-0598

Self Regulation Systems Inc (SRS)
14770 NE 95th St
Redmond, WA 98052
800/345-5642
206/882-1101
FAX: 206/882-1935

Tekdyne Corp
550-3 California Rd
Quakertown, PA 18951
800/747-1824
215/538-1826
FAX: 215/338-3059

Thera-Kinetics Inc
1300 Rte 73
Mount Laurel, NJ 08054
800/234-0900

Universal Gym Equipment Inc
PO Box 1270
Cedar Rapids, IA 52406
800/843-3906
319/365-7561

Verimed Inc
1401 E Broward Blvd
Ste 200
Ft Lauderdale, FL 33301
800/999-9797
305/768-9990

CRYOTHERAPY
Ice Packs, Disposable

Austin Medical Equipment Inc
5947 S Oak Park Ave
Chicago, IL 60638
800/382-0300

Biomark Inc
PO Box 340
Edmonds, WA 98040
800/633-3034
206/745-9200

DeRoyal Orthopedic Group
200 DeBusk Ln
Powell, TN 37849
800/251-9864

Medical Science Products Inc
PO Box 381
Canal Fulton, OH 44614
800/456-1971

Mueller Sports Medicine Inc
One Quench Dr
Prairie du Sac, WI 53578
800/356-9522
608/643-8530

Pelton Shepherd Industries
PO Box 30218
Stockton, CA 95213
800/BLUEICE
209/983-0893

Rolliture Systems
4231 Pacific St, #31
Rocklin, CA 95677
916/652-7887
FAX: 916/652-8188

Rothhammer International
PO Box 5579
Santa Maria, CA 93456
800/235-2156
See ad on page 120.

Slim Ez/Mr America Mfg Inc
Ooltewah Industrial Park
Ooltewah, TN 37363
800/251-6040

Southwest Technologies Inc
2018 Baltimore
Kansas City, MO 64108
800/247-9951

Ice Packs, Reusable

Anodyne Inc
7300 France Ave S, Ste 403
Edina, MN 55435
800/736-8367
612/831-6130

Aqua-Cel Corp
PO Box 26827
Santa Ana, CA 92799
714/962-2776

Biomark Inc
PO Box 340
Edmonds, WA 98040
800/633-3034
206/745-9200

Bird & Cronin Inc
2601 E 80th St
Minneapolis, MN 55425
800/328-1095
612/854-5626

Bodyline Comfort Systems
3730 Kori Rd
Jacksonville, FL 32257
800/874-7715
904/262-4068

Chattanooga Group Inc
4717 Adams Rd
PO Box 489
Hixson, TX 37343
800/592-7329
615/870-2281

DePuy Inc
700 Orthopaedic Dr
PO Box 988
Warsaw, IN 46581-0988
800/366-8143

Dura-Kold Corp
1117 Cornell Pkwy
Oklahoma City, OK 73108
405/943-8811

Elgin Exercise Equipment Corp
270 N Eisenhower Ln
Unit 4-A
Lombard, IL 60148
800/279-3762
708/268-1000

Medical Science Products Inc
PO Box 381
Canal Fulton, OH 44614
800/456-1971

Mueller Sports Medicine Inc
One Quench Dr
Prairie du Sac, WI 53578
800/356-9522
608/643-8530

**Northwest Orthopaedic
Products Corp**
12300 SW Sidney Rd
Port Orchard, WA 98366
800/331-8188

**Orthopedic Physical
Therapy Products**
PO Box 47009
Minneapolis, MN 55447-0009
800/367-7393
612/553-0452
FAX: 612/553-9355

Pelton Shepherd Industries
PO Box 30218
Stockton, CA 95213
800/BLUEICE
209/983-0893

JA Preston Corp
PO Box 89
Jackson, MI 49204
800/631-7277
517/787-1600

Rich-Mar Corp
PO Box 879
Inola, OK 74036
800/762-4665
918/543-2222

Rothhammer International
PO Box 5579
Santa Maria, CA 93456
800/235-2156
See ad on page 120.

Slim Ez/Mr America Mfg Inc
Ooltewah Industrial Park
Ooltewah, TN 37363
800/251-6040

Southwest Technologies Inc
2018 Baltimore
Kansas City, MO 64108
800/247-9951

Sports Supports Inc
400 Union Bower Ct, #410
Irving, TX 75061
800/527-5273
214/554-1174

Sportsware West
415 E Figueroa St, Ste A
Santa Barbara, CA 93101
805/962-7454
FAX: 805/966-3631

SUB IP Inc
1545 N Verdugo Rd
Glendale, CA 91208
818/242-7546

Sutter Corp
9425 Chesapeake Dr
San Diego, CA 92123
800/854-2216
619/569-8148

Therabite Corp
6 S Bryn Mawr Ave
Ste 100
Bryn Mawr, PA 19010
800/322-2650

TMD, A Division of Staodyn Inc
3625 Queen Palm Dr
PO Box 30244
Tampa, FL 33630-3244
800/343-0488

Uni-Patch Inc
1313 Grant Blvd W
PO Box 271
Wabasha, MN 55981
800/328-9454
612/565-2601

Sprays, Vapocoolants

Austin Medical Equipment Inc
5947 S Oak Park Ave
Chicago, IL 60638
800/382-0300

Gebauer Co
9410 St Catherine Ave
Cleveland, OH 44104
216/271-5252

Mueller Sports Medicine Inc
One Quench Dr
Prairie du Sac, WI 53578
800/356-9522
608/643-8530

THERMOTHERAPY
Fluidotherapy

AquaSoothe International Inc
2016 Concord Lake Rd
Kannapolis, NC 28083
704/784-4620

**Henley International, A
Division of Maxxim Medical**
104 Industrial Blvd
Sugar Land, TX 77478
800/477-7342
FAX: 713/240-2577

Thera-Kinetics Inc
1300 Rte 73
Mount Laurel, NJ 08054
800/234-0900

Heating Pads

American Imex
16520 Aston St
Irvine, CA 92714
800/521-8286
714/553-8885

Battle Creek Equipment Co
307 W Jackson St
Battle Creek, MI 49017-2385
800/253-0854

Southwest Technologies Inc
2018 Baltimore
Kansas City, MO 64108
800/247-9951

Hot Packs

American Imex
16520 Aston St
Irvine, CA 92714
800/521-8286
714/553-8885

Aqua-Cel Corp
PO Box 26827
Santa Ana, CA 92799
714/962-2776

Austin Medical Equipment Inc
5947 S Oak Park Ave
Chicago, IL 60638
800/382-0300

Battle Creek Equipment Co
307 W Jackson St
Battle Creek, MI 49017-2385
800/253-0854

Biomark Inc
PO Box 340
Edmonds, WA 98040
800/633-3034
206/745-9200

Bird & Cronin Inc
2601 E 80th St
Minneapolis, MN 55425
800/328-1095
612/854-5626

Bodyline Comfort Systems
3730 Kori Rd
Jacksonville, FL 32257
800/874-7715
904/262-4068

Contour Form Products
12 N Diamond St
PO Box 328
Greenville, PA 16125
800/223-8808
412/588-4452

**Ferno Ille, A Division of
Ferno-Washington Inc**
70 Weil Way
Wilmington, OH 45177
513/382-1451

Ideal Medical Products Inc
County Rd 623
Rte 1, PO Box 56
Broseley, MO 63932
800/321-5490
314/686-0003

Logan Inc
3041 S Shannon St
Santa Ana, CA 92704
714/556-6441

Medical Science Products Inc
PO Box 381
Canal Fulton, OH 44614
800/456-1971

**Orthopedic Physical Therapy
Products**
PO Box 47009
Minneapolis, MN 55447-0009
800/367-7393
612/553-0452
FAX: 612/553-9355

Pelton Shepherd Industries
PO Box 30218
Stockton, CA 95213
800/BLUEICE
209/983-0893

JA Preston Corp
PO Box 89
Jackson, MI 49204
800/631-7277
517/787-1600
See ad on page 45.

Re-Heater Inc
15828 S Broadway
Garden, CA 90248
310/719-9582

Paraffin Baths

American Imex
16520 Aston St
Irvine, CA 92714
800/521-8286
714/553-8885

Austin Medical Equipment Inc
5947 S Oak Park Ave
Chicago, IL 60638
800/382-0300

Bird & Cronin Inc
2601 E 80th St
Minneapolis, MN 55425
800/328-1095
612/854-5626

Complete Medical Products Inc
2052 N Decatur Rd
Decatur, GA 30033
800/525-4119

**Ferno Ille, A Division of
Ferno-Washington Inc**
70 Weil Way
Wilmington, OH 45177
513/382-1451

Grimm Scientific Industries Inc
Newport Pike
PO Box 2143
Marietta, OH 45750
800/223-5395
614/374-3412

The Hygenic Corp
1245 Home Ave
Akron, OH 44310-2575
800/321-2135
216/633-8460
See ad on page 96.

I-REP Inc
29885 Second St, #G
Lake Elsinore, CA 92532
800/828-0852

William B McBeth Co
PO Box 267
Telford, PA 18969
800/346-2171
215/723-0824

JA Preston Corp
PO Box 89
Jackson, MI 49204
800/631-7277
517/787-1600
See ad on page 45.

Thermo-Electric Co
455 Rte 30
Imperial, PA 15126
800/633-8088
412/695-1890

WR Medical Electronics Co
123 N Second St
Stillwater, MN 55082
800/321-6387
612/430-1200

HYDROTHERAPY
Hydrotherapy Equipment

AquaSoothe International Inc
2016 Concord Lake Rd
Kannapolis, NC 28083
704/784-4620

AquaTherapeutics™
PO Box 5775
Asheville, NC 28813
800/237-0469

Bailey Manufacturing Co
118 Lee St
PO Box 130
Lodi, OH 44254
800/321-8372
216/948-1080
FAX: 216/948-4439

Ferno Ille, A Division of Ferno-Washington Inc
70 Weil Way
Wilmington, OH 45177
513/382-1451

GNR Health Systems Inc
1203 SW 12th St
Bldg H
Ocala, FL 32674
800/523-0912

Good Sports
6031 Broad St Mall
Pittsburgh, PA 15206
412/661-9500

Hospital Therapy Products Inc
757 N Central Ave
Wood Dale, IL 60191
708/766-7101

I-REP Inc
29885 Second St, #G
Lake Elsinore, CA 92532
800/828-0852

Jetta Products Inc
217 Altamonte Commerce Blvd, #1218
Altamonte Springs, FL 32714
800/775-3882
FAX: 407/774-7260

Rothhammer International
PO Box 5579
Santa Maria, CA 93456
800/235-2156
See ad on page 120.

Sportmaster
PO Box 5000
Pittsburgh, PA 15206
412/441-0200

Stewart Medical
70 NE Loop 410
Ste 675
San Antonio, TX 78216
800/437-8216

Stranco
PO Box 389
Bradley, IL 60915
800/882-6466
815/932-8154

Whitehall Manufacturing Inc
15058 Proctor Ave
City of Industry, CA 91746
818/968-6681

ULTRASOUND
Gels

AloeTran Products Inc
PO Box 337
Farmerville, LA 71241
800/328-8367
318/368-7266

Anodyne Inc
7300 France Ave S, Ste 403
Edina, MN 55435
800/736-8367
612/831-6130

Ari-Med Pharmaceuticals
1615 W University Dr
Ste 125
Tempe, AZ 85281
800/527-4923
602/966-9802
FAX: 602/966-9806
See ad on page 136.

AR Davis Co Inc
PO Box 219
Irvington, AL 36544
800/872-5804
205/957-3214
FAX: 205/957-2031

Echo Ultrasound
RR 2, PO Box 118
Reedsville, PA 17084-9772
800/233-0261
See ad on page 36.

ELMED Inc
60 W Fay Ave
Addison, IL 60101
312/543-2792

Excel Tech Ltd
1200-11 Aerowood Dr
Mississauga, Ontario, Canada
L4W 2S7
800/387-7516

Fairway King Co
3 E Main St
Oklahoma City, OK 73104
405/528-8571

Ideal Medical Products Inc
County Rd 623
Rte 1, PO Box 56
Broseley, MO 63932
800/321-5490
314/686-0003

William B McBeth Co
PO Box 267
Telford, PA 18969
800/346-2171
215/723-0824

Mettler Electronics Corp
1333 S Claudina St
Anaheim, CA 92805
800/854-9305
714/533-2221
FAX: 714/635-7539

North Coast Medical Inc
187 Stauffer Blvd
San Jose, CA 95125-1042
800/821-9319
408/283-1900
FAX: 408/283-1950

Parker Laboratories Inc
307 Washington St
Orange, NJ 07050
201/676-5000
FAX: 201/676-0784
See ad on page 138.

Pelton Shepherd Industries
PO Box 30218
Stockton, CA 95213
800/BLUEICE
209/983-0893

Pharmaceutical Innovations Inc
897 Frelinghuysen Ave
Newark, NJ 07114
201/242-2900
FAX: 201/242-0578

Rich-Mar Corp
PO Box 879
Inola, OK 74036
800/762-4665
918/543-2222

Third Millennium Science
2195 Faraday Ave, Ste F
Carlsbad, CA 92008
619/431-7181

Uni-Patch Inc
1313 Grant Blvd W
PO Box 271
Wabasha, MN 55981
800/328-9454
612/565-2601

Ultrasound Equipment

Anodyne Inc
7300 France Ave S, Ste 403
Edina, MN 55435
800/736-8367
612/831-6130

Arjo-Century Inc
8130 Lehigh Ave
Morton Grove, IL 60053
800/323-1245
708/967-0360

Austin Medical Equipment Inc
5947 S Oak Park Ave
Chicago, IL 60638
800/382-0300

Chattanooga Group Inc
4717 Adams Rd
PO Box 489
Hixson, TN 37343
800/592-7329
615/870-2281

Complete Medical Products Inc
2052 N Decatur Rd
Decatur, GA 30033
800/525-4119

Dynatronics
470 W Lawndale Dr
Bldg D
Salt Lake City, UT 84115
801/485-4739

ELMED Inc
60 W Fay Ave
Addison, IL 60101
312/543-2792

Excel Tech Ltd
1200-11 Aerowood Dr
Mississauga, Ontario, Canada
L4W 2S7
800/387-7516

GNR Health Systems Inc
1203 SW 12th St
Bldg H
Ocala, FL 32674
800/523-0912

Good Sports
6031 Broad St Mall
Pittsburgh, PA 15206
412/661-9500

Huntleigh Healthcare
227 Rte 33 E
Manalapan, NJ 07726
800/223-1218

Ideal Medical Products Inc
County Rd 623
Rte 1, PO Box 56
Broseley, MO 63932
800/321-5490
314/686-0003

I-REP Inc
29885 Second St, #G
Lake Elsinore, CA 92532
800/828-0852

William B McBeth Co
PO Box 267
Telford, PA 18969
800/346-2171
215/723-0824

Mettler Electronics Corp
1333 S Claudina St
Anaheim, CA 92805
800/854-9305
714/533-2221
FAX: 714/635-7539

Nemectron Medical Inc
28069 Diaz Rd, Unit A
Temecula, CA 92590
800/428-4010

Promatek Medical Systems Inc
1851 Black Rd
Joliet, IL 60435
800/327-3422
815/725-6766

PTI
PO Box 19005
Topeka, KS 66619-0005
800/255-3554

Rich-Mar Corp
PO Box 879
Inola, OK 74036
800/762-4665
918/543-2222

Rothhammer International
PO Box 5579
Santa Maria, CA 93456
800/235-2156

PHOTOTHERAPY
Infrared Lamps

I-REP Inc
29885 Second St, #G
Lake Elsinore, CA 92532
800/828-0852

Lasers, Helium-Neon

Dynatronics
470 W Lawndale Dr
Bldg D
Salt Lake City, UT 84115
801/485-4739

I-REP Inc
29885 Second St, #G
Lake Elsinore, CA 92532
800/828-0852

North Coast Medical Inc
187 Stauffer Blvd
San Jose, CA 95125-1042
800/821-9319
408/283-1900
FAX: 408/283-1950

Smith & Nephew Rolyan Inc
N93W14475 Whittaker Way
PO Box 555
Menomonee Falls, WI 53051
800/558-8633

Ultraviolet Lamps

I-REP Inc
29885 Second St, #G
Lake Elsinore, CA 92532
800/828-0852

DIATHERMY
Microwave Diathermy

Nemectron Medical Inc
28069 Diaz Rd, Unit A
Temecula, CA 92590
800/428-4010

Shortwave Diathermy

ELMED Inc
60 W Fay Ave
Addison, IL 60101
312/543-2792

**International Medical
Electronics Ltd**
3939 Broadway
Ste 100
Kansas City, MO 64111-2516
800/432-8003

I-REP Inc
29885 Second St, #G
Lake Elsinore, CA 92532
800/828-0852

Mettler Electronics Corp
1333 S Claudina St
Anaheim, CA 92805
800/854-9305
714/533-2221
FAX: 714/635-7539

TRACTION EQUIPMENT

**Akron Therapy Products/Electro-
Medical Equipment Inc**
PO Box 7671
Marietta, GA 30065
800/235-2952

AliMed Inc
297 High St
Dedham, MA 02026
617/329-2900

AquaSoothe International Inc
2016 Concord Lake Rd
Kannapolis, NC 28083
704/784-4620

Austin Medical Equipment Inc
5947 S Oak Park Ave
Chicago, IL 60638
800/382-0300

Ballert International Inc
3645 Woodhead Dr
Northbrook, IL 60062-1816
800/345-3456
FAX: 312/480-1088

Care · a · peutics
10850 White Oak Ave
Granada Hills, CA 91344
818/831-1361

INTERMITTENT COMPRESSION UNITS

Chattanooga Group Inc
4717 Adams Rd
PO Box 489
Hixson, TN 37343
800/592-7329
615/870-2281

Complete Medical Products Inc
2052 N Decatur Rd
Decatur, GA 30033
800/525-4119

Huntleigh Healthcare
227 Rte 33 E
Manalapan, NJ 07726
800/223-1218

The Jobst Institute Inc
653 Miami St
PO Box 653
Toledo, OH 43697
419/698-1611

Ideal Medical Products Inc
County Rd 623
Rte 1, PO Box 56
Broseley, MO 63932
800/321-5490
314/686-0003

Sammons
145 Tower Dr, Dept 966
Burr Ridge, IL 60521
708/325-1700

Schaefer Products
PO Box 450208
Garland, TX 75045
214/238-9368

Sportsware West
415 E Figueroa St, Ste A
Santa Barbara, CA 93101
805/962-7454
FAX: 805/966-3631

SUB IP Inc
1545 N Verdugo Rd
Glendale, CA 91208
818/242-7546

MASSAGERS

AquaSoothe International Inc
2016 Concord Lake Rd
Kannapolis, NC 28083
704/784-4620

Battle Creek Equipment Co
307 W Jackson St
Battle Creek, MI 49017-2385
800/253-0854

Foot Management Inc
Rte 1, 30-A Friendship Rd
PO Box 100
Pittsville, MD 21850-0100
800/468-3668
301/835-3668

General Physiotherapy Inc
13222 Lakefront Dr
St Louis, MO 63045-1504
800/237-1832
314/291-1442

GMG Enterprises Inc
3536 Ctr Circle Dr
Fort Mill, SC 29715
800/848-3985
803/548-1131

Units of Measure

C

Milliseconds (msec) $= \frac{1}{1000}$ of a second
Microseconds (μsec) $= \frac{1}{1,000,000}$ of a second
Nanosecond (nsec) $= \frac{1}{1,000,000,000}$ of a second
Milliamp (mamp) $= \frac{1}{1,000}$ of an amp
Microamp (μamp) $= \frac{1}{1,000,000}$ of an amp
Angstrom (Å) $= \frac{1}{10,000,000,000}$ of a meter
Nanometer (nm) $= \frac{1}{1,000,000,000}$ of a meter
Hertz (Hz) $= 1$ cycle per second
Kilohertz (KHz) $= 1,000$ cycles per second
Megahertz (MHz) $= 1,000,000$ cycles per second

Glossary

A

absolute refractory period Brief time period (.5 μsec) after membrane depolarization during which the membrane is incapable of depolarizing again.

absorption Energy that stimulates a particular tissue to perform its normal function.

accommodation Adaptation by the sensory receptors to various stimuli over an extended period of time.

acidic reaction The accumulation of negative ions under the positive pole, which produces hydrochloric acid.

acoustic impedance Determines the amount of ultrasound energy reflected at tissue interfaces.

acoustic microstreaming The unidirectional movement of fluids along the boundaries of cell membranes, resulting from the mechanical pressure wave in an ultrasonic field.

acoustic spectrum The range of frequencies and wavelengths of sound waves.

ACTH Adrenocorticotropic hormone. This hormone stimulates the release of glucocorticoids (cortisol) from the adrenal glands.

action potential A recorded change in electrical potential between the inside and outside of a nerve cell, resulting in muscular contraction.

active electrode The smaller of the two electrodes under which greatest current density occurs or the electrode that is used to drive ions into the tissues.

acupressure The technique of using finger pressure over acupuncture points to decrease pain.

acute Pain of sudden onset often associated with physical trauma.

acute injury An injury in which active inflammation is present that includes the classic symptoms of tenderness, swelling, redness, and so on.

afferent Conduction of a nerve impulse toward an organ.

air space plate A capacitor type electrode in which the plates are separated from the skin by the space in a glass case. Used with shortwave diathermy.

alkaline reaction The accumulation of positive ions under the negative electrode, which produces sodium hydroxide.

all-or-none response The depolarization of nerve or muscle membrane is the same once a depolarizing intensity threshold is reached; further increases in intensity do not increase the response. Stimuli at intensities less than threshold do not create a depolarizing effect.

alternating current Current that periodically changes its polarity or direction of flow.

ampere Unit of measure that indicates the rate at which electrical current is flowing.

amplifier A device using electrical components to increase electrical power.

amplitude Describes the magnitude of the vibration in a wave. It is the maximum distance from equilibrium that any particle reaches. It is also referred to as the intensity of current flow as indicated by the height of the waveform from baseline.

analgesia Loss of sensibility to pain.

anesthesia Loss of sensation.

annulus fibrosus The interlacing cross-fibers of fibroelastic tissue that are attached to adjacent vertebral bodies that contain the nucleus pulposus.

anode Positively charged electrode in a direct current system.

anoxia Reduction of oxygen in body tissues below physiologic levels.

applicator The electrode used to transfer energy in microwave diathermy.

Arndt-Schultz Principle No reactions or changes can occur in the body if the amount of energy absorbed is not sufficient to stimulate the absorbing tissues.

attenuation A decrease in energy intensity while the ultrasound wave is transmitted through various tissues caused by scattering and dispersion.

average current The amount of current flowing per unit of time.

avulsion fracture A fracture in which a small piece of bone is torn away by an attached tendon or ligament.

B

bacteriostatic A chemical environment in which bacteria is destroyed.

bandwidth A specific frequency range in which the amplifier will pick up signals produced by electrical activity in the muscle.

beam nonuniformity ratio (BNR) Indicates the amount of variability of intensity within the ultrasound beam and is determined by the maximal point intensity of transducer to the average intensity across the transducer surface.

beat Distinct wave pattern created by combining two distinct circuit electrical waves that blend into a gradual rising and falling wave.

β-endorphin A neurohormone derived from proopiomelanocortin (POMC). It is similar in structure and properties to morphine. β-endorphin has a half-life of 4 hours.

Bindegewebsmassage Reflex zone massage; uses a pulling stroke across connective tissue to effect change.

bioelectromagnetics The study of biologic tissues' electrical and magnetic properties.

biphasic current Another name for alternating current, in which the direction of current flow reverses direction.

bipolar arrangement Two active recording electrodes placed in close proximity to one another.

bursts A combined set of three or more pulses; also referred to as packets or envelopes.

C

cable electrodes An inductance type electrode in which the electrodes are coiled around a body part, creating an electromagnetic field.

capacitor electrodes Air space plates or pad electrodes that create a stronger electrical field than a magnetic field.

cathode Negatively charged electrode in a direct current system.

cavitation The formation of gas-filled bubbles that expand and compress because of ultrasonically induced pressure changes in tissue fluids.

central biasing A theory of pain modulation where higher centers such as the cerebral cortex influence the perception of and response to pain.

chronaxie The duration of time necessary to cause observable tissue excitation, given a current intensity of two times rheobasic current.

chronic injury An injury in which the normal cellular response in the inflammatory process is altered, replacing leukocytes with macrophages and plasma cells, along with degeneration of the injured structure.

chronic pain Pain lasting more than 6 months.

circuit The path of current from a generating source through the various components back to the generating source.

coherence Property of identical phase and time relationship. All photons of laser light are the same wavelength.

collimate To make parallel.

collimated beam A focused, less divergent beam of ultrasound energy produced by a large-diameter transducer.

common mode rejection ratio (CMRR) The ability of the differential amplifier to eliminate the common noise between the active electrodes.

compressions Regions of high molecular density (i.e., a great amount of ultrasound energy) within the longitudinal wave.

conductance The ease with which a current flows along a conducting medium.

conduction Heat loss or gain through direct contact.

conductors Materials that permit the free movement of electrons.

congestion Presence of an abnormal amount of blood in the vessels resulting from an increase in blood flow or obstructed venous return.

consensual heat vasodilation Vasodilation and increased blood flow will spread to remote areas, causing increased metabolism in the unheated area.

constructive interference The combined amplitude of two distinct circuits increases the amplitude.

continuous wave An uninterrupted beam of laser light as opposed to pulsed.

continuous wave ultrasound The sound intensity remains constant throughout the treatment and the ultrasound energy is being produced 100% of the time.

contrast bath Hot (106° F) and cold (50° F) treatments in a combined sequence to stimulate superficial capillary vasodilation or vasoconstriction.

convection Heat loss or gain through the movement of water molecules across the skin.

conversion Changing from one energy form into another.

cosine law Optimal radiation occurs when the source of radiation is at right angles to the center of the area being radiated.

coulomb Measurement indicating the number of electrons flowing in a current.

coupling medium A substance used to decrease the acoustic impedance at the air-skin interface and thus facilitate the passage of ultrasound energy.

cryokinetics The use of cold and exercise in the treatment of pathology or disease.

cryotherapy The use of cold in the treatment of pathology or diseases.

current density Amount of current flow per cubic area.

current of injury A bioelectric current produced by any type of cellular trauma that plays a key role in stimulating healing.

D

decay time The time required for a waveform to go from peak amplitude to 0 V.

depolarization Process or act of neutralizing the cell membrane's resting potential.

destructive interference Combined amplitude of two distinct circuits decreases the amplitude.

diathermy The application of high-frequency electrical energy that is used to generate heat in body tissues resulting from tissue resistance to the passage of energy. It may also be used to produce nonthermal effects.

differential amplifier Monitors the two separate signals from the active electrodes and amplifies the difference, thus eliminating extraneous noise.

diode laser A solid-state/semiconductor used as a lasing medium.

dipoles Molecules whose ends carry opposite charges.

disk herniation The protrusion of the nucleus pulposus through a defect in the annulus fibrosus.

disk material Cartilaginous material from vertebral body surfaces, disk nucleus, or annulus fibrosus.

disk nucleus The protein polysaccharide gel that is contained between the cartilaginous end plates of the vertebrae and the annulus fibrosus.

disk protrusion The abnormal projection of the disk nucleus through some or all of the annular rings.

direct current Galvanic current that always flows in the same direction and may flow in either a positive or a negative direction.

divergence The bending of light rays away from each other, the spreading of light.

DNA Deoxyribonucleic acid; the substance found in the chromosomes of the cell nucleus that carries the genetic code of the cell.

drum electrodes Induction electrodes that produce a strong magnetic field. Primarily used with pulsed short-wave diathermy.

duration Sometimes referred to as pulse width. Indicates the length of time the current is flowing.

duty cycle The percentage of time that ultrasound is being generated (pulse duration) over one pulse period, which is also referred to as the mark:space ratio.

dynorphin An endogenous opioid derived from the pro-hormone prodynorphin.

E

eddy currents Small circular electrical fields induced when a magnetic field is created that result in intramolecular oscillation (vibration) of tissue contents, causing heat generation.

edema The presence of abnormal amounts of fluid in the extracellular tissue spaces of the body.

effective radiating area The total area of the surface of the transducer that actually produces the sound wave.

efferent Conduction of a nerve impulse away from an organ.

effleurage To stroke; any stroke that glides over the skin without attempting to move the deep muscle masses. The hand is molded to the part, stroking with more or less constant pressure, usually upward. Any degree of pressure may be applied, varying from the lightest possible touch to very deep pressure.

electrets Insulators carrying a permanent charge similar to a permanent magnet.

electrical current The net movement of electrons along a conducting medium.

electrical field The lines of force exerted on charged ions in the tissues by the electrodes that cause charged particles to move from one pole to the other.

electrical impedance The opposition to electron flow in a conducting material.

electrical potential The difference between charged particles at a higher and lower potential.

electrolytes Solutions in which ionic movement occurs.

electromagnetic spectrum The range of frequencies and wavelengths associated with radiant energy.

electromyographic biofeedback A therapeutic procedure that uses electronic or electromechanical instruments to accurately measure, process, and feedback reinforcing information via auditory or visual signals.

electron Fundamental particle of matter possessing a negative electrical charge and small mass.

electrophoresis The movement of ions in solution.

electropiezo activity Changing electric surface charges of a structure forces the structure to change shape.

endogenous opioids Opiate- like substances made by the body.

endorphins Endogenous opioids whose actions have analgesic properties (i.e., β-endorphin).

endothelial cell Cells that line the cavities of vessels.

endothelial-derived relaxing factor Relaxes smooth muscle and stimulates blood flow rates in veins.

enkephalin Neurotransmitter proteins that block the passage of noxious stimuli from first-order to second-order afferents. These proteins inhibit the release of substance P and are produced by enkephalinergic neurons.

enkephalinergic interneurons Neurons with short axons that release enkephalin. They are widespread in the central nervous system and are found in the substantia gelatinosa, raphe nucleus, and periaqueductual grey matter.

erythema Redness of the skin; inflammation. A redness of the skin caused by capillary dilation.

excited state State of an atom that occurs when outside energy causes it to contain more energy than normal.

F

facet joints Articular joints of the spine.

faradic current An asymmetric biphasic waveform seldom used on modern electrical generators.

Federal Communications Commission (FCC) Federal agency charged with assigning frequencies for all radio transmitters including diathermies.

fiberoptic A solid glass or plastic tube that conducts light along its length.

fibrils Connective tissue fibers supporting the lymphatic capillaries.

fibroplasia The period of scar formation that occurs during the fibroblastic-repair phase.

fibrosis The formation of fibrous tissue in the injury repair process.

filter Changes pulsating DC current to smooth DC.

filters Devices that help to reduce external noise that essentially makes the amplifier more sensitive to some incoming frequencies and less sensitive to others.

fluidotherapy A modality of dry heat using a finely divided solid suspended in a stream with the properties of liquid.

fluorescence The capacity of certain substances to radiate when illuminated by a source of a given wavelength; a light of a different wavelength (color) than that of the irradiating source when illuminated by a given wavelength.

focusing Narrowing attention to the appropriate stimuli in the environment.

free nerve endings Receptors that are sensitive to extreme mechanical, chemical, or thermal energy.

frequency The number of cycles or pulses per second.

frequency window selectivity Cellular responses may be triggered by a certain electrical frequency range.

friction massage A technique that affects fibrositic adhesions in tendon, muscle, or ligament. It is performed by small circular movements that penetrate into the depth of a muscle, not by moving the finger on the skin, but by moving the tissues under the skin.

G

gap junctions Specialized junction areas connecting cells of like structure, which contain channels for ionic, electrical, and small molecule signaling that pass messages from cell to cell.

ground A wire that makes an electrical connection with the earth.

ground-fault interruptors (GFI) A safety device that automatically shuts off current flow and reduces the chances of electrical shock.

ground state The normal, unexcited state of an atom.

H

heterodyns Cyclic rising and falling waveform of interferential current.

high-voltage current Current in which the waveform has an amplitude of greater than 150 V with a relatively short pulse duration.

hot spots Areas at tissue interfaces that may become overheated.

Hubbard tank An immersion tank for the whole body, it may have vertical depth for walking or supine treatment.

hunting response A reflex vasodilation that occurs in response to cold approximately 15 minutes into the treatment. This has been demonstrated to be only an increase in temperature and not necessarily a change in blood flow.

hybrid currents Currents that have waveforms containing parameters that are not classically alternating or direct.

hydrocollator A synthetic hot (170° F) or cold (0° F) gel used as an adjunctive modality to stimulate a rise or fall in tissue temperature.

hydrotherapy Cryotherapy and thermotherapy techniques that use water as the medium for heat transfer.

hyperemia Presence of an increased amount of blood in part of the body.

hyperplasia An increase in the size of a tissue; in the skin, an increased thickness of the epidermis.

I

impedance The resistance of the tissue to the passage of electrical current.

indication The reason to prescribe a remedy or procedure.

indifferent or dispersive electrode Large electrode used to spread out electrical charge and decrease current density at that electrode site.

induction electrodes Cable or drum electrodes that create a stronger magnetic field than electrical field.

infrared That portion of the electromagnetic spectrum associated with thermal changes; located adjacent to the red portion of the visible light spectrum. That part of the electromagnetic spectrum dealing with infrared wavelengths.

insulators Materials that resist current flow.

integration An EMG signal processing technique that measures the area under the curve for a specified period of time, thus forming the basis for quantification of EMG activity.

intensity A measure of the rate at which energy is being delivered per unit area.

intermolecular oscillation (vibration) Movement between molecules that produces friction and thus heat.

interneurons Neurons contained entirely in the central nervous system. They have no projections outside the spinal cord. Their function is to serve as relay stations within the central nervous system.

interpulse interval The interruptions between individual pulses or groups of pulses.

intrapulse interval The period of time between individual pulses.

inverse square law The intensity of radiation striking a particular surface varies inversely with the square of the distance from the radiating source.

ion A positively or negatively charged particle.

ion transfer A technique of transporting chemicals across a membrane using an electrical current as a driving force.

ionization A process by which soluble compounds such as acids, alkaloids, or salts dissociate or dissolve into ions that are suspended in some type of solution.

iontophoresis A therapeutic technique that involves introducing ions into the body tissues by means of a continuous direct electrical current.

J

joint capsule Ligamentous structure that surrounds and encapsulates a joint.

joint swelling Accumulation of blood and joint fluid within the joint capsule.

K

Kehr's sign Referred pain pattern involving pain in the left jaw, shoulder, and arm.

keratin The fibrous protein that forms the chemical basis of the epidermis.

keratinocytes A cell that produces keratin.

L

laser A device that concentrates high energies into a narrow beam of coherent, monochromatic light (Light Amplification by the Stimulated Emission of Radiation).

Law of Grotthus-Draper Energy not absorbed by the tissues must be transmitted.

ligament deformation Lengthening distortion of ligament caused by traction loading.

longitudinal wave The primary waveform in which ultrasound energy travels in soft tissue, with the molecular displacement along the direction in which the wave travels.

low-voltage current Current in which the waveform has an amplitude of less than 150 V.

lymph A transparent slightly yellow liquid found in the lymphatic vessels.

lymphedema Swelling of subcutaneous tissues as a result of accumulation of excessive lymph fluid.

M

macroshock An electrical shock that can be felt and has a leakage of electrical current of greater than 1 mA.

macrotears Significant damage to soft tissues caused by acute trauma that result in clinical symptoms and functional alterations.

magnetic field Field created when current is passed through a coiled cable that affects surrounding tissues by inducing localized eddy currents within the tissues.

massage The act of rubbing, kneading, or stroking the superficial parts of the body with the hand or with an instrument for the purpose of modifying nutrition, restoring power of movement , or breaking up adhesions.

maximum voluntary isometric contraction Peak torque produced by a muscular contraction.

medical galvanism Creation of either an acidic or alkaline environment that may be of therapeutic value.

melanin A group of dark brown or black pigments that occur naturally in the eye, skin, hair, and other animal tissues.

meniscoid structures A cartilage tip found on the synovial fringes of some facet joints.

metabolites Waste products of metabolism or catabolism.

microcurrent electrical nerve stimulator (MENS) Used primarily in tissue healing, the current intensities are too small to excite peripheral nerves.

microshock An electrical shock that is imperceptible because of a leakage of current of less than 1 mA.

microtears Minor damage to soft tissue most often associated with overuse.

minimal erythemal dose The amount of time of exposure to UVR necessary to cause a faint erythema 24 hours after exposure.

modulation Refers to any alteration in the magnitude or any variation in the duration of an electrical current.

monochromaticity When a light source produces a single color or wavelength.

monophasic current Another name for direct current, in which the direction of current flow remains the same.

muscle guarding A protective response in muscle that occurs because of pain or fear of movement.

myofascial pain A type of referred pain associated with trigger points.

myofascial release A group of techniques used to relieve soft tissue from the abnormal grip of tight fascia.

N

nerve root impingement Abnormal encroachment of some body tissue into the space occupied by the nerve root.

neuromuscular electrical stimulator (NMES) Also called an electrical muscle stimulator (EMS), it is used to stimulate muscle directly as would be the case with denervated muscle where peripheral nerves are not functioning.

neurotransmitter Substance that passes information between neurons. It is released from one neuron terminal (presynaptic membrane), enters the synaptic cleft, and attaches (binds) to a receptor on the next neuron (postsynaptic membrane). Substance P, enkephalins, serotonin, methionine, and leucine enkephalin are neurotransmitters.

nociceptors Pain information or signals of pain stimuli.

noise Extraneous electrical activity that may be produced by any source other than the contracting muscle.

norepinephrine A neurotransmitter.

nutrients Essential or nonessential food substance.

O

ohm A unit of measure that indicates resistance to current flow.

Ohm's law The current in an electrical circuit is directly proportional to the voltage and inversely proportional to the resistance.

opiate receptors Neurons that have receptors that bind to opiate substances.

oscillator Used to produce and output a specific waveform, which may be different from that used to power or drive the stimulating unit.

output amplifier Used to magnify or increase the amplitude of the voltage output of the generator and control it at a specific level.

P

pad electrodes Capacitor type electrode used with short-wave diathermy to create an electrical field.

pain An unpleasant sensory and emotional experience associated with actual or potential tissue damage.

paraffin bath A combined paraffin and mineral oil immersion technique in which the paraffin substance is heated to 126° F for conductive heat gains; commonly used on the hands and feet for distal temperature gains in blood flow and temperature.

parallel circuit A circuit in which two or more routes exist for current to pass between the two terminals.

periaqueductal grey A midbrain structure that plays an important role in descending tracts that inhibit synaptic transmission of noxious input in the dorsal horn.

periosteum A highly vascularized and innervated membrane lining the surface of bone.

petrissage Massage technique that is a kneading manipulation. Consists of repeatedly grasping and releasing the tissue with one or both hands or parts thereof in a lifting, rolling, or pressing movement. The outside characteristic of this movement as contrasted to stroking movements is that the pressure is applied intermittently.

phases That portion of the pulse that rises above or below the baseline for some period of time.

phonophoresis A technique in which ultrasound is used to drive a topical application of a selected medication into the tissues.

photokeratitis An inflammation of the eyes caused by exposure to UVR.

photon The basic unit of light; a packet or quanta of light energy.

piezoelectric activity Changing electric surface charges of a structure forces the structure to change shape.

piezoelectric effect When an alternating electrical current generated at the same frequency as the crystal resonance is passed through the piezoelectric crystal, the crystal will expand and contract or vibrate at the frequency of the electrical oscillation, thus generating ultrasound at a desired frequency.

pitting edema A type of swelling that leaves a pitlike depression when the skin is compressed.

polyphasic current Current that contains three or more grouped phases in a single pulse and that is used in interferential and "Russian" currents.

population inversion A condition where more atoms exist in a high energy, excited state than those atoms that are in a normal ground state. This is required for lasing to occur.

power The total amount of ultrasound energy in the beam. Power is expressed in watts.

proprioceptive nervous system System of nerves that provides information on joint movement, pressure, and muscle tension.

pulse An individual waveform.

pulse charge The total amount of electricity being delivered to the athlete during each pulse.

pulse period The combined time of the pulse duration and the interpulse interval.

pulsed shortwave diathermy Created by simply interrupting the output of continuous shortwave diathermy at consistent intervals, it is used primarily for nonthermal effects.

pulsed ultrasound The intensity is periodically interrupted with no ultrasound energy being produced during the off period. When using pulsed ultrasound, the average intensity of the output over time is reduced.

R

radiating pain Pain that moves away from the site of a lesion, usually associated with some pressure in the area of injury.

radiation The process of emitting energy from some source in the form of waves. A method of heat transfer through which heat can be either gained or lost.

ramping Another name for surging modulation, in which the current builds gradually to some maximum amplitude.

raphe nucleus Part of the brain that is known to inhibit pain impulses being transmitted through the ascending system.

rarefactions Regions of lower molecular density (i.e., a small amount of ultrasound energy) within a longitudinal wave.

rate of rise How quickly a waveform reaches its maximum amplitude.

raw EMG A form in which the electrical activity produced by muscle contraction may be displayed or recorded before the signal is processed.

rectification A signal processing technique that changes the deflection of the waveform from the negative pole to the positive pole, essentially creating a pulsed direct current.

rectifier Converts AC current to pulsating DC current.

reference electrode Also referred to as the ground electrode, serves as a point of reference to compare the electrical activity recorded by the active electrodes.

referred pain (referred myofascial pain) When nociceptive impulses reach the dorsal grey matter, they converge and their summation can depolarize internuncial neurons over several spinal segments, causing the individual to feel pain in distal areas innervated by these segments.

reflection The bending back of light or sound waves from a surface that they strike.

refraction The change in direction of a sound wave or radiation wave when it passes from one medium or type of tissue to another.

regulator Produces a specific controlled voltage output.

resistance The opposition to electron flow in a conducting material.

resting potential The potential difference between the inside and outside of a membrane.

rheobase The intensity of current necessary to cause observable tissue excitation given a long current duration.

RNA Ribonucleic acid; an acid found in the cell cytoplasm and nucleolus. It is intimately involved in protein synthesis.

Rolfing A system devised to correct inefficient structure by balancing the body within a gravitational field through a technique involving manual soft tissue manipulation.

Russian current A medium frequency (2,000 to 10,000 Hz) polyphasic AC wave generated in 50 burst per second envelopes.

S

sclerotome A segment of bone innervated by a spinal segment.

series circuit A circuit in which there is only one path for current to get from one terminal to another.

sensitization Prolonged depolarization of nociceptive neurons that results in continuous stimulation. Most sensory receptors are rendered less sensitive after prolonged stimulations. This is not the case with nociceptive neurons.

serotonin A neurotransmitter found in neurons descending in the dorsolateral tract. The dorsolateral tract is thought to play a significant role in pain control. Serotonin is found in the vesicles in nerve endings that bind when released to postsynaptic membranes. Its action is terminated by reuptake into presynaptic membranes. It is probably involved in both endogenous pain control and opiate analgesia. Increased levels of serotonin in the central nervous system are generally associated with increased analgesia.

signal gain Determines the signal sensitivity. If a high gain is chosen the biofeedback unit will have a high sensitivity for the muscle activity signal.

smoothing An EMG signal processing technique that eliminates the high frequency fluctuations that are produced with a changing electrical signal.

spondylolisthesis Forward displacement of one vertebra over another.

spontaneous emission When an atom in a high energy state emits a photon and drops to a more stable ground state.

standing wave As the ultrasound energy is reflected at tissue interfaces with different acoustic impedances, the intensity of the energy is increased as the reflected energy meets new energy being transmitted, forming waves of high energy that can potentially damage surrounding tissues.

stereodynamic interference current Three distinct circuits blending and creating a distinct electrical wave pattern.

stimulated emission When a photon interacts with an atom already in a high energy state and decay of the atomic system occurs, releasing two photons.

strain related potentials Tissue based electric potentials generated in response to strain of the tissue.

strength-duration curve A graphic illustration of the relationship between current intensity and duration in causing depolarization of a nerve or muscle membrane.

substance P A peptide believed to be the neurotransmitter of small-diameter primary afferent. It is released from both ends of the neuron.

substantia gelatinosa Lamina 2 of the dorsal horn of the gray matter. Melzack and Wall[21] proposed that it is responsible for closing the gate to painful stimuli.

summation of contractions Shortening of muscle myofilaments caused by increasing the frequency of muscle membrane depolarization.

synovial fringes Folds of synovial tissue that move in and out of the joint space.

T

tapotement A percussion massage; any series of brisk blows following each other in a rapid alternating fashion: hacking, cupping, slapping, beating, tapping, and pinchment. It is used when stimulation is the objective.

tetanization When individual muscle twitch responses can no longer be distinguished and the responses force maximum shortening of the stimulated muscle fiber.

tetany Muscle condition that is caused by hyperexcitation and results in cramps and spasms.

thermal Pertaining to heat.

thermopane An insulating layer of water next to the skin.

thermotherapy The use of heat in the treatment of pathology or disease.

traction Drawing tension applied to a body segment.

Trager A technique that attempts to establish neuromuscular control so that more normal movement patterns can be routinely performed.

transcutaneous electrical nerve stimulator (TENS) A transcutaneous electrical stimulator used to stimulate peripheral nerves.

transcutaneous electrical stimulator All therapeutic electrical generators regardless of whether they deliver AC, DC, or pulsed currents through electrodes attached to the skin.

transformer Reduces the amount of voltage from the power supply.

transmission The propagation of energy through a particular biologic tissue into deeper tissues.

transverse wave Occurring only in bone, the molecules are displaced perpendicular to the direction in which the ultrasound wave is moving.

trigger point Localized deep tenderness in a palpable firm band of muscle. When stretched, a palpating finger can snap the band like a taut string, which produces local pain, a local twitch of that portion of the muscle, and a jump by the patient. Sustained pressure on a trigger point reproduces the pattern of referred pain for that site.

twitch muscle contraction A single muscle contraction caused by one depolarization phenomenon.

U

ultrasound A portion of the acoustic spectrum located above audible sound.

ultraviolet The portion of the electromagnetic spectrum associated with chemical changes located adjacent to the violet portion of the visible light spectrum.

unilateral foramen opening Enlargement of the foramen on one side of a vertebral segment.

V

vasconstriction Narrowing of the blood vessels.

vasodilation Dilation of the blood vessels.

vibration A shaking massage technique; a fine tremulous movement made by the hand or fingers placed firmly against a part that will cause the part to vibrate. Often used for a soothing effect; may be stimulating when more energy is applied.

viscoelastic properties The property of a material to show sensitivity to rate of loading.

volt The electromotive force that must be applied to produce a movement of electrons.

voltage The force resulting from an accumulation of electrons at one point in an electrical circuit, usually corresponding to a deficit of electrons at another point in the circuit.

voltage sensitive permeability The quality of some cell membranes that makes them permeable to different ions based on the electric charge of the ions. Nerve and muscle cell membranes allow negatively charged ions into the cell while actively transporting some positively charged ions outside the cell membrane.

W

watt A measure of electrical power. Mathematically, Watts = Volts − Amperes.

waveform The shape of an electrical current as displayed on an oscilloscope.

wavelength The distance from one point in a propagating wave to the same point in the next wave.

Wolff's law Bone remodels itself and provides increased strength along the lines of the mechanical forces placed on it.

Index